KT-475-817

UICC
International Union Against Cancer
Union Internationale Contre le Cancer

Springer
Berlin
Heidelberg
New York
Barcelona
Budapest
Hong Kong
London
Milan
Paris
Tokyo

Prognostic Factors in Cancer

Edited by
P. Hermanek, M.K. Gospodarowicz,
D.E. Henson, R.V.P. Hutter, L.H. Sobin

With 14 Figures and 60 Tables

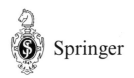 Springer

UICC
3, rue du Conseil-Général, CH-1205 Geneva, Switzerland

Editors:

Professor Dr. Dr. h.c. P. Hermanek
Vorstand der Abteilung für Klinische Pathologie i. R.
Chirurgische Universitätsklinik Erlangen
Krankenhausstr. 12, 91054 Erlangen, FRG

Dr. Mary K. Gospodarowicz
Princess Margaret Hospital, Department of Radiation Oncology
University of Toronto, 500 Sherbourne Street
Toronto, Ontario M4X 1K9, Canada

Dr. D.E. Henson
Early Detection Branch, Division of Cancer Prevention and Control
National Cancer Institute, EPN Building, Room 305
9000 Rockville Pike, Bethesda, MD 20892, USA

Dr. R.V.P. Hutter
Clinical Professor of Pathology
University of Medicine and Dentistry
New Jersey Medical School, Newark, NJ
Department of Pathology, Saint Barnabas Medical Center
Old Short Hills Road, Livingston, NJ 07039, USA

Dr. L.H. Sobin
Professor of Pathology
Uniformed Services University of the Health Sciences
Bethesda, MD
Division of Gastrointestinal Pathology
Armed Forces Institute of Pathology, Washington, DC 20306, USA

Library of Congress Cataloging-in-Publication Data

Prognostic factors in cancer / edited by P. Hermanek ... [et al.]. p. cm.
  "UICC, International Union Against Cancer – Union Internationale Contre le Cancer" --P. preceding t. p.
  Includes bibliographical references and index.   ISBN 3-540-58688-1
  1. Cancer--Prognosis. I. Hermanek, Paul. II. International Union against Cancer.
  [DNLM: 1. Neoplasms--diagnosis. 2. Prognosis. 3. Neoplasm Staging. 4. Survival Rate. QZ 241 P964 1996]
  RC262.P688 1995   616.99'4075--dc20   95-19216

ISBN 3-540-58688-1 Springer-Verlag Berlin Heidelberg New York

This work is subject to copyright. All rights are reserved, whether the whole or part of the material is concerned, specifically the rights of translation, reprinting, reuse of illustrations, recitation, broadcasting, reproduction on microfilm or in any other way, and storage in data banks. Duplication of this publication or parts thereof is permitted only under the provisions of the German Copyright Law of September 9, 1965, in its current version, and permission for use must always be obtained from Springer-Verlag. Violations are liable for prosecution under the German Copyright Law.

© International Union Against Cancer, Geneva 1995
Printed in Germany

The use of general descriptive names, registered names, trademarks, etc. in this publication does not imply, even in the absence of a specific statement, that such names are exempt from the relevant protective laws and regulations and therefore free for general use.

Product liability: The publishers cannot guarantee the accuracy of any information about dosage and application contained in this book. In every individual case the user must check such information by consulting the relevant literature.

Typesetting: Thomson Press (India) Ltd, New Delhi
SPIN: 10572164   31/3111/SPS – 5 4 3 2 1 – Printed on acid-free paper

Preface

This monograph is the result of an effort by the International Union Against Cancer (UICC) to study prognostic factors related to cancer. It is an extension of the long-term work on the TNM classification, the most widely used "staging" classification and the strongest prognostic factor for most cancer.

Although anatomic extent of disease (TNM) is generally the most important indicator of prognosis for cancer patients and provides the main criterion for selection of therapy, anatomic extent coupled with other factors could provide an even more powerful system for prognostic assessment and choice of therapy.

The purpose of this monograph is to compile information on prognostic factors for most tumour sites and selected tumour types. Each site- or tumour-specific chapter provides a general overview of the relevant literature on prognostic factors. Where possible, the authors have attempted to assess these factors in terms of their strength and independence to influence prognosis and their clinical relevance.

The TNM classification, which describes the anatomic extent of disease, is the most time proven prognostic classification. As such, TNM serves as a standard against which other prognostic factors and classifications are measured.

We hope that the present compilation of prognostic factors will aid in: (1) portraying the scope of this field; (2) stimulating the study of these and other prognostic factors; and (3) bringing some perspective to those working on specific factors.

March 1995

P. Hermanek, Erlangen
M.K. Gospodarowicz, Toronto
D.E. Henson, Bethesda, MD
R.V.P. Hutter, Livingston, NJ
L.H. Sobin, Washington, DC

Acknowledgement

Reviewer

Bielach S, MD, Hamburg, Germany
Diehl V, MD, Prof., Köln, Germany
Dold UW, MD, Priv. Doz., Freiburg, Germany
Gebhardt Ch, MD, Prof., Nürnberg, Germany
Höffken K, MD, Prof., Jena, Germany
Hohenberger W, MD, Prof., Erlangen, Germany
Kindermann G, MD, Prof., München, Germany
König HJ, MD, Prof., Erlangen, Germany
Laperriere NJ, MD, Toronto, Ontario, Canada
Meister P, MD, Prof., München, Germany
Mennel HD, MD, Prof., Marburg/Lahn, Germany
Payne DG, MD, Toronto, Ontario, Canada
Schlag P, MD, Prof., Berlin, Germany
Schrott KM, MD, Prof., Erlangen, Germany
Siewert JR, MD, Prof., München, Germany
Steiner W, MD, Prof., Göttingen, Germany
Wigand ME, MD, Prof., Erlangen, Germany
Winkler K, MD, Prof., Hamburg, Germany
Wustrow TPU, MD, Prof., München, Germany

The editors have much pleasure in acknowledging the great help received from the reviewers listed above.

Contents

List of Contributors

Antonaci, A.
Department of Clinical Surgery IV,
University "La Sapienza" di Roma, 00161 Rome, Italy

Asamura, H.
Division of Thoracic Surgery, Department of Surgery,
National Cancer Center Hospital, 1-1, Tsukiji 5-Chome,
Chuo-ku, Tokyo 104, Japan

Bacchi, G.
Division of Otorhinolaryngology, Ospedale Civile Regionale,
33100 Udine, Italy

Badellino, F.
Division of Surgical Oncology, National Institute for Cancer
Research-IST, 10132 Genoa, Italy

Benedet, J.L.
Department of Gynaecology, Vancouver General Hospital,
805 West 12th Avenue, Vancouver, BC, Canada V5Z 1M9

Blinov, N.N.
N.N. Petrov Research Institute of Oncology, 68 Leningradskaya St.,
Pesochny 2, St. Petersburg 189646, Russia

Breuninger, H.
Universitätshautklinik, 72076 Tübingen, Germany

Brierley, J.
Department of Radiation Oncology, University of Toronto,
Princess Margaret Hospital, 500 Sherbourne Street, Toronto,
Ontario, Canada M4X 1K9

Burke, B.
Department of Medicine, New York Medical College, Valhalla,
NY 10595, USA

Calearo, C.
Department of Otolaryngology, University of Ferrara,
Arcispedale S. Anna, 44100 Ferrara, Italy

Canavese, G.
Division of Surgical Oncology, National Institute for Cancer
Research-IST, 10132 Genoa, Italy

Carriaga, M.T.
Department of Pathology, Georgetown University School
of Medicine, Washington, DC 20007, USA

Catton, P.A.
Department of Radiation Oncology, University of Toronto,
Princess Margaret Hospital, 500 Sherbourne Street, Toronto,
Ontario, Canada M4X 1K9

Consoli, C.
Department of Clinical Surgery IV, University "La Sapienza"
di Roma, 00161 Rome, Italy

Consorti, F.
Department of Clinical Surgery IV, University "La Sapienza"
di Roma, 00161 Rome, Italy

Cummings, B.J.
Department of Radiation Oncology, University of Toronto,
Ontario Cancer Institute/Princess Margaret Hospital,
500 Sherbourne Street, Toronto, Ontario, Canada M4X 1K9

Denis, L.J.
Department of Urology, A.Z. Middelheim, 2020 Antwerp,
Belgium

Di Paola, M.
Department of Clinical Surgery IV, University "La Sapienza"
di Roma, 00161 Rome, Italy

Ehlen, T.G.
Department of Gynaecology, Vancouver General Hospital,
805 West 12th Avenue, Vancouver, BC, Canada V5Z 1M9

Ficulccilli, F.
Department of Clinical Surgery IV, University "La Sapienza"
di Roma, 00161 Rome, Italy

Fukuma, H.
Department of Orthopedic Surgery, National Cancer Center Hospital,
1-1, Tsukiji 5-Chome, Chuo-ku, Tokyo 104, Japan

Fyles, A.
Department of Radiation Oncology, University of Toronto,
Princess Margaret Hospital, 500 Sherbourne Street, Toronto,
Ontario, Canada M4X 1K9

Gospodarowicz, M.K.
Department of Radiation Oncology, University of Toronto,
Princess Margaret Hospital, 500 Sherbourne Street, Toronto,
Ontario, Canada M4X 1K9

Hayat, M.
Department of Oncology, Institut Gustave Roussy,
rue Camille Desmoulin, 94805 Villejuif, France

Hedlund, P.O.
Department of Urology, Karolinska Hospital, 10401 Stockholm,
Sweden

Henk, J.M.
Royal Marsden Hospital, Sutton, Surrey SM2 5PT, UK

Henson, D.E.
Early Detection Branch, Division of Cancer Prevention and Control,
National Cancer Institute, EPN Building, Room 305,
9000 Rockville Pike, Bethesda, MD 20892, USA

Hermanek, P.
Department of Surgical Pathology, University of Erlangen,
Krankenhausstr. 12, 91054 Erlangen, Germany

Hohenberger, W.
Chirurgische Klinik und Poliklinik, University of Erlangen,
Krankenhausstr. 12, 91054 Erlangen, Germany

Hutter, R.V.P.
St. Barnabas Medical Center, Old Short Hills Road, Livingston,
NJ 07039, USA

Karim, A.B.M.F.
Department of Radiation Oncology, Academisch Ziekenhuis,
Vrije Universiteit, 1007 MB Amsterdam, The Netherlands

Kasdorf, H.
Academia Nazional de Medicine, Montevideo 11000, Uruguay

Kirkbride, P.
Department of Radiation Oncology, University of Toronto,
Princess Margaret Hospital, 500 Sherbourne Street, Toronto,
Ontario, Canada M4X 1K9

Klein, M.J.
Donauspital, Department of Oncology, 1200 Vienna, Austria

Kovacs, E.
Department of Obstetrics and Gynecology, University of Basel,
4031 Basel, Switzerland

Lang, G.K.
University Eye Hospital and Clinic, University of Ulm,
Prittwitzstr. 43, 89075 Ulm, Germany

Ludwig, H.
Department of Obstetrics and Gynecology, University of Basel,
4031 Basel, Switzerland

Manzini, A.
Department of Clinical Surgery IV, University "La Sapienza"
di Roma, 00161 Rome, Italy

Maruyama, K.
Division of Gastric Surgery, Department of Surgery, National Cancer
Center Hospital, 1-1, Tsukiji 5-Chome, Chuo-ku, Tokyo 104, Japan

Menichelli, F.
Department of Clinical Surgery IV, University "La Sapienza"
di Roma, 00161 Rome, Italy

Miani, C.
Divisione of Otorhinolaryngology, Ospedale Civile Regionale,
33100 Udine, Italy

Miani, P.
Divisione of Otorhinolaryngology, Ospedale Civile Regionale,
33100 Udine, Italy

Miller, D.M.
Division of Gynaecologic Oncology, Vancouver General Hospital,
British Columbia Cancer Agency, 805 West 12th Avenue, Vancouver,
BC, Canada V5Z 1M9

Montie, J.E.
Department of Urology, Wayne State University, Harper Hospital,
Detroit, MI 48201, USA

Mostofi, F.K.
Department of Genitourinary Pathology, Armed Forces Institute of
Pathology, Washington, DC 20306, USA

Murphy, G.P.
Pacific Northwest Research Foundation, Seattle, WA 98122, USA

Naruke, T.
Division of Thoracic Surgery, Department of Surgery,
National Cancer Center Hospital, 1-1, Tsukiji 5-Chome,
Chuo-ku, Tokyo 104, Japan

Naumann, G.O.H.
University Eye Hospital and Clinic, University of Erlangen-
Nürnberg, Schwabachanlage 6, 91054 Erlangen, Germany

Nicolò, G.
Service of Pathology and Cytology, National Institute for Cancer
Research-IST, 10132 Genoa, Italy

Nomura, K.
Division of Surgical Oncology, National Cancer Centre Hospital,
1-1, Tsukiji 5-Chome, Chuo-ku, Tokyo 104, Japan

Palumbo, R.
Department of Medical Oncology, National Institute for Cancer
Research-IST, 10132 Genoa, Italy

Pastore, A.
Department of Otolaryngology, University of Ferrara,
Arcispedale S. Anna, 44100 Ferrara, Italy

Pfleiderer, A.
Universitätsfrauenklinik, Klinikum der Universität, 79106 Freiburg,
Germany

Piemonte, M.
Division of Otorhinolaryngology, Ospedale Civile Regionale,
33100 Udine, Italy

Roder, J.D.
Chirurgische Klinik und Poliklinik, Klinikum rechts der Isar,
TU München, Ismaninger Str. 22, 81675 Munich, Germany

Rosen, A.C.
Donauspital, Department of Gynaecology, 1200 Vienna, Austria

Saitoh, Y.
1st Department of Surgery, Kobe University School of Medicine,
Kobe City 650, Japan

Schmidt, O.
Department of Surgery, Universitätsklinikum, 93053 Regensburg,
Germany

Siewert, J.R.
Chirurgische Klinik und Poliklinik, Klinikum rechts der Isar,
TU München, Ismaninger Str. 22, 81675 Munich, Germany

Sobin, L.H.
Division of Gastroenterology, Armed Forces Institute of Pathology,
Washington, DC 20306, USA

Specht, L.
Department of Oncology, Rigshospitalet, University of Copenhagen,
2100 Copenhagen, Denmark

Spraul, C.W.
University Eye Hospital and Clinic, University of Ulm,
Prittwitzstr. 43, 89075 Ulm, Germany

Stein, H.J.
Chirurgische Klinik und Poliklinik, Klinikum rechts der Isar,
TU München, Ismaninger Str. 22, 81675 Munich, Germany

Strong, E.W.
Head and Neck Service, Memorial Sloan Kettering Cancer Centre,
New York, NY 10021, USA

Sturgeon, J.F.G.
Department of Medicine, University of Toronto,
Princess Margaret Hospital, 500 Sherbourne Street,
Toronto, Ontario, Canada M4X 1K9

Sutcliffe, S.B.
Department of Radiation Oncology, University of Toronto,
Princess Margaret Hospital, 500 Sherbourne Street, Toronto,
Ontario, Canada M4X 1K9

Tagliaferri, M.
Department of Clinical Surgery IV, University "La Sapienza"
di Roma, 00161 Rome, Italy

Toma, S.
Department of Medical Oncology, National Institute for Cancer
Research-IST, 10132 Genoa, Italy

Wittekind, C.
Institute of Pathology, Department of Surgery and Urology,
Friedrich-Alexander-University Erlangen, Krankenhausstr. 12,
91054 Erlangen, Germany

Yamamoto, M.
1st Department of Surgery, Kobe University School of Medicine,
Kobe City 650, Japan

1 Introduction

M.K. Gospodarowicz, P. Hermanek, and D.E. Henson

Attention to innovations in cancer treatment has tended to eclipse the importance of prognostic assessment. However, the recognition that prognostic factors often have a greater impact on outcome than available therapies and the proliferation of biochemical, molecular, and genetic markers have resulted in renewed interest in this field. The outcome in patients with cancer is determined by a combination of numerous factors. Presently, the most widely recognized are the extent of disease, histologic type of tumor, and treatment. It has been known for some time that additional factors also influence outcome. These include histologic grade, lymphatic or vascular invasion, mitotic index, performance status, symptoms, and most recently genetic and biochemical markers. It is the aim of this volume to compile those prognostic factors that have emerged as important determinants of outcome for tumors at various sites. This compilation represents the first phase of a more extensive process to integrate all prognostic factors in cancer to further enhance the prediction of outcome following treatment. Certain issues surrounding the assessment and reporting of prognostic factors are also considered.

Importance of Prognostic Factors

Prognostic factors in cancer often have an immense influence on outcome, while treatment often has a much weaker effect. For example, the influence of the presence of lymph node involvement on survival of patients with metastatic breast cancer is much greater than the effect of adjuvant treatment with tamoxifen in the same group of patients [5].

Prognostic factors serve many purposes (Tables 1 and 2). They are used to understand the natural history of cancer, to predict the results of therapeutic interventions, to identify homogeneous patient populations, to compare results of treatment, to identify subsets of patient with unfavorable outcome, and to plan follow-up strategies [7, 31, 32]. Most prognostic factors evaluated at the time of diagnosis are used to predict the outcome. However, in the contemporary era of clinical intervention, an assessment of factors reflecting the natural course of the disease is rarely possible, and outcomes generally reflect the impact of the disease in the context of specific therapeutic interventions.

Prognostic factors also permit treatment to be individualized. Intensive treatment can be reserved for those patients with adverse prognostic factors, and

Table 1. Use of prognostic factors in clinical practice

To understand the course of the disease
To predict the outcome for an individual patient
To select appropriate treatment modality
To explain variation in treatment outcome
To alleviate patient anxiety
To plan specific therapeutic intervention

Table 2. Use of prognostic factors in clinical trials

To characterize and predict patient outcome
To examine interrelationship and degree of dependence among important factors
To insure comparability of patients groups in randomized trials
To allow more precise analysis of the differences in outcome
To identify subgroups for novel treatment approaches
To serve as an intermediate endpoint in early detection

less intensive therapy for those identified as having favorable outcomes. On the basis of prognostic factors, patients for whom standard therapy is ineffective and who may benefit from experimental approaches, may be identified before treatment is started (Table 1). In randomized clinical trials, knowledge of important prognostic factors can help to ensure a better balance between treatment arms (Table 2) [31]. An understanding of prognostic factors may facilitate analysis in the context of stage migration and reduce the biologic heterogeneity inherent in stage assignment [13]. Furthermore, an accurate assessment of prognosis can relieve uncertainties for cancer patients, thereby enhancing the humane aspects of the care we can provide [7].

Prognostic Factors Groups

Prognostic factors may be classified in several ways, including mechanism of action or function. However, the TNM Project Committee has employed a classification based on the origin of the prognostic factors. Factors are divided into three groups – those related to the patient (including the effects of the tumor on the host), those related to the tumor, and those related to treatment.

Patient-Related Prognostic Factors

Patient-related factors are clinical factors. They depend on variables attributed to or found in the patient. Age, gender, race, genetic background, immune status, and local or systemic complications from the cancer are typical examples. While often used for estimating outcome, their role is less well established in predicting response to therapy.

Most patient-related prognostic factors have not undergone extensive study. While age and performance status have been identified as important independent prognostic factors in many cancers [11, 14], the mechanisms by which they affect outcome are not clear. Weight loss, hemoglobin level, and serum albumin may also be relevant for specific tumor types. Less well documented are clinical manifestations prior to treatment including the presence of symptoms, the severity of illness, the rate of progression of clinical manifestations, and the severity of associated co-morbidity [11]. The duration and severity of symptoms may predict an aggressive tumor behavior and have been used for estimating outcome for patients with lung cancer [12, 35]. Although the clinical manifestations, functional effects, and associated co-morbidity of a cancer are recognized as having major prognostic importance, they have not been widely studied in prospective trials nor considered in any system of formal staging. Patient related prognostic factors, when investigated, were found to have a profound influence on outcome which in some instances outweighed the effects of therapy and, as such, are essential in the comprehensive evaluation of patients. In a study of patients with advanced lung cancer, the survival with inoperable cancer varied between 6 weeks to more than a year, depending on the initial performance status, extent of disease, and prior weight loss [35]. Reporting of results without considering such strong prognostic factors severely impedes any comparisons of the effect of therapy on survival.

Tumor-Related Prognostic Factors

Prognostic factors that predict the response to treatment are usually tumor related. They include traditional features such as the classification of the primary tumor, histologic type, histologic grade, and the presence, location and extent of metastases. The primary tumor description includes the anatomic extent of disease at the initial site, invasion of other structures, and the size of the primary lesion. Other factors including hormone receptors, biochemical markers, oncogene expression, expression of proliferation-related antigens, and other molecular markers have also been recognized widely [18, 19, 27]. The UICC (International Union Against Cancer) TNM classification and stage grouping [26], and the identical AJCC (American Joint Committee on Cancer) TNM classification, are based primarily on the anatomic extent of disease. Therefore, the classification deals only with one domain of tumor-associated prognostic factors.

Treatment-Related Prognostic Factors

The prognosis and outcomes observed in most studies reflect the impact of the disease in the context of specific therapeutic interventions. Consequently, putative prognostic factors that are under investigation must be considered in the context of the specific treatment applied. It is accepted that therapeutic intervention will, in most instances, affect outcome. Thus the impact of the choice of therapy, usually discussed in detail in standard textbooks, will not be considered further in the discussion that follows.

The term "treatment related prognostic factors" as used in this book relates to variation within a given treatment policy, such as differences in techniques employed and mode of treatment delivery that may also vary in quality. Whereas the impact of the overall treatment selection has been extensively studied in prospective randomized trials, and the quality of treatment delivery is accepted as important, there is insufficient information about the impact of specific treatment related issues on outcome. Specific treatment issues, such as chemotherapy, dose, intensity and overall treatment time in radiotherapy have been reported recently, but the magnitude of their impact remains unknown [3, 20]. Prognostic factors affecting the outcome of surgical treatment have not been studied to the same extent, presumably because of difficulties with standardization and audit. However, it is becoming increasingly clear that surgeons vary in the ability to produce a given result. This "surgeon-related variability" relates to the short-term outcome (postoperative morbidity and mortality) as well as to long-term prognosis [15, 16, 25, 29].

After surgical treatment, the outcome is decisively determined by the residual tumor status as determined by the residual tumor (R) classification. While TNM and pTNM consider the anatomic extent of disease before treatment, the R classification describes the tumor status after treatment. It influences further therapeutic procedures and is a strong predictor of prognosis [18, 26]. In general, a favourable prognosis after surgery can be expected only in case of R0 (no residual tumor) while the prognosis for R1 and R2 (microscopic and gross residual tumor) is extremely poor [28]. There are correlations between TNM/pTNM and R because R0 resections are less frequently possible in higher tumor stages. To a certain degree, the R classification reflects the quality of surgery: in some stages R0 resection is achieved only by very experienced surgeons while some surgeons consider such cases as unresectable or not completely resectable. However, in most cases, the inability to achieve R0 status is related to the extent of disease at the time of surgery.

Response to nonsurgical treatment has not the same significance as R0 after surgery. In particular, in comparing the survival of responders and non-responders the bias caused by the so-called guarantee time for responders has to be considered [1]. Patients with poor survival prognosis who die early will not have an opportunity to enter the responders group and are automatically in-cluded in the nonresponse group, resulting in a poorer survival for the non-response group. Therefore, longer survival for responders does not imply that response causes longer survival. In such cases, the significance of response has to be analysed by special biometric techniques, e.g., the Mantel-Byar or the land-mark method [1].

Prognostic Factors – Statistical Considerations

In statistical terminology, potential prognostic factors are referred to as covariates. Potential factors may be classified as "time-dependent" covariates, that change over time during the course of the disease, or as "fixed" covariates that remain constant. Certain prognostic factors, such as recurrence, may be expressed only at a certain time during the course of the disease. For example, in patients with localized prostate cancer the PSA level 6 months following radiation therapy was an important prognostic factor for relapse [37]. Performance status, pain and size of the primary tumor 6 months following institution of hormonal therapy were also found to be of prognostic value for survival in patients with prostate cancer [36]. The problem in considering time-dependent covariates is that the covariate itself may be affected by treatment and its interpretation may be difficult, as it may act simply as a surrogate for response to treatment. Time-dependent covariates may not be identified at diagnosis and thus the following review will consider only fixed covariates. Some covariates may be monotonic, that is, are linearly related to outcome, while others that are non-monotonic are not linearly related. For breast cancer, age is a non-monotonic prognostic factor since age is not linearly related to outcome. Women less than 40 years of age and women over 85 years of age have a less favorable outcome than women between 40 years and 85 years [22].

The second method of defining covariates is based on the statistical nature of the covariates. Two types can be distinguished: continuous or discrete. Continuous covariates, such as hemoglobin level or age, have a consecutive range of values. Discrete covariates have a limited range of values and may be ordered or unordered. An unordered discrete covariate, such as race or gender, is beyond the control of the investigator. An ordered variable, such as stage or histologic grade, is allocated according to a system defined by the investigator.

Definition of Outcomes

Treatment outcome can be measured in various ways and these definitions are critical in studies on prognostic factors. It can be defined in a binary form: alive versus dead or as recurrence versus recurrence free. Alternatively, time-dependent measures such as survival (overall, cause-specific, disease-free), or relapse rate may be used. Outcome measures are usually clinically relevant since they often influence decisions about treatment. In a comparison of prognostic factors defined in different patient cohorts, the outcome measure must be the same. However, the limitations of evaluating prognostic factors in relation to outcome must also be considered. A factor that is prognostic for recurrence-free survival, may have no prognostic value in terms of overall survival. Alternatively, some prognostic factors may predict response to therapy, but have no predictive role in estimating survival. The usefulness of any given factor may depend on the clinical setting or on the specific treatment used [17, 27]. For some tumors a factor may apply to all patients or only to those assigned specific TNM or pTNM categories. In addition, a factor that is prognostically useful for patients treated with radiotherapy may be unimportant for patients treated surgically. Furthermore, the prognostic factors are usually different for patients with no residual tumor after initial treatment (R0) and those with remaining residual tumor (R1, 2) [27].

The most reliable and relevant end point in the study of cancer is survival. However, since survival studies may take many years to complete, intermediate end points representing events occurring earlier in the course of disease may be used as surrogates for survival. It should be noted that the use of surrogate end points is associated with risks, since the earlier end points may not accurately predict the ultimate survival [9, 10].

Analysis of Prognostic Factors – Univariate and Multivariate Methods

The first step in an analysis of prognostic factors is the identification of the individual covariates that relate to the outcome variable. This is known as univariate analysis. However, in most cases, prognosis is influenced by a variety of factors. There may be a multitude of associations of different strengths among the different prognostic factors. For this reason, the influence of a particular factor on prognosis can be misleading when considered alone, as this factor may depend entirely on another stronger and unrelated factor [18, 19, 27]. As a consequence, a reliable interpretation of prognostic factors requires the use of multivariate analysis such as the Cox model or logistic regression analysis with simulation of nonproportional hazards. The Cox model and logistic regression simultaneously evaluate the independent effects of several factors and show the relative risk associated with each covariate [2, 8, 30, 32, 34]. Model-based approaches are especially useful for assessing the effects of reciprocal adjustments amongst covariates.

Prognostic Index

Studies of prognostic factors offer the possibility of developing mathematical models that predict the course of disease. These models, which include prognostic indices and other scoring systems, can be derived from information available at the time of diagnosis [17, 18, 24, 27, 34]. A prognostic index applies a constant weight to each prognostic variable. As a result, all variables contribute to a single statement of outcome. The organization of prognostic factors into predictive systems, for example prognostic indices, should serve the same purpose as anatomic staging but would provide more accurate estimates of outcome. While important for research, prognostic indices have not been systematically used in practice.

Limitations of Prognostic Factor Analysis

One of the main difficulties in studying prognostic factors is dealing with missing data [21, 23]. The simplest method is to eliminate all subjects with missing data from analysis. However, this will, by reducing sample size, impair the sensitivity of the analysis. Also, if the data are not randomly missing, bias will be introduced. Unless the proportion of missing data is quite small, the conclusions may be misleading. Any conclusion regarding a covariate that results from the analysis of a data set with less than 80% complete data on that covariate should be viewed with suspicion. Multivariate analyses are particularly vulnerable to this problem since the effects of missing data are multiplicative. It is of paramount importance to realize that multivariate analysis will not reconcile differences observed which may have arisen as a function of bias.

The identification of prognostic factors is subject to certain caveats [33]. The most important point concerns the interpretation of the results of the statistical procedures. The techniques used fall into the general category of explanatory data analysis. One should always temper the results of statistical analyses with clinical and biologic knowledge. Multivariate studies often overemphasize the statistical significance of results and fail to adequately evaluate the clinical importance or magnitude of effects represented by the factor [32]. There are many problems in evaluating the importance of prognostic factors reported in the literature. Many published studies are based on small numbers of patients and are therefore unreliable, and there is generally little attempt to assess the predictive accuracy of a given factor or prognostic model by data splitting or cross-validation or by testing on independent data. Testing for predictive accuracy on independent data is essential to establish the value of a prognostic factor. Whenever possible, an entirely new data set should be used to validate findings. An additional difficulty with prognostic factor analysis is the lack of standardization in selection of variables for assessment, the manner in which data is collected, assessment of treatment effect, and outcome. Thus, separate studies identifying or failing to confirm the independent value of a given covariate may not be comparable, rendering the comparison between studies difficult.

Multivariate studies often overemphasize the statistical significance of the results and fail to evaluate adequately the importance or magnitude of effects represented by the factor. A striking new result should therefore be reviewed and validated carefully [25]. Additional data will usually resolve the issue, but a cautious interpretation of unlikely results is advised until appropriate confirmation is obtained. Accurate and reliable multivariate analyses for the generation of prognostic factors and indices require carefully planned prospective studies. Data must be collected methodically and uniformly and ideally should be obtained from more than one center. Strictly speaking, the prognostic index derived from a multivariate analysis should only be applied to the data from which it was generated. Prospective testing, either by splitting the data or by cross-validation, is essential before an index can be used generally. Statistical techniques in this field are continually evolving but, as yet, there is no universally accepted correct method applicable to all circumstances [18, 23, 27].

To classify studies, the study phase from which data are derived should be defined, for example, pilot, definitive, or confirmatory types of clinical studies [19].

Review of Literature

The review of the literature on prognostic factors in clinical oncology has been an arduous process. In many areas there is a lack of reliable information. There are no accepted standards of analysis for defining prognostic factors or for integrating prognostic factors into a system of staging. Three criteria, however, have been established by the AJCC for prognostic factors [6]. According to the AJCC, factors must be significant, independent, and clinically important. Significance implies that the prognostic factor rarely occurs by chance; independent means that the prognostic factor retains its prognostic value despite the addition of new prognostic factors; and clinically important implies clinical relevance, such as being capable of influencing patient management and thus outcome.

In this review, the authors have attempted to emphasize the prognostic factors that were identified by analysis of large data sets and generally accepted in clinical practice. In addition, there are those that may be considered important, but were supported by insufficient data; and finally there are promising new prognostic factors under investigation. The accepted prognostic factors should be proven to be independent by the use of multivariate analysis of data from at least two separate studies. Factors considered important are based either on a single study with multivariate analysis or on a large body of evidence. The lack of standardization for the selection of factors for assessment means that a rigid application of the selection criteria might hinder the recognition of the importance of some prognostic factors. Factors that have not been extensively studied may be overlooked if assessment is in favor of fashionable covariates, which, therefore, undergo more frequent study. For some cancers, there will be exceptions dictated by specific tumor characteristics and/or the state of current knowledge. An additional important consideration, especially for centers in which the latest technology may not be easily available, is that most accepted prognostic factors are readily available by careful clinical assessment, conventional imaging, and careful examination of pathology specimens. The assessment of prognostic factors is further improved by the availability of endoscopic and fine needle aspiration biopsy techniques combined with improved pathologic examination techniques and the use of special histologic stains and markers.

The utility of a prognostic factor is partly artifactual. In a disease that is routinely curable (or conversely rapidly fatal) identification of prognostic factors is of no assistance. However, the heterogeneity of human cancer is very apparent to clinicians treating this disease. Furthermore, prognostication is inherent in the practice of medicine. Therefore, the identification of prognostic factors is an essential part of patient assessment and decision making in oncology. Reduced patient heterogeneity will allow small but important treatment effects to be detected in clinical trials [6].

Many valuable prognostic factors have been identified and are currently used in clinical practice. As treatment improves, the importance of a given prognostic factor may change, necessitating reassessment of its impact with the new treatment. Furthermore, if treatment alters the natural history, new prognostic factors are needed to predict the outcomes. Up to this point factors that have been identified explain relatively little of the biologic heterogeneity observed in cancer and, in many diseases, new, influential, and fundamental covariates including distinct biologic and molecular prognostic factors remain to be identified.

Plan for the Future

The ultimate goal of prognostic factor identification is to provide a so-called prognostic system [6], i.e. an accurate system of predicting outcome for individual patients so that physicians can plan therapeutic interventions at any time during the course of disease. The currently used statistical methods are poorly equipped to handle the vast amount of data necessary for comprehensive evaluation and integration of prognostic factors. Newer computer-based technology such as neural networks hold promise for evaluating clinical data with superior efficiency and precision [4]. The goals of any such system should be a high predictive accuracy so that clinicians can customize treatment and investigators can identify homogenous patient populations in order to detect small but important treatment effects [6].

Summary

Accepting the limitations of current methodology for prognostic factor analysis, the UICC TNM Project Committee has recognized the need to consider prognostic factors other than the anatomic extent of disease. In the series of chapters that follow, the authors attempt to describe the prognostic factors that are generally accepted. In view of the complexity of assessing the impact of prognostic factors, this monograph aims to provide an overview of the present knowledge of factors in addition to the extent of disease. Part of the intention of this overview is to highlight the use of prognostic factors in the planning and evaluation of treatments and clinical trials. A further goal is to assist the interpretation of retrospective studies through standardization of prognostic factors and uniform categorization of individual variables.

References

1. Anderson JR, Cain KC, Gelber RD (1983) Analysis of survival by tumour response. J Clin Oncol 1: 710–719
2. Armitage P (1973) Statistical methods in medical research. Blackwell, Oxford,
3. Barton MB, Keane TJ, Gadalla T et al (1992) The effect of treatment time and treatment interruption on tumour control following radical radiotherapy of laryngeal cancer. Radiother Oncol 23: 137–143
4. Baxt W (1991) Use of an artificial neural network for the diagnosis of myocardial infarction. Ann Intern Med 115: 843–848
5. Boyd NF (1992) Guide to studies of diagnostic tests, prognosis, and treatment. In: Tannock IF, Hill R (eds)The basic science of oncology. McGraw Hill, New York, pp 379–394
6. Burke HB, Henson DE (1993) Criteria for prognostic factors and for an enhanced prognostic system. Cancer 72: 3131–3135
7. Byar DP (1984) Identification of prognostic factors. In: Buyse ME, Staquet MJ, Sylvester RJ (eds) Cancer clinical trials. Oxford University Press, New York, pp 423–443
8. Cox DR (1972) Regression models and life tables (with discussion). J Stat Soc B 34: 187–220
9. Ellenberg SS, Hamilton JM (1989) Surrogate endpoints in clinical trials: cancer. Stat Med 8: 405–413
10. Ellenberg SS (1991) Surrogate end points in clinical trials. Br Med J 302: 63–64
11. Feinstein AR (1985) On classifying cancers while treating patients. Arch Intern Med 145: 1789–1791
12. Feinstein AR, Gelfman NA, Yesner R (1970) Observer variability in histopathologic diagnosis of lung cancer. Am Rev Respir Dis 101: 671–684
13. Feinstein AR, Sosin DM, Wells CK (1985) The Will Rogers phenomenon. Stage migration and new diagnostic techniques as a source of misleading statistics for survival in cancer. N Engl J Med 312: 1604–1608
14. Feinstein AR, Wells CK (1990) A clinical severity staging system for patients with lung cancer. Medicine 69: 1–33
15. Fielding LP (1988) Surgeon-related variability in the outcome of cancer surgery. J Clin Gastroenterol 10: 120–132
16. Fielding LP, Stewart-Brown S, Dudley HA (1978) Surgeon-related variables and the clinical trial. Lancet ii: 778–779
17. Fielding LP, Arsenault PA, Chapuis PH et al (1991) Clinicopathological staging for colorectal cancer: An international documentation system (IDS) and an international comprehensive anatomical terminology (ICAT). J Gastroenterol Hepatol 6: 325–344
18. Fielding LP, Fenoglio-Preiser CM, Freedman LS (1992) The future of prognostic factors in outcome prediction for patients with cancer. Cancer 70: 2367–2377
19. Fielding LP, Henson DE (1993) Multiple prognostic factors and outcome analysis in patients with cancer. Communication from the American Joint Committee on Cancer. Cancer 71: 2426–2429
20. Fyles A, Keane TJ, Barton M et al (1992) The effect of treatment duration in the local control of cervix cancer. Radiother Oncol 25: 273–279
21. George SL (1988) Identification and assessment of prognostic factors. Semin Oncol 5: 462–471
22. Gloeckler LA, Henson DE, Harras A (1994) Survival from breast cancer according to tumour size and nodal status. Surg Oncol Clin North Am 3: 35–53
23. Harrell FE Jr, Lee KL, Matchar DB et al (1985) Regression models for prognostic predictions: advantages, problems and suggested solution. Cancer Treat Rep 69: 1071–1077
24. Henson DE (1992) Future directions for the American Joint Committee on Cancer. Cancer 69: 1639–1644
25. Hermanek P (1993) Long-term results of a German prospective multicenter study on colo-rectal cancer. In: Takahashi T (ed) Recent advances in management of digestive cancers. Springer, Berlin Heidelberg New York
26. Hermanek P, Sobin LH (eds) (1992) UICC TNM classification of malignant tumours, 4th edn, 2nd rev. Springer, Berlin Heidelberg New York
27. Hermanek P, Hutter RVP, Sobin LH (1990) Prognostic grouping: the next step in tumour classification. J Cancer Res Clin Oncol 116: 513–516

28. Hermanek P, Wittekind C (1994) Residual tumor (R) classification and prognosis. Semin Surg Oncol 10: 12–20
29. Hermanek P Jr, Wiebelt H, Riedl S, Staimmer D, Hermanek P und die Studiengruppe Kolorektales Karzinom (SGKRK) (1994) Langzeitergebnisse der chirurgischen Therapie des Coloncarcinoms. Ergebnisse der Studiengruppe Kolorektales Karzinom. Chirurg 65: 287–297
30. Kalbfleisch JD, Prentice RL (1980) The statistical analysis of failures time data. Wiley, New York
31. Sather HN (1986) The use of prognostic factors in clinical trials. Cancer 58: 461–467
32. Simon R (1984) Importance of prognostic factors in cancer clinical trials. Cancer Treat Rep 68: 185–192
33. Simon R, Altman DG (1994) Statistical aspects of prognostic factor studies in oncology. Br J Cancer 69: 979–985
34. Soong S-J (1992) A computerized mathematical model and scoring system for predicting outcome in patients with localized melanoma. In: Balch CM, Houghton AN, Milton GW et al (eds) Cutaneous melanoma. Lippincott, Philadelphia, pp 200–212
35. Stanley KE (1980) Prognostic factors for survival in patients with inoperable lung cancer. J Natl Cancer Inst 65: 25–32
36. Suciu S, Sylvester RJ, Yamanaka H (1990) Time-dependent prognostic factors in advanced prostatic cancer. In: Newling DWW, Jones WG, (eds) Prostate cancer and testicular cancer. Wiley-Liss, New York, pp 203–215 (EORTC Genitourinary Group monograph 7)
37. Zagars GK (1993) The prognostic significance of a single serum prostate-specific antigen value beyond six months after radiation therapy for adenocarcinoma of the prostate. Int J Radiat Oncol Biol Phys 27: 39–45

2 Squamous Cell Carcinoma of the Head and Neck

E.W. Strong, H. Kasdorf, and J.M. Henk

Introduction

A wide variety of tumor types arising from different tissues are included under the heading of "head and neck cancer." This review is concerned with squamous cell carcinomas arising from the surface epithelium of the upper respiratory and alimentary tract, which includes the oral cavity, pharynx, larynx, and paranasal sinuses. In excess of 95% of head and neck cancers are squamous cell carcinomas; their behavior differs according to the topographic site of origin but they have many prognostic factors in common. Undifferentiated carcinoma of nasopharyngeal type (UCNT), although arising from respiratory epithelium, has a different behavior from squamous cell carcinoma and will not be considered here.

Patient-Related Factors

Age

The prognosis of squamous cell carcinoma of the head and neck worsens with increasing age at presentation. In a multivariate analysis of over 3000 patients, Gamel and Jones [18] found that age had a small effect on probability of tumor cure which only just reached statistical significance ($p < 0.05$). However, there was marked effect on survival ($p < 0.001$). In an analysis of prognostic factors in laryngeal cancer, Stell [40] showed that older patients were less likely to receive radical treatment and had a higher mortality from intercurrent disease and second primaries. When allowance was made for these other factors, age ceased to be significant. Patients under the age of 40 have a significantly better prognosis with respect to both tumor cure and survival [7]. Age in excess of 40 seems to have only a minor influence on treatment outcome. Cancer of the oral tongue in patients less than 40 years of age may be an exception. While rare, its behavior may be aggressive. One collected series of retrospective reports indicates higher local regional recurrence and cancer-associated mortality than in older patients with similarly staged oral tongue cancers [35].

Gender

Squamous cell carcinoma at most head and neck sites has a considerably higher incidence in males than in females. A number of authors have reported a better prognosis for females compared with males, for example glottic (but not supraglottic) carcinoma [42], oral cavity [25], and oropharynx [4]. Many other reports fail to show this difference, although there are hardly any reports of a better outcome in males. The multivariate analysis by Gamel and Jones [18] found a significantly higher tumor cure rate in females but no effect on survival. In cancer females generally fare somewhat better than males [44] and squamous cell carcinoma of the head and neck is almost certainly no exception.

Performance Status

In most multivariate analyses of head and neck squamous cell carcinoma, performance status, when included, has proved to be one of the most significant independent patient-related prognostic factors. This is true whether the Karnovsky or the WHO scale is used. Performance status is a significant factor for both tumor cure and survival. It has been shown to have a profound effect on the probability of local control of primary tumors by radiotherapy [19]. Mick et al. [28] studied the effect of weight loss, which can be claimed to be a more specific and measurable variable than performance status and which also reflects the patient's general health. Loss of more than 10% of body weight prior to treatment was the most potent adverse prognostic factor in a multivariate analysis of patients with advanced squamous cell carcinoma of the head and neck undergoing multi-modality therapy.

Hemoglobin

Anemia is known to prejudice the success of radical radiotherapy. Hemoglobin concentration has been shown to correlate strongly with local tumor control by radiotherapy [4,31], but has not been demonstrated to be an independent prognostic factor for survival.

Immunologic Factors

Numerous immunologic parameters have been investigated hoping to link them with prognosis and survival of patients with squamous cell carcinoma of the head and neck. Absolute lymphocyte counts, T cell subsets, natural killer cell population, and humoral and cellular immunity have been studied. In general the prognostic value and clinical utility of the known immunologic parameters remain unclear and do not justify their use in routine clinical care [12]. Further investigation is necessary and warranted.

Life-Style

Tobacco and alcohol consumption are potent etiological factors for head and neck cancer. It is the impression of clinicians treating head and neck cancer that patients who continue to smoke and drink heavily after treatment have a poor outcome, but these factors have rarely been included in multivariate analyses. Mick et al. [28] demonstrated an effect of alcohol consumption ($p = 0.012$) on survival. Pradier et al. [33], using multivariate analysis of prognostic factors in 296 males with larynx cancer, demonstrated that alcohol intake as well as lymph node enlargement and vocal cord mobility were the only statistically significant variables impacting upon survival. It has been shown that patients who continue to smoke during radiotherapy have a lower local tumor cure rate [6].

Tumor-Related Factors

Site of Origin

Squamous cell carcinomas have differing prognoses according to the site of origin within the upper air and food passages. This is in some measure because tumors at some sites tend to present when smaller and at an earlier stage than at other sites. Anatomical differences also contribute to the varying prognoses. Some areas have a richer blood supply and lymphatic drainage than others, and in some sites there are anatomical barriers to spread which confine the tumor to the organ of origin for a considerable period. For example, carcinoma of the vocal cord has the most favorable prognosis of all. This is largely because a tumor on the vocal cord gives rise to recognizable symptoms at a very early stage and is therefore usually treated when quite small, but also because the framework of the larynx provides a barrier to local spread and the relative lack of lymphatic vessels means that nodal involvement is uncommon. As a result, in most series the overall 5-year survival rate for glottic carcinoma is at least 80%. By contrast, tumors of the adjacent hypopharynx are rarely diagnosed when less than 2 cm in diameter and readily invade adjacent structures and metastasize to lymph nodes, so that overall survival rates are only about 20%.

Local Spread of Primary Tumor

As a general principle *T category* correlates well with prognosis, patients with lower T faring better as would be expected. However, in considering head and neck cancer globally, T categories cannot be grouped together, because at some sites the T category is based mainly on the measurements of the tumor while at other sites it is based on local spread to adjacent structures. Consequently, tumors can have the same T category but very different prognoses. For example, the 5-year survival rates for T2 tumors of the vocal cord and base of tongue are 80% and 40%, respectively. In many multivariate analyses of large series of head and neck cancer T status is one of the less significant prognostic factors.

Tumor volume correlates better with prognosis than T status. In analyses which have considered the size of the primary tumor, it has proved one of the most significant factors [9]. Primary size and T status are especially important in determining local tumor control rates by radiotherapy [19]. These factors have relatively less impact on survival than nodal stage (see below).

Depth of infiltration/tumor thickness of the primary tumor may be prognostically significant, probably more so than the surface extent of the lesion (T status). Spiro et al. [39] showed that depth of invasion of early floor of mouth and oral tongue cancers (any T, N0) was directly related to the risk of subsequent regional nodal metastases and ultimate survival. Baredes et al. [1] similarly demonstrated that tumor thickness in soft palate carcinoma correlated more directly with nodal metastases than T status. Thicker lesions were also associated with poorer survival, as were tumors of more advanced T and stage grouping categories.

N Status

In most analyses involvement of lymph nodes by tumor is the most significant factor predicting for survival. The presence of nodal metastases reduces survival rates by approximately half in both oral [11,19,25] and supraglottic [21] carcinoma. The effect is less in carcinoma of the oropharynx, possibly because oropharyngeal carcinoma is more often treated by radical radiotherapy [22].

The current TNM staging system for lymph nodes is based mainly on the size of the nodes and correlates well with prognosis. In most series the presence of one involved node 3 cm or less in diameter (N1) has only a small effect on survival and scarcely any effect on locoregional control, whereas larger nodes have a pronounced effect on both these outcomes. Radiocurability of lymph node metastases is strongly related to nodal size [2].

Bilateral or contralateral node involvement is generally believed to indicate an unfavorable prognosis, but so far this observation has not been definitely confirmed statistically. Jones and Stell [23] reported that 5-year survival rates were 9% lower in patients with bilateral or contralateral nodes compared with those with only unilateral nodes, but this difference did not reach statistical significance on multivariate analysis unless only nodes greater than 6 cm in diameter were considered.

When nodal metastases are treated by radical neck dissection, histologic findings in the operative specimen correlate well with outcome. Snow et al. [37] found extracapsular spread to be the most important single prognostic factor for local recurrence in the neck. Nodal fixation, the number of positive nodes, and histologic grade were also significant factors for local recurrence.

One of the reasons often quoted for the worse survival of patients with nodal involvement is the higher frequency of distant metastases. Leemans et al. [26] studied results in 511 patients undergoing neck dissection; those patients with histopathologic evidence of nodal involvement were twice as likely to develop distant metastases as those without nodal involvement. Those with more than three positive nodes were at highest risk of distant metastases; extracapsular spread also predicted a significant increase in distant metastases. On the other hand, a multivariate analysis of 500 patients with advanced head and neck cancer treated by radiotherapy failed to show any influence of nodal stage on the development of distant metastases [15]. The inference is that pathologic findings in lymph nodes are better predictors of outcome than clinical findings.

Histologic Features

There are conflicting data on the prognostic significance of histologic grading. Gamel and Jones [18] found that the degree of differentiation was second only to nodal stage as a prognostic factor for tumor cure, but its influence on survival was not significant. Langdon et al. [25] were unable to demonstrate any effect of histologic grade on local recurrence, but noted that poorly differentiated tumors were more likely to give rise to lymph node metastases.

Crissman et al. [9] studied biopsy specimens from 77 patients with carcinoma of the oropharynx treated by a uniform policy. They evaluated the specimens for degree of keratinization, nuclear pleomorphism, frequency of mitoses, inflammatory response, vascular invasion, and patterns of invasion. They performed multivariate analysis to relate these factors to survival. The pattern of invasion proved to be the only significant factor: tumors invading as large cohesive aggregates indicated a better prognosis than those invading as thin irregular cords or individual cells. In a smaller study looking critically at the histologic grading of the deep invasive margins of lingual squamous cell carcinomas, Odell et al. [29] concluded that local recurrence correlated with Broder's grade, keratinization, and pattern of invasion. Distant metastases had a highly significant correlation with Broder's grade, pattern of invasion, and invasive front-grading total score. Zatterstrom et al. [45], reporting their analysis of histologic grading and DNA ploidy as prognostic factors in 72 squamous cell carcinomas of the head and neck, concluded that with multivariate analysis the combination of grading score and nodal status were the strongest predictors for survival and that DNA ploidy did not contribute further prognostic information. Soo et al. [38] found perineural spread in the primary to be independent of tumor size, nodal involvement, or histologic grade, but was associated with a statistically significant increase in local recurrence and decrease in survival. Close et al. [8] demonstrated that the presence of squamous cell carcinoma within capillaries and/or venules in the immediate vicinity of T2 and larger primary lesions of the oral cavity and oropharynx resulted in statistically significant increased frequency of regional nodal metastases over those patients without such vascular invasion, independent of clinical appearance, differentiation, depth of invasion, and perineural invasion of the primary. In a multivariate analysis of 181 patients with oropharyngeal carcinoma treated by radiotherapy, Bentzen et al. [4] demonstrated that well-differentiated primary tumors were significantly less likely to be cured by radical radiotherapy than moderately or poorly differentiated tumors.

The prognostic value of histologic grading is uncertain. It is partly a matter of individual interpretation, and in any case a biopsy specimen may not be representative of the whole tumor. The histologic grading system employed by Crissman [9] may give a more representative assessment of the biologic aggressiveness of the tumor than more limited grading by Broder's system. Histologic grading may thus be of some value in estimating tumor behavior and response to therapy, especially in the more anaplastic, aggressive varieties of squamous cell carcinoma. Histologic grade, however, is of limited prognostic usefulness when isolated and separate from clinical and other factors.

Ploidy

Ploidy is another subject on which conflicting data have been published. Most series suggest that diploid tumors have the best prognosis, but some have suggested that aneuploid tumors are more responsive to radiotherapy and chemotherapy. Stell [41] reviewed 26 publications on the subject. He concluded that both survival and local cure rates were higher in diploid tumors and that ploidy did not affect the response to radiotherapy. Nondiploid tumors were more likely to be poorly differentiated and to give rise to lymph node metastases. Kearsley et al. [24] studied 172 biopsy specimens for DNA content. A multivariate analysis taking into account all other known significant prognostic factors revealed that the death rate from cancer was approximately three times higher with aneuploid tumors compared with diploid. Ensley and Maciorowaki [14] have shown that significant differences in clinical and treatment outcome as well as the biology of tumors result from evolution of DNA ploidy in head and neck squamous cell carcinomas from diploid to aneuploid status. This may result from many different molecular events, including loss of wild-type p53 function and higher tumor epidermal growth factor receptor (EGFR) protein levels, among many other events. The aneuploid tumors have acquired certain more "malignant" advantages, including increased cell motility, inhibition of host stromal and inflammatory responses, increased proliferative activity, and local invasiveness and metastatic potential. In their series of more than 200 patients with stage III and IV resectable squamous cell carcinoma of the head and neck undergoing multidisciplinary treatment, recurrence rate was lower (19% versus 63%) and the 2-year survival rate better (63% versus 32%) in the DNA diploid group; 81% of those with diploid tumors remained disease free compared to 40% of those with DNA aneuploid tumors. Complete response to neoadjuvant chemotherapy was much higher in those patients with DNA aneuploid tumors (80%) than in those with pure DNA diploid tumors (3%). This favorable responsiveness to preliminary chemotherapy by aneuploid tumors has been confirmed by other investigators. The correlation of DNA content parameters and response to conventionally administered radiation therapy for head and neck squamous cell carcinoma is less clear. Favorable response to chemotherapy is usually indicative of favorable response to conventional radiotherapy. Nonresponders are much less likely to be cured by radiotherapy. However, these DNA diploid tumors may have a better response to concurrent radiation and high-dose cisplatin chemotherapy. This has implications in treatment selection for diploid tumors.

It seems that diploid tumors do have a better prognosis, but the relation of ploidy to response to various forms of treatment is less clear. Further investigation of ploidy status using optimum techniques is appropriate and correlation with prognosis can only be made with suitable numbers of patients followed for adequate time intervals. Certain aspects of DNA ploidy may have some prognostic significance. Significant differences of opinion still exist.

Tumor Cell Kinetics

It is believed that fast-growing tumors have a worse prognosis than slow-growing tumors. The potential doubling time of a tumor, which is a measure of cell proliferation rate, can be estimated by labeling tumor cells in vivo with 5-bromodeoxyuridine (BUdR) or iododeoxyuridine (IUdR) and examining biopsy specimens by flow cytometry. The preliminary results of Begg et al. [3] suggested that local control rates from radiotherapy are related to potential doubling time, but statistically significant results have yet to be obtained. There is much current interest in variations of fractionation of radiation therapy to achieve optimum treatment results with acceptable morbidity. Fowler [17] has correlated calculated log cell kill as a function of effective cell doubling time (T_{eff}) for a number of radiation fractionation schedules. He concluded that neither hyperfractionation nor accelerated fractionation were "panacea" treatments. Use of kinetic data may be helpful in indicating more effective fractionation, but the fact that pretreatment tumor doubling time (T_{pot}) may be different from actual doubling time (T_{eff}) of tumors during treatment may detract from its value. As yet no precise data on the effects of varied fractionation schedules based upon large groups of patients with similar tumors exists. We need further experience with kinetic data before using it routinely in clinical practice. Its greater relevance to radiotherapy and chemotherapy than surgery is apparent.

Receptors

In one study of laryngeal cancer, the EGFR level in tumors was shown to be related to survival and risk of distant metastases [27]. The relative mortality risk was three times higher in tumors with a positive EGFR status than in those with a negative EGFR status. This difference proved to be highly significant on multivariate analysis.

Tumor Markers

An ever-increasing number of tumor markers are being identified and studied. Those having relevance to head and neck cancer include carcinoembryonic antigen (CEA), squamous cell carcinoma antigen (SCC-Ag), ferritins, glycoprotein cancer-associated antigens (CA-50, CA-19–9), serum enzymes including alkaline phosphatase, serum phosphohexose isomerase (PH1), serum adenosine deaminase (ADA), erythrocyte polyamines, prostaglandins, prostacyclines, and derivatives of sialic acid including lipid-associated sialic acid (LASA) and protein-bound sialic acid (PBSA) [5,12,13,20]. Studies of patients with head and neck cancer have shown increased levels of LASA and PBSA correlating with extent of disease. Serial determinations of PBSA in one study [5] showed excellent correlation with progression of disease or response to treatment in patients with advanced disease. In the same group of patients SCC-Ag showed less correlation with disease extent and response to treatment. There are no serologic markers shown to have prognostic value for patients with squamous cell carcinoma of the head and neck [13]. All have disadvantages, usually with limited sensitivity and low degree of specificity, thus limiting their diagnostic usefulness in screening. Measuring more than one marker may enhance diagnostic accuracy, as may serial determination of marker levels. The latter may provide information on reponse to therapy / tumor status, but will not be usually adequate to provide reliable prognostic information [5,12,13,20].

Genetic Abnormalities

Tumors arise from a series of genetic events / mutations involving various cellular genes. These genetic alterations may include deletions, amplifications, or translocations. Such point mutations are common in squamous cell carcinomas of the head and neck with a clustering of chromosomal breakpoints particularly in the regions of 1p22 and 11q13 [16,32]. These point mutations occur in proto-oncogenes and in tumor suppressor genes and are detectable in clinical tissues. They act as markers for the specific cancers and may be of assistance in detecting the cancer in screening, indicating those at risk of developing the cancer, and may also be of prognostic and therapeutic value [30,36]. Genetic alterations in squamous cell carcinoma of the head and neck are multiple. Mutants of the *ras* gene family have been noted in multiple human cancers but are rarely seen in head and neck cancer in Europe or in the United States. In general, high levels of *ras* p21 were associated with poor prognosis. Amplification and rearrangement of the *myc* gene family in head and neck cancer has been shown not to be an important feature in the Western world, but is more common in India. Overexpression of c-*myc* is thought to be correlated with a poor prognosis. Epidermal growth factor (EGF) amplification has not been a consistent feature of head and neck squamous cell carcinomas or cell lines. The proto-oncogene product p53 is one of the most common genetic features in a wide variety of human cancers, but the specific relationship of p53 to head and neck cancer is not clear [16]. Mutation of p53 prevents control of cell cycle and allows spontaneous or environmentally induced mutations to go unrepaired. Alterations in the p53 gene may be one of the early events in head and neck squamous cell carcinoma. Cigarette smoking and p53 overexpression may be related to head and neck squamous cell carcinoma. As yet, these and other genetic markers have not been sufficiently studied or their effects sufficiently documented to be of value as indicators of prognosis.

Treatment-Related Factors

Although it is generally recognized that the quality of treatment is of paramount importance, most analyses of prognostic factors have failed to show any relationship between treatment and survival. This is probably because most series studied were treated according to a uniform policy.

There are some data relating radiotherapy treatment parameters to outcome. The American Patterns of Care Studies showed that local control of early oral cavity carcinoma was higher using interstitial rather than external beam radiation [43]. A number of studies have shown the importance of treatment time, with a significantly increased risk of radiotherapy failure if the treatment time is prolonged beyond 6 weeks.[19,34]

References

1. Baredes S, Leeman DJ, Chen TS et al (1993) Significance of tumor thickness in soft palate carcinoma. Laryngoscope 103: 389–393
2. Bataini JP, Bernier J, Asselain B et al (1988) Primary radiotherapy of squamous cell carcinoma of the oropharynx and pharyngolarynx: tentative multivariate modeling system to predict the radiocurability of neck nodes. Int J Radiat Oncol Biol Phys 14: 635–642
3. Begg AC, Hofland I, Moonen L, et al (1990) The predictive value of cell kinetic measurements in a European trial of accelerated fractionation in advanced head and neck tumours: an interim report. Int J Radiat Oncol Biol Phys 19: 1449–1453
4. Bentzen SM, Johansen LV, Overgaard J, Thames HD (1991) Clinical radiobiology of squamous carcioma of the oropharynx. Int J Radiat Oncol Biol Phys 20: 1197–1206
5. Bhalavdekar JM, Patel DD, Vora HH et al (1991) Squamous cell carcinoma antigen and protein bound sialic acid in the management of head and neck cancer. Int J Biol Markers 6: 237–240
6. Bowman GP, Wong G, Hodson I et al (1993) Influence of cigarette smoking on the efficacy of radiation therapy in head and neck cancer. N Engl J Med 328: 159–163
7. Clarke RW, Stell PM (1992) Squamous carcinoma of the head and neck in the young adult. Clin Otolaryngol 17: 18–23
8. Close LG, Burus DK, Reisch J et al (1987) Microvascular invasion in cancer of the oral cavity and oropharynx. Arch Otolaryngol Head Neck Surg 113: 1191–1195
9. Crissman JD, Liu WY, Gluckman JL, Cummings G (1984) Prognostic value of histopathologic parameters in squamous cell carcinoma of the oropharynx. Cancer 54: 2995–3001

10. Davidson BJ, Hsu TC, Schantz SP (1993) The genetics of tobacco induced malignancy. Arch Otolaryngol Head Neck Surg 119: 1198–1205
11. Decroix Y, Ghossein NA (1981) Experience of the Curie Institute in treatment of cancer of the mobile tongue. Cancer 47: 496–502
12. Dreyfuss AI, Clark JR (1991) Analysis of prognostic factors in squamous cell carcinomas of the head and neck. Hemat/Oncol Clin N Am 5: 701–712
13. Dreyfuss AI, Clark JR, Andersen JW (1992) Lipid associated sialic acid, squamous cell carcinoma antigen, carcino-embryonic antigen and lactic dehydrogenase levels as tumor markers in squamous cell carcinoma of the head and neck. Cancer 70: 2499–2503
14. Ensley JF, Maciorowaki Z (1994) Clinical applications of DNA content parameters in patients with squamous carcinoma of the head and neck. Sem Oncol 21: 330–339
15. Fazekas JT, Sommer C, Kramer S (1983) Tumor regression and other prognosticators in advanced head and neck cancers: a sequel to the RTOG methotrexate study. Int J Radiat Oncol Biol Phys 9: 957–964
16. Field JK (1992) Oncogenes and tumor suppressor genes in squamous cell carcinoma of the head and neck. Oral Oncol Eur J Cancer 28B: 67–76
17. Fowler JF. (1992) Intercomparisons of new and old schedules in fractionated radiotherapy. Sem Radiat Oncol 2: 67–72
18. Gamel JW, Jones AS (1993) Squamous carcinoma of the head and neck: cured fraction and median survival time as functions of age, sex, histologic type, and node status. Br J Cancer 67: 1071–1075
19. Griffin TW, Pajak TF, Gillespie BW et al (1984) Predicting the response of head and neck cancers to radiation therapy with a multivariate modeling system: an analysis of the RTOG head and neck registry. Int J Radiat Oncol Biol Phys 10: 481–487
20. Hanna EYN, Papay FA, Gupta MK et al (1990) Serum tumor markers of head and neck cancer: current status. Head Neck 12: 50–59
21. Harwood AR (1982) Cancer of the larynx – the Toronto experience. J Otolaryngol [Suppl] 11: 1–21
22. Henk JM, A'Hern RP, Taylor K (1993) Carcinoma of the oropharynx in the United Kingdom. In: Johnson ST, Didolkar MS (eds) Head and neck cancer, vol. III. Excerpta Medica, Amsterdam, pp 779–784
23. Jones AS, Stell PM (1991) Is laterality important in neck node metastases? Clin Otolaryngol 16: 221–225
24. Kearsley JH, Bryson G, Battistuta D, Collins RJ (1991) Prognostic importance of cellular DNA content in head and neck squamous cell cancers: a comparison of retrospective and prospective series. Int J Cancer 47: 31–37
25. Langdon JD, Harvey PW, Rapidis AD et al (1977) Oral cancer; the behavior and response to treatment of 194 cases. J Maxillofac Surg 5: 221
26. Leemans CR, Tiwari R, Nauta JJP et al (1993) Regional lymph node involvement and its significance in the development of distant metastases in head and neck carcioma. Cancer 71: 452–456
27. Maurizi M, Scambria G, Benedetti-Pancici P et al (1992) EGF receptor expression in primary laryngeal cancer: correlation with clinicopathological features and prognostic significance. Int J Cancer 52: 862–866
28. Mick R, Vokes EE, Weichselbaum RR, Panje WR (1991) Prognostic factors in advanced head and neck cancer patients undergoing multimodality therapy. Otolaryngol Head Neck Surg 105: 62–73
29. Odell EW, Jani P, Ahluwalia SM et al (1994) The prognostic value of individual histologic grading parameters in small lingual squamous cell carcinomas. Cancer 74: 89–94
30. O'Malley BW, Ledley FD (1993) Somatic gene therapy in otolaryngology – head and neck surgery. Arch Otolaryngol Head Neck Surg 119: 1191–1197
31. Overgaard J, Sand Hansen H, Andersen AP et al (1986) Misonidazole combined with split-course radiotherapy in the treatment of invasive carcinoma of the larynx and pharynx. Int J Radiat Oncol Biol Phys 12: 516–521
32. Owens W, Field JK, Howard PJ et al (1992) Multiple cytogenetic aberrations in squamous cell carcinomas of the head and neck. Oral Oncol Eur J Cancer 28B: 17–21
33. Pradier R, Gonzalez A, Matos E et al (1993) Prognostic factors in laryngeal carcinoma; experience in 296 male patients. Cancer 71: 2472–2476
34. Robertson AG, Robertson C, Boyle P et al (1993) The effect of differing radiotherapeutic schedules on the response of glottic carcinoma of the larynx. Eur J Cancer 29A: 501–510

35. Sarkarice JN, Harari PM (1993) Oral tongue cancer in young adults less than 40 years of age: rationale for aggressive therapy. Head Neck 16: 107–111
36. Sideransky D, Boyle J, Koch W (1993) Molecular screening. Prospects for a new approach. Arch Otolaryngol Head Neck Surg 119: 1187–1190
37. Snow GB, Annyas AA, van Slooten EA et al (1982) Prognostic factors of neck node metastases. Clin Otolaryngol 7: 185–192
38. Soo KC, Carter RL, Barr L et al (1986) Prognostic implications of perineural spread in squamous carcinomas of the head and neck. Laryngoscope 96: 1145–1149
39. Spiro RH, Huvos AG, Wong GY et al (1986) Predictive value of tumor thickness in squamous carcinoma confined to the tongue and floor of mouth. Am J Surg 152: 345–350
40. Stell PM (1988) Prognostic factors in laryngeal carcinoma. Clin Otolaryngol 13: 399–409
41. Stell PM (1991) Ploidy in head and neck cancer: a review and metaanalysis. Clin Otolaryngol 16: 510–516
42. Till JE, Bruce WR, Elwan A et al (1975) A preliminary analysis of end results for cancer of the larynx. Laryngoscope 85: 259–275
43. Wallner PE, Hanks GE, Kramer S, McLean CJ (1986) Patterns of care study: analysis of outcome survey data – anterior two-thirds of tongue and floor of mouth. Am J Clin Oncol 9: 50–57
44. Waterhouse JAH (1974) Cancer handbook of epidemiology and prognosis. Churchill Livingstone, Edinburgh
45. Zatterstrom UK, Wennerberg J, Evers SB et al (1991) Prognostic factors in head and neck cancer: histologic grading, DNA ploidy and nodal status. Head Neck 13: 477–487

3 Parotid Carcinoma

C. Calearo and A. Pastore

Introduction

Primary parotid gland epithelial malignancies are rare, accounting for approximately 1%–3% of all head and neck carcinomas. The histological variety of such tumours, their different natural history and the peculiar anatomy of the region can make diagnosis, prognosis and therapeutic strategy quite controversial. Appropriate parotid gland carcinoma management requires up-to-date information regarding those prognostic factors able to affect local, regional or distant recurrences and survival. The event which determines therapeutic failure in parotid gland malignancies is most notably the appearance of recurrences: local, regional and/or distant [13]. Therefore, it appeared reasonable to perform a statistical assessment of prognostic factors by considering recurrences as the end point. In this contribution, the results of an analysis of the prognostic factors for parotid carcinomas are described based on personal data and reports published on this topic.

Not included is a discussion on choice of treatment and the controversies with regard to the extent of surgery (radical versus conservative) and indications for radiotherapy.

Tumour-Related Factors

Anatomical Extent of Disease

In all the works in which the covariants T and pT [1, 23] were present, these appeared to be highly related both to recurrence and disease-free survival [9, 10, 19, 21, 22, 24]. The T and pT categories are subdivided according to the absence or presence of local extension, i.e. clinical or macroscopic evidence of invasion of skin, soft tissues, bone or nerve. Local extension proves strongly related to prognosis [16], particularly for patients with T1 and T2 tumours (personal data). In these locally extended tumours, survival rates drop to less than 50% of those found in the same categories without local extension.

Facial nerve involvement is an extremely important prognostic factor for both recurrence and survival since very few patients presenting with facial paralysis survive their disease [5–7, 9, 13, 16, 20, 21]. In a study on 378 malignant parotid tumours, Eneroth and Hamberger [8] found 100% mortality in patients with facial nerve paralysis. The same was observed by Pedersen et al. [16]. According to all the authors reviewed, survival for patients with spontaneous facial nerve palsy is at most between 10% and 30%.

The presence of local–regional adenopathies proves highly significant for a bad prognosis [9, 20, 21]. According to Spiro et al. [20], stage and nodal status at diagnosis are the most significant prognostic variables in a Cox regression analysis.

Frankenthaler et al. [9] assert that positive cervical nodes, tumour size greater than 3 cm and nerve invasion are the factors having the greatest effect on survival rate. In fact, when these factors were all present at the same time, the patient ran a 67 times greater risk of dying of disease than did the study population as a whole. Our personal data on 57 malignant epithelial tumours revealed a highly significant correlation between recurrence and T category ($p < 0.01$), pT ($p < 0.001$), N ($p < 0.05$) and facial nerve involvement ($p < 0.001$).

Histological Type

Histological tumour type appears to be a relevant prognostic factor, particularly in terms of different biological tumour behaviour [3, 4, 8, 11, 12, 15, 16, 20, 22]. Although there is no absolute agreement between the various authors, it is evident that there are different "degrees" of malignancy. In this light, undifferentiated, squamous, malignant mixed, adenoid cystic carcinomas and adenocarcinomas have the worst prognosis, while mucoepidermoid and acinic cell carcinomas have the best. The slow tumour kinetics of some histological types (e.g. adenoid cystic carcinoma) require follow-up in excess of 10 years [3] to assess prognosis.

According to Spiro et al. [20], about 85% of all patients with acinic cell carcinoma are alive at 10 years, whereas this is true for only about 44%–50% of those with malignant mixed tumour, adenocarcinoma, or adenoid cystic carcinoma. Patients with squamous carcinoma have survival rates of less than 30% at 10 years. Mucoepidermoid tumour survival rates appear strictly linked to tumour grading; thus low-grade tumours have 10-year survival rates of up to 85%, while intermediate or high-grade lesions have a rate of only 45%.

Bjorklund and Eneroth [3] confirm a 10-year survival rate of approximately 85% for mucoepidermoid and acinic cell carcinomas, while the worst prognosis, down to less than 25% at 15 years, is found with poorly differentiated solid carcinomas, malignant mixed tumours and adenoid cystic carcinoma. The same authors stress the fact that for acinic cell carcinoma, and above all for adenoid cystic carcinoma, prognosis cannot be based on a follow-up of less than 10–15 years.

Kane et al. [14] found good 5-year survival rates for low-grade mucoepidermoid carcinoma (higher than 90%) and fairly good survival rates (about 80%) for acinic cell and adenoid cystic carcinoma. On the other hand, while the figures for mucoepidermoid carcinoma appear to change only slightly during the course of an extended follow-up, with adenoid cystic and acinic cell carcinomas they found a dramatic drop in the survival rate from 5 to 15 years. These authors stress the fact that the latter are the only histotypes capable of causing death after a 10-year disease-free interval. High-grade mucoepidermoid and squamous cell carcinomas have intermediate survival rates (approximately 40% at 10 years), whereas for all the other carcinomas prognosis is poor.

Pedersen et al. [16] note that the longest recurrence time is found in cases of acinic cell carcinomas, followed by mucoepidermoid and adenoid cystic carcinoma; the shortest time to recurrence (10 months) was found in patients with malignant mixed tumours. The reported 10-year survival rates were similar to those published by Spiro et al. [20].

Calearo et al. [4], in their therapeutic planning for malignant epithelial tumours, recognised different classes of local or regional risk of recurrence; thus a better prognosis is recognised for mucoepidermoid and acinic cell tumours. Adenoid cystic carcinoma has a good 5-year follow-up prognosis which worsens after 10–15 years of follow-up study. All the other carcinomas show poor results within the first 3 years.

Histological Grade

Only in the case of the highest grade does tumour grading appear significant in the prognosis of both recurrence and survival [9, 15-18]. Kane et al. [14] consider grading the most reliable prognostic factor, especially for mucoepidermoid carcinoma. On the other hand, Conley et al. [5] claim this also holds true for adenocarcinomas and acinic cell tumours. While Spiro et al. [20] do confirm that grading can provide some prognostic information in cases of mucoepidermoid or acinic cell carcinoma, they found no reliable correlation in cases of adenoid cystic carcinoma. Some authors [14, 24] found that grade and stage had a significant correlation with survival, while others did not [15]. Grade and tumour size have also been considered key factors in predicting distant metastases [9].

Patient-Related Factors

Age has been considered a prognostic factor by some authors ([9], personal data), but this may be explained by the fact that older patients tend to have a higher percentage of high-grade and advanced-stage lesions [20]. Male gender has been identified as an independent prognostic factor [14], while other authors [20] rule gender out of the prognostic factors. Prognostic significance has been attributed to pain and paresthesia as well as to rapid enlargement of the lesion at the time of presentation [2, 10, 14], although there is no general agreement on this topic.

Conclusions

The most relevant prognostic factors in parotid gland carcinomas are anatomic extent expressed by TNM/pTNM including local invasion (especially local nerve involvement), histological tumour type and histological grade. These factors, along with other information (i.e. age, sex, symptoms, delay of diagnosis, etc.), should always be submitted to statistical analysis in order to reliably predict the patient's chances of survival.

References

1. Beahrs OH, Woods JE, Weiland LH (1978) Surgical management of cancer of parotid tumours. Adv Surg 12: 301–326
2. Beahrs OH, Henson DE, Hutter RVP, Kennedy BJ (eds) (1992) American Joint Committee on Cancer (AJCC): manual for staging of cancer, 4th edn. Lippincott, Philadelphia
3. Bjorklund A, Eneroth CM (1980) Management of parotid gland neoplasm. Am J Otolaryngol 1: 155–167
4. Calearo C, Magno L, Bignardi L (1985) Therapeutic planning for malignant epithelial parotid tumours. Acta Otorhinolaryngol Ital 5: 206–209
5. Conley J, Hamaker RD (1975) Prognosis of malignant tumours of the parotid gland with facial paralysis. Arch Otolaryngol 101: 39–41
6. Eneroth CM, Andreasson L, Beran M et al (1977) Preoperative facial paralysis in malignant parotid tumours. ORL 39: 272–277
7. Eneroth CM (1972) Facial nerve paralysis: a criterion of malignancy in parotid tumours. Arch Otolaryngol 95: 300–304
8. Eneroth CM, Hamberger CA (1974) Principles of treatment of different types of parotid tumours. Laryngoscope 84: 1732–1740
9. Frankenthaler RA, Luna MA, Sangsook L et al (1991) Prognostic variables in parotid gland cancer. Arch Otolaryngol Head Neck Surg 117: 1251–1256
10. Fu KK, Leibel SA, Levine ML et al (1977) Carcinoma of the major and minor salivary glands. Cancer 40: 2882–2890
11. Guillamondegui OM, Byers RM, Luna MA et al (1975) Aggressive surgery in treatment for parotid cancer: the role of adjunctive post-operative radiotherapy. Am J Roentgenol 123: 49–54
12. Hermanek P, Sobin LH (eds) (1992) UICC TNM classification of malignant tumours, 4th edn, 2nd rev. Springer, Berlin Heidelberg New York
13. Hunter RM, Davis BW, Gray GF et al (1983) Primary malignant tumours of salivary gland origin. Am Surg 49: 82–89
14. Kagan AR, Nussbaum H, Handler S et al (1976) Recurrences from malignant parotid salivary gland tumor. Cancer 37: 2600–2604
15. Kane WJ, McCaffrey TV, Olsen KD et al (1991) Primary parotid malignancies. Arch Otolaryngol Head Neck Surg 117: 307–316
16. Matsuba HM, Thawley SE, Devineni VR et al (1985) High grade malignancies of the parotid gland: effective use of planned combined surgery and irradiation. Laryngoscope 95: 1059–1063
17. Pedersen D, Overgaard J, Sogaard H et al (1992) Malignant parotid tumours in 110 consecutive patients: treatment results and prognosis. Laryngoscope 102: 1064–1069
18. Perzin KH, Gullane P, Clairmont AC (1978) Adenoid cystic carcinomas arising in salivary glands. A correlation of histologic features and clinical course. Cancer 42: 265–282
19. Rafla S (1977) Malignant parotid tumours: natural history and treatment. Cancer 40: 136–144
20. Shidnia H, Hornbach NP, Hamaker R et al (1980) Carcinoma of major salivary glands. Cancer 45: 693–697
21. Spiro RH, Armstrong J, Harrison L et al (1989) Carcinoma of major salivary glands. Recent trends. Arch Otolaryngol Head Neck Surg 115: 316–321

22. Spiro RH, Huvos AG, Strong EW (1975) Carcinoma of the parotid gland: a clinicopathologic study of 288 primary cases. Am J Surg 130: 452–459
23. Tu G, Hu Y, Jiang P et al (1982) The superiority of combined therapy in parotid cancer. Arch Otolaryngol 108: 710–713
24. Witten J, Hybert F, Hansen HS (1990) Treatment of malignant tumours in the parotid glands. Cancer 65: 2515–2520

4 Thyroid Carcinoma

A. Antonaci, J. Brierley, G. Bacchi, F. Consorti, C. Consoli,
A. Manzini, M. Tagliaferri, F. Ficulccilli, F. Menichelli, C. Miani,
P. Miani, M. Di Paola, and M. Piemonte

One of the earliest studies on prognostic factors in thyroid cancer involved a multivariate analysis of the EORTC (European Organisation for Research on Treatment of Cancer) Thyroid Cancer Cooperative Group [9]. This study combined all histologies and found survival to depend on histological types. The 5-year survival ranged from 80% in differentiated carcinoma (papillary and follicular), to 55% in medullary carcinoma to 10% in anaplastic carcinoma. This was incorporated in the EORTC prognostic index. Subsequently, most studies of prognostic factors in thyroid cancer were developed for these histological types separately. Recently, the Italian Association of Surgical Oncology (SICO) [2, 15] has confirmed the significance of histological types. They found a similar survival for both papillary and follicular carcinoma, 97% and 95% at 4 years, a slightly lower survival for medullary carcinoma (91.3%) and an extremely poor survival for anaplastic carcinoma. Medullary carcinoma is derived from the parafollicular cells. The differentiated papillary and follicular carcinomas and the anaplastic carcinoma are derived from the follicular epithelium. In view of differences in treatment approaches, natural history and outcome, papillary–follicular, medullary and anaplastic carcinomas will be considered separately in this review.

Papillary – Follicular (Differentiated) Thyroid Carcinoma

Patient-Related Factors

The age of the patient at diagnosis has been found to be a significant variable in several multivariate analyses of prognostic factors in differentiated thyroid carcinoma [8, 9, 14, 20, 24, 28, 40, 42, 45], with survival decreasing with advancing age. In the original report of the EORTC [8], data for all histological types of thyroid cancer showed that survival decreased with progressively older age groups, i.e. 20–40, 40–60, 60–70, and over 70 years of age. The SICO study [2, 15] confirmed this trend reporting a 4-year survival rate of almost 100% for patients under 60 years, compared to 84.6% for patients over 65 years of age. In papillary thyroid carcinoma, Hay reported decreasing cause-specific survival with increasing age for each decade over age 50 [20]. In their Canada-wide study, Simpson et al. [40] found a similar effect of age on cause-specific survival in both papillary and follicular thyroid carcinomas. When examined separately, the 20-year cause-specific survival for patients less than 40 was 95% for papillary carcinoma and 88% for follicular carcinoma, but only 39% and 32%, respectively, for patients over 60 years old. In an analysis from the Institute Gustave-Roussy, Tubiana et al. [45] reported that patients younger than 45 years old with papillary and follicular tumours had the lowest relapse and best survival rate. In follicular carcinoma, Brennan et al. showed age greater than 50 to be associated with poorer survival [7]. In contrast to other multivariate analyses, however, Schelfhoutl [36] did not find age to be a significant prognostic factor in papillary and follicular tumours. Although age at the time of diagnosis has been found to be a major prognostic factor in differentiated thyroid carcinoma, various studies use different age cut-off points. Patients less than 40 or 50 years old have been reported to have a favourable prognosis. It is likely that there is no strict cut-off point at which prognosis changes suddenly, but rather the prognostic influence of age changes progressively. In the AMES (Age, Metastasis, Extension, Size) prognostic index, a different age cut-off point is used for female patients (50 years) than for male patients (40 years) [9].

Although several univariate analyses have found a lower survival rate in male patients, this has not always been confirmed in multivariate analysis. For instance, in the EORTC report [8], gender was a significant factor in the univariate but not in the multivariate analysis. However, in the Mayo Clinic report, male gender was associated with poorer survival in papillary carcinoma [20], but not follicular carcinoma [7]. Tubiana et al. [45] found male gender to be associated with increased risk of both relapse and death in papillary and follicular tumours. Although many investigators have documented a negative effect of male gender [1, 4, 13, 14, 28, 34], several other studies showed no effect of gender on survival [40, 42, 43].

Benign thyroid disease frequently co-exists with malignancy. In an analysis of patients with papillary carcinomas from the Mayo Clinic, Hay [20] found 40% of patients with pre-existing or concurrent benign thyroid conditions. Of these, 41% had benign nodular goitre and 20% chronic lymphocytic thyroiditis. In the Mayo Clinic series, the presence of thyroiditis or benign nodular thyroid disease did not affect the outcome. The frequency of carcinoma among patients undergoing surgery for toxic goitre ranges between 0.06% and 8.7% [37, 41]. In most cases the neoplastic lesion is less than 1 cm [48]. Belfiore et al. [5] reported increased aggressiveness of thyroid cancer in patients with Graves disease with an increase in multifocality, invasion of the extrathyroid tissue, lymph node involvement and an increased incidence of distant metastases. This has also been noted by others [16, 27]. Although the association of previous radiation therapy and thyroid carcinoma is well established, the prognosis in patients who have been exposed to radiation does not appear to differ from those with no history of radiation [10, 14, 28].

Tumour-Related Factors

Anatomic Extent Of Disease

In differentiated thyroid carcinoma, the T category is an important prognostic factor. In the EORTC study [8], survival declined with increasing T category from T0 (no palpable tumour) to T1 (mobile tumour limited to the thyroid gland without deformity), T2 (single or multiple mobile tumours deforming the thyroid gland) and T3 (tumours extending beyond the thyroid gland with fixation to or infiltration of adjacent structures) [46]. Extrathyroid extension of the tumour has been found to be a poor prognostic factor in many multivariate analyses [9, 14, 20, 24, 28, 34, 40, 42, 43]. In papillary carcinoma, Hay [20] reported a 20-year cause-specific survival rate of 98% for patients with tumours confined to the thyroid gland, compared to 28% for those with locally invasive tumours. Hay also found a progressive decrease in survival in papillary thyroid carcinoma with increasing tumour size. Tumour-related mortality was only 0.2% for carcinomas less than 1 cm in size, 0.8% for lesions 1 cm to less than 2 cm in size and 6% for lesions 2 cm to less than 6 cm, but increased to 16% for lesions between 6 and 7 cm in size and was greater than 50% for lesions over 7 cm. Simpson et al. found tumours greater than 4 cm to be associated with poorer survival, but tumour size was not an independent prognostic factor in multivariate analysis [40]. However, extrathyroid extension was an unfavourable factor in both univariate and multivariate analyses. In his most recent multivariate analysis of patients with well-differentiated thyroid carcinoma, Mazzaferri found the size of tumour predictive for local recurrence, but not for survival [28]. Extrathyroid invasion was a significant factor for both local recurrence and for cause-specific survival.

There is no agreement regarding the prognostic significance of cervical lymph node metastases at diagnosis. In the EORTC analysis, Byar et al. [8] reported a lower survival for patients with mobile positive lymph nodes and even lower for those with fixed lymph node metastasis. Simpson et al. [40] reported the presence of cervical lymph node metastases to be associated with decreased survival in follicular, but not in papillary carcinoma. In a multivariate analysis from the Institute Gustave-Roussy, Tubiana et al. [45] found a shorter disease-free interval and a lower survival rate in patients with positive cervical lymph nodes in both papillary and follicular tumours. This is in contrast to other reports [7, 12, 14, 20]. Although Coborn and Wanebo [9] did not find a difference in relapse or survival rates with cervical lymph node involvement, they reported extrathyroid invasion, age greater than 45, and mediastinal lymph node involvement as being associated with poor survival.

The presence of distant metastases at diagnosis is associated with a markedly decreased survival in both papillary and follicular tumours [1, 8, 9, 15, 20, 28, 40, 43]. The location of the metastases is also of importance. In an analysis by Casara et al. [11], there was a 53% and 52% 10-year survival in patients with lung or mediastinal metastases, respectively, but only a 15% 10-year survival in those with bone metastases. The site of metastases remained significant in a multivariate analysis. Other investigators [20, 23, 40] have confirmed the importance of the site of metastases.

Other Pathological Features

Prognostic features in papillary and follicular tumours are often analyzed together. Tubiana et al. [45] reported similar relapse-free and overall survival rates in papillary and well-differentiated follicular carcinoma. However, moderately differentiated follicular carcinoma was associated with a reduced survival and an increased recurrence rate. There are several reports [1, 14, 20, 36, 40] indicating the degree of differentiation to be an independent prognostic factor for survival in papillary thyroid carcinoma. Johnson [25] described a variant of papillary thyroid carcinoma characterized by the presence of columnar cells, wherein the height is at least twice the width. When matched with patients with similar tumour size and lymph node characteristics, there was an increased instance of local and distant relapse and reduced survival in patients with this tall cell variant. In follicular carcinoma, the presence of vascular invasion has been reported to be an independent adverse prognostic factor [7, 40]. However, in papillary carcinoma this was not confirmed in multivariate analyses [20, 40].

In a univariate analysis of papillary carcinoma, Carcangiu et al. [10] reported an increased frequency of lymph node and pulmonary metastases and a reduced disease-free survival in multifocal tumours. Simpson et al. [40] found that multifocal tumour had no deleterious effect on recurrence or survival.

Biological and Molecular Factors

Quantitative analysis of cellular DNA content has become increasingly available in recent years. In an analysis of papillary tumours, Backdahl [3] claimed ploidy to be more important than the other prognostic factors. Hrafnkelsson [22] reported an aneuploid DNA profile in 12% of patients, of whom 47% eventually died of thyroid carcinoma; aneuploidy was more common among male patients and older patients. In Hrafnkelsson's multivariate analysis, age was the most important significant prognostic factor, but ploidy was an independent prognostic factor for survival. Hay [20] found the highest mortality rate for tumours with an aneuploid pattern, intermediate for tumours with tetraploid–polyploid pattern and smallest for those with diploid profiles ($p < 0.0001$). Hamming et al. [19] confirmed the diagnostic potential of these results, showing an abnormal DNA content with multiple aberrant profiles to be the only significant factor in patients with disease limited to thyroid. Joensuu [24] found aneuploidy to correlate with a lower survival rate, but in a multivariate analysis DNA ploidy was not significant, whereas age, differentiation and invasion through the thyroid capsule remained important.

In follicular tumours, Grant et al. [18] found aneuploidy in benign as well as malignant lesions and was unable to demonstrate any prognostic effect of ploidy when the Hurtle cell variant was excluded; however, when included, aneuploidy was a significant factor for reduced cause-specific survival. They also found that in patients without metastases DNA ploidy was the only significant factor for reduced survival.

Serum thyroglobulin has become an established marker for differentiated thyroid carcinoma in patients who had total thyroidectomy or radioiodine ablation of the thyroid. Its level is increased in any thyroid disease associated with increased thyroid mass or activity, i.e. goitre, Graves disease, thyroiditis, thyroid adenoma as well as thyroid carcinoma. Thyroglobulin does not differentiate between benign or malignant conditions and therefore has no prognostic value in initial evaluation of thyroid carcinoma [31].

Prognostic Indexes

In an attempt to stratify patients into different risk groups in terms of predicting survival, and thereby guiding therapy, a variety of prognostic indices have been formulated. The initial index from the EORTC [8] identified gender, histological pattern, tumour extent and presence or absence of metastases as important factors used to develop the index. The EORTC index, unlike subsequent indices, was developed for differentiated, medullary and anaplastic tumours. The AGES (Age, Grading, Extension, Size) score [20], which uses age, histological grade, extent and size of tumour, was developed at the Mayo Clinic for papillary carcinoma. The AMES scale [9] for papillary and follicular carcinoma includes age at diagnosis, presence or absence of metastases, tumour extension and size. The TNM (4th edn.) classification depends on age, histology, tumour size, tumour extent and the presence or absence of metastases [21]. It is important to note that for papillary carcinoma the AGES score incorporates the histological grade of papillary tumours and this is not always reported. However, a comparison of AGES, AMES, TNM and EORTC indexes revealed that the AGES and AMES scores identified a good prognostic group better than the EORTC and TNM staging classifications [20]. Young patients (less than 40 years in men and less than 50 years in women in the AMES score) with small tumours, no extrathyroid extension and either well-differentiated papillary histology (AGES) or no metastases (AMES) fall in the good prognostic group with a cause-specific survival rate greater than 98% at 20 years. For the poor prognostic group, the 20-year cause-specific survival rate is only about 60%. Akslen [1] has proposed a prognostic score dependent on gender, age and grade in papillary thyroid carcinoma which he described as being superior in identifying a good prognostic group compared to the AGES score.

Summary

The most important prognostic factor for survival in differentiated papillary and follicular thyroid carcinomas is age at diagnosis. Other independent prognostic factors include: the presence of metastases, extrathyroid extension, tumour size and histological grade. The influence of gender is less clear, but male patients tend to do less well than female patients. The impact of lymph node involvement is uncertain and may not be significant in papillary tumours but is an adverse factor in patients with follicular cancer. The use of prognostic indices allows the identification of patients with a very good prognosis and enables treatment to be suitably tailored.

Anaplastic Carcinoma

In the analysis of the EORTC thyroid cancer study group, the presence of any element of anaplasia within a well-differentiated thyroid carcinoma or anaplastic features throughout the tumour were associated with a 1-year survival rate of 10%. Any anaplastic features in thyroid carcinoma have been found to be associated with poor prognosis by many authors [2, 8, 15, 36].

Within anaplastic thyroid carcinoma, Nel et al. [29] have described a better prognostic group of patients with small tumours (less than 5 cm), no extrathyroid invasion and no lymph node involvement. Age has not been found to be a prognostic factor in this study or in the SICO group, but Venkatesh et al. [47] reported age and stage to be significant factors for survival in anaplastic thyroid carcinoma. Gender has not been shown to affect the outcome in these tumours.

The presence of the so-called small cell variant of anaplastic thyroid carcinoma has been reported in the past to be a good prognostic feature. Immuno-histological studies have now shown that most, if not all of these tumours are lymphomas or medullary thyroid carcinomas [38].

In general, patients with anaplastic thyroid carcinoma present with advanced-stage disease and invariably have a poor prognosis [23, 29].

Medullary Thyroid Carcinoma

The prognosis in patients with medullary thyroid carcinoma may be related to its hereditary or sporadic nature. It has been reported that the familial medullary thyroid carcinoma, with or without the association of multiple endocrine neoplasia (MEN) IIA syndrome, is associated with a better survival rate than the sporadic medullary thyroid carcinoma, which in turn has a better survival rate than that associated with the MEN IIB syndrome [26, 30]. However, Saaman found that in patients matched for age, extent of tumour and lymph node involvement, survival was similar for those with the hereditary and sporadic medullary thyroid carcinomas [35]. This implied that any differences in survival of patients with hereditary and sporadic carcinomas may have been due to the earlier diagnosis of the hereditary medullary thyroid cancers. They also found no difference between patients with MEN IIA or MEN IIB syndromes.

Age less than 40 and female gender have been reported as favourable prognostic indicators. Lymph node involvement in medullary thyroid carcinoma may not necessarily affect survival adversely, unlike extension through the thyroid capsule [32, 33, 42].

Calcitonin is a tumour marker for medullary thyroid carcinoma. The basal levels of calcitonin are proportional to the tumour burden. However, a decrease in the calcitonin level may indicate progression to a poorly differentiated tumour [44]. In a univariate analysis, a high frequency of calcitonin-immunoreacting tumour cells, presence of amyloid, intact tumour capsule and euploidy were associated with an increased overall survival rate, but only calcitonin immunoreactivity and positive amyloid staining were independent prognostic factors [6]. The most important use of calcitonin is in the screening of relatives of patients with the familial form of the disease to enable early detection and therapy [17, 39]. Carcinoembryonic antigen (CEA) has also been used as a marker for disease progression in medullary thyroid carcinoma. A rapidly progressive disease was reported to be associated with a short CEA doubling time [33].

References

1. Akslen LA (1993) Prognostic importance of histologic grading in papillary thyroid carcinoma. Cancer 72: 2680–2685
2. Antonaci A, Amanti C, Consoli C, et al (1993) La ripresa di malattia nell'ambito della ricerca multicentrica SICO sul trattamento chirurgico del carcinoma della tiroide. Atti XVII Congr Naz SICO, Naples, Italy, 19–21 September, 1992
3. Bäckdahl M, Carstensen J, Auer G et al (1986) Statistical evaluation of the prognostic value of nuclear DNA content in papillary, follicular, and medullary thyroid tumours. World J Surg 10: 974–980
4. Bacourt F, Asselain B, Savoie JC et al (1986) Multifactorial study of prognostic factors in differentiated thyroid carcinoma and a re-evaluation of the importance of age. Br J Surg 73: 274–277
5. Belfiore A, Garofalo MR, Giuffrida D et al (1990) Increased aggressiveness of thyroid cancer in patients with Graves' disease. J Clin Endocrinol Metab 70: 830–835
6. Bergholm U, Adami HO, Auer G et al (1989) Histopathologic characteristics and nuclear DNA content as prognostic factors in medullary thyroid carcinoma. A nationwide study in Sweden. The Swedish MTC Study Group. Cancer 64: 135–142
7. Brennan MD, Bergstralh EJ, van Heerden JA et al (1991) Follicular thyroid cancer treated at the Mayo clinic, 1946 through 1970: initial manifestations, pathologic findings, therapy, and outcome. Mayo Clin Proc 66: 11–22
8. Byar DP, Green SB, Dor P et al (1979) A prognostic index for thyroid carcinoma. A study of the E.O.R.T.C. Thyroid Cancer Cooperative Group. Eur J Cancer 15: 1033–1041
9. Cady B, Rossi R (1988) An expanded view of risk-group definition in differentiated thyroid carcinoma. Surgery 104: 947–953
10. Carcangiu ML, Zampi G, Pupi A et al (1985) Papillary carcinoma of the thyroid. A clinicopathologic study of 241 cases treated at the University of Florence, Italy. Cancer 55: 805–828
11. Casara B, Petronio R et al (1991) Risultati a lungo termine e analisi statistica uni-e multivariata dei fattori prognostici per il carcinoma della tiroide in fase avanzata. Atti XV Cong Naz SICO. Padua, Italy, 1990
12. Coburn MC, Wanebo HJ (1992) Prognostic factors and management considerations in patients with cervical metastases of thyroid cancers. Am J Surg 164: 671–676
13. Crile G, Pontius KI, Hawk WA (1985) Factors influencing the survival of patients with follicular carcinoma of the thyroid gland. Surg Gynecol Obstet 160: 409–413

14. Cunningham MP, Duda RB, Recant W et al (1990) Survival discriminants for differentiated thyroid cancer. Am J Surg 160: 344–347
15. Di Paola M, Antonaci A, Consoli C, et al (1992) I resultati della terapia chirurgica dei carcinoma della tiroide Atti XVI Congr Naz SICO. Trieste, Italy, 19–21 November 1991
16. Farbota LM, Calandra DB, Lawrence AM et al (1985) Thyroid carcinoma in Graves' disease. Surgery 98: 1148–1153
17. Gagel RF, Tashjian AH Jr, Cummings T (1988) The clinical outcome of prospective screening for multiple endocrine neoplasia type 2a. An 18 year experience. N Engl J Med 318: 478–484
18. Grant CS, Hay ID, Ryan JJ et al (1990) Diagnostic and prognostic utility of flow cytometric DNA measurements in follicular thyroid tumors. World J Surg 14: 283–289
19. Hamming JF, Schelfhout LJ, Cornelisse CJ et al (1988) Prognostic value of nuclear DNA content in papillary and follicular thyroid cancer. World J Surg 12: 503–508
20. Hay ID (1990) Papillary thyroid carcinoma. Endocrinol Metab Clin North Am 19: 545–576
21. Hermanek P, Sobin LH (eds) (1992) UICC TNM classification of malignant tumours, 4th edn, 2nd rev. Springer, Berlin Heidelberg New York
22. Hrafnkelsson J, Stal O, Enestrom S et al (1988) Cellular DNA pattern, S-phase frequency and survival in papillary thyroid cancer. Acta Oncol 27: 329–333
23. Jensen MH, Davis RK, Derrick L (1990) Thyroid cancer: a computer-assisted review of 5287 cases. Otolaryngol Head Neck Surg 102: 51–65
24. Joensuu H, Klemi P, Eerola E et al (1986) Influence of cellular DNA content on survival in differentiated thyroid cancer. Cancer 58: 2162–2167
25. Johnson TL, Lloyd RV, Thompson NW et al (1988) Prognostic implications of the tall cell variant of papillary thyroid carcinoma. Am J Surg Pathol 12: 22–27
26. Kakudo K, Carney J, Sizemore GW (1985) Medullary carcinoma of thyroid: biologic behaviour of the sporadic and familial neoplasm. Cancer 55: 2818–2821
27. Livadas D, Psarras A, Koutras DA (1976) Malignant cold nodules in hyperthyroidism. Br J Surg 63: 726–728
28. Mazzaferri EL (1991) Radiodine and other treatments and outcomes. In: Braverman LE, Utiger RD (eds) Werner and Ingbar's The Thyroid: a fundamental and clinical text. Lippincott, Philidelphia, pp 1138–1165
29. Nel CJ, van Heerden JA, Goellner JR et al (1985) Anaplastic carcinoma of the thyroid: a clinicopathologic study of 82 cases. Mayo Clin Proc 60: 51–58
30. Raue F, Späth-Röger M, Winter J et al (1990) A registry of medullary thyroid cancer in West Germany. Med Klin 85: 113–116
31. Refetoff S, Lever EG (1983) The value of serum thyroglobulin measurement in clinical practice. J Am Med Assoc 250: 2352–2357
32. Rougier P, Parmentier C, Laplanche A et al (1983) Medullary thyroid carcinoma: prognostic factors and treatment. Int J Radiat Oncol Biol Phys 9: 161–169
33. Saad MF, Ordonez NG, Rashid RK et al (1984) Medullary carcinoma of the thyroid: a study of the clinical features and prognostic factors in 161 patients. Medicine 63: 319–342
34. Salvesen H, Njolstad PR, Akslen LA et al (1992) Papillary thyroid carcinoma: a multivariate analysis of prognostic factors including an evaluation of the p-TNM staging system. Eur J Surg 158: 583–589
35. Samaan NA, Schultz PN, Hickey RC (1988) Medullary thyroid carcinoma: prognosis of familial versus sporadic disease and the role of radiotherapy. J Clin Endocrinol Metab 67: 801–805
36. Schelfhout LJ, Creutzberg CL, Hamming JF et al (1988) Multivariate analysis of survival in differentiated thyroid cancer: the prognostic significance of the age factor. Eur J Cancer Clin Oncol 24: 331–337
37. Shapiro SJ, Friedman NB, Perzik SL et al (1970) Incidence of thyroid carcinoma in Graves' disease. Cancer 26: 1261–1270
38. Shvero J, Gal R, Avidor I et al (1988) Anaplastic thyroid carcinoma. A clinical, histologic, and immunohistochemical study. Cancer 62: 319–325
39. Simpson WJ, Carruthers JS, Malkin D (1990) Results of a screening program for C cell disease (Medullary thyroid cancer and C cell hyperplasia). Cancer 65: 1570–1576
40. Simpson WJ, McKinney SE, Carruthers JS et al (1987) Papillary and follicular thyroid cancer. Prognostic factors in 1,578 patients. Am J Med 83: 479–488

41. Sokal JE (1954) Incidence of malignancy in toxic and nontoxic nodular goiters. J Am Med Assoc 154: 1321–1325
42. Tennvall J, Biorklund A, Möller T et al (1985) Prognostic factors of papillary, follicular and medullary carcinomas of the thyroid gland. Retrospective multivariate analysis of 216 patients with a median follow-up of 11 years. Acta Radiol 24: 17–24
43. Thoresen SO, Akslen LA, Glattre E et al (1989) Survival and prognostic factors in differentiated thyroid cancer – a multivariate analysis of 1055 cases. Br J Cancer 59: 231–235
44. Trump DL, Mendelsohn G, Baylin SB (1979) Discordance between plasma calcitonin and tumor-cell mass in medullary thyroid carcinoma. N Engl J Med 301: 253–255
45. Tubiana M, Schlumberger M, Rougier P et al (1985) Long-term results and prognostic factors in patients with differentiated thyroid carcinoma. Cancer 55: 794–804
46. UICC (1974) TNM classification of malignant tumours, 2nd edn. UICC, Geneva
47. Venkatesh YS, Ordonez NG, Schultz PN et al (1990) Anaplastic carcinoma of the thyroid: a clinicopathologic study of 121 cases. Cancer 66: 321–330
48. Zarrilli L (1989) Ipertiroidismo e cancro della tiroide. Atti IV Congr SIFIPAC e XVIII. SICO, Naples, Italy, 1988

5 Oesophageal Carcinoma

J.D. Roder, H.J. Stein, and J.R. Siewert

Introduction

Prognostic factors in patients with cancer can broadly be classified into three categories: (1) tumour-related prognostic factors, (2) patient-related factors and (3) factors that relate to therapeutic measures. In contrast to other tumours of the gastrointestinal tract, prognostic factors are only just beginning to be identified in patients with oesophageal carcinoma. This is because most studies assessing the prognosis of patients with oesophageal cancer are retrospective univariate analyses of small patient populations that were usually not treated according to standardized protocols. Due to interrelations between various patient- and tumour-related factors and their alterations by therapeutic strategies, an independent prognostic effect of individual parameters cannot be deducted from these analyses. This can only be achieved by multiple stepwise regression analysis applied to a sufficiently large patient population that has undergone standardized treatment and has been followed for a sufficiently long period of time. Only very recently have studies that meet these criteria become available. The currently available literature on prognostic factors in patients with oesophageal cancer is critically reviewed in the present article.

Tumour-Related Prognostic Factors

A variety of tumour characteristics have been implicated as predictors of a good or poor prognosis in patients with oesophageal carcinoma. These include tumour location, length and depth of invasion of the primary tumour, lymph node metastasis, systemic metastases, histological tumour type, differentiation of the tumour, DNA distribution pattern and a number of other factors including growth factors, growth factor receptors, oncogenes and tumour suppressor genes. Reliable and reproducible identification of tumour characteristics which may influence survival is only possible by an accurate histological assessment of the resected specimen according to the guidelines given in the TNM classification system [13]. Only patients who have had complete tumour removal together with an adequate lymph node dissection and who survived the resection should be included in such analyses.

Tumour Location

Due to the proximity to the trachea and main stem bronchi, extensive resection cannot usually be performed in patients with oesophageal carcinoma located in the proximal part of the oesophagus. The prognosis of patients with proximal oesophageal tumours is therefore generally thought to be poor. In multivariate analyses, the location of the primary tumour could not, however, be identified as an independent prognostic marker [9,46].

Tumour Length and Depth of Invasion

In most univariate analyses the tumour length and depth of invasion are major prognostic factors. On multivariate analysis, tumour length uniformly does not show any independent prognostic significance and should consequently be abandoned as a factor that influences therapeutic decisions. In contrast, depth of invasion, i.e. the pT category, has been identified as an independent prognostic factor in some [9,31], but not all multivariate analyses [4,33,37,46,47]. Of particular interest is the fact that the pT category can be predicted with a high degree of certainty by endoscopic ultrasonography. This new technology should consequently be used to guide therapeutic decisions [42].

Lymph Node Metastases

At the time of resection, lymph node metastases are present in the majority patients with oesophageal carcinoma even with early-stage tumours. Most univariate and multivariate analyses show the presence or absence of lymph node metastases as a major and independent predictor of survival in patients with oesophageal carcinoma [4,31,33,37,47,50]. However, the presence of positive mediastinal lymph nodes alone does not lead to a sudden deterioration of the survival probability. Rather, survival decreases in a stepwise fashion as the number of involved lymph nodes increases [17,33]. This indicates that with a limited number of involved mediastinal lymph nodes, long-term survival may still be possible following a radical resection with adequate lymphadenectomy.

Distant Metastases

Haematogenous systemic metastases in patients with oesophageal carcinoma are an ominous prognostic marker. The median survival time of these patients is below 6 months in most series. Consequently, only palliative measures improving the quality of life are indicated in this situation.

   With the current TNM classification of oesophageal carcinoma, metastasis to non-regional lymph nodes, e.g. celiac axis nodes or cervical nodes, is also considered as distant tumour spread and classified as M1LYM [13]. Prognostically this situation is more favourable than metastases to distant organs [16,17,41] and probably does not constitute true systemic disease. This will have to be taken into consideration when compiling the next revision of the TNM classification system.

Histological Tumour Type

In recent years the prevalence of adenocarcinoma of the oesophagus has shown a marked increase in the Western world, while the prevalence of squamous cell oesophageal carcinoma has remained steady [21]. The reasons for this change in the histological spectrum of oesophageal carcinoma are unclear.

Overall, there is no prognostic difference between squamous cell carcinoma and adenocarcinoma of the oesophagus in most studies. Only patients with early adenocarcinoma, i.e. T1 tumours, appear to have a survival advantage as compared to patients with early squamous cell tumours [43].

Tumour Differentiation and DNA Pattern

Tumour differentiation is an important prognostic factor in many gastrointestinal tumours and has also been suggested as a predictor of survival in oesophageal carcinoma [32]. An independent prognostic effect of tumour differentiation could, however, not be shown in most multivariate analyses [4,33,47].

The prognostic role of DNA ploidy in patients with oesophageal carcinoma is presently not clear. While some authors report an independent prognostic effect of the DNA distribution pattern on tumour recurrence and survival [2,23,27,47,51], this could not be shown in multivariate analyses by others [31,32,35,37]. Prospective studies with sufficiently large patient populations are required to clarify this issue.

Oncogenes, Tumour Suppressor Genes, Growth Factors and Growth Factor Receptors

Oncogenes, tumour suppressor genes, growth factors and their receptors are increasingly being implicated in the pathogenesis and progression of a variety of human cancers including oesophageal carcinoma. In contrast to other gastrointestinal cancers, the ras oncogene family (c-H-*ras*, c-Ki-*ras*, and c-N-*ras*) does not appear to play a major role in the pathogenesis of oesophageal carcinoma [14]. Amplification of the proto-oncogenes *int*-2 and *hst*-1 [19,24] and mutations in the tumour suppressor gene p53 have been reported in a substantial percentage of patients with squamous cell carcinoma and adenocarcinoma of the oesophagus and appear to indicate a poor prognosis [8,39]. Amplification of the epidermal growth factor receptor gene and overexpression of the epidermal growth factor receptor, the oncoprotein c-erbB-2 and the transforming growth factor alpha have also been observed in patients with squamous cell carcinoma or adenocarcinoma of the oesophagus, and all have been related to poor survival [14,15,26,27,30]. The evaluated populations in these studies were usually small and the clinical role of these observations is not clear at the present time. Prospective long-term follow-up studies of large patient populations are clearly required to clarify the prognostic impact of these exciting, though preliminary observations.

Other Tumour-Related Prognostic Markers

In a recent multivariate analysis, venous invasion and the number of nucleolar organizer regions were shown to have an independent prognostic effect on survival in patients undergoing resection of oesophageal carcinoma [25,50]. In univariate analyses, the potential of cancer cells for growth in cell culture, the presence of intramural metastases and the endoscopic growth pattern have also been suggested as prognostic indicators [28,38,48]. These observations, however, still need to be confirmed by other investigators.

Patient-Related Prognostic Factors

Age and Sex

Oesophageal carcinoma is a disease which affects mostly male patients over 60 years of age. On univariate analysis of more than 8000 patients with oesophageal cancer collected in the Japanese Cancer Registry, female sex was associated with a better prognosis than male sex [16]. This observation has not been confirmed in Western countries or in several multivariate analyses of large Japanese series [4,9,31,33,46,47].

Because of an anticipated limited life expectancy, a potentially curative resection is frequently not considered in patients who present with oesophageal carcinoma at an advanced age. Although perioperative mortality increases with increasing age, multivariate analysis shows that survival following resection for oesophageal carcinoma is not determined by the age of the patient [33,47]. The benefits of a potentially curative resection should therefore not be denied just because of advanced age. Rather, the decision to perform a resection should be guided by the presence of a resectable tumour and a detailed analysis of cardiac, pulmonary, hepatic and renal function to limit perioperative mortality [41].

Nutritional Status

Patients with oesophageal carcinoma frequently present with a deteriorated nutritional status. However, prospective studies could not show an impact of the nutritional status or preoperative weight loss on perioperative morbidity, mortality or long-term survival [3,9]. Consequently, routine preoperative nutritional therapy appears unjustified in patients with oesophageal carcinoma.

Physiological Status

Due to the advanced age and the factors predisposing to the development of oesophageal squamous cell carcinoma, i.e. alcohol abuse and smoking, the co-morbidity of patients with oesophageal carcinoma is high. Pulmonary, cardiac, hepatic and renal function, general physiological status and the co-operation of the patient are the major parameters that determine the severity and length of the postoperative course [41]. A detailed preoperative analysis of these patient-dependent risk factors and subsequent improvements in patient selection for surgical resection, combined with standardization of resection techniques and individualized perioperative management, has in recent years led to a marked reduction in operative mortality and morbidity in many centres. However, the physiological status of the patient does not predict long-term survival time after a curative surgical resection.

Prognostic Factors That Relate to Therapeutic Measures

Tumour- and patient-related prognostic markers are given at the time of presentation and cannot be altered by therapeutic intervention. Prognostic factors associated with therapeutic measures therefore have the most important impact on the management of patients with oesophageal carcinoma. Of all the therapeutic measures available, oesophageal resection remains the mainstay of curative therapy in patients with resectable tumours. There is broad agreement that radiation, chemotherapy, combined radio-chemotherapy or local measures should be considered as primary treatment options only in patients with irresectable tumours or in patients whose physiological status does not permit major surgery. In patients undergoing surgical resection, the prognostic impact of the residual tumour status after resection, the extent of resection and the effect of perioperative adjuvant or additive therapy have been most widely assessed.

Residual Tumour Status and Extent of Resection

In most uni- and multivariate analysis, the presence of residual tumour after surgical resection is the factor with the strongest independent prognostic impact [4,31,33,46]. In the experience of the Technische Universität München, Germany, the 5-year survival time is 31% for patients with complete macroscopic and microscopic tumour resection (R0 resection) compared to 7% for patients with residual microscopic disease (R1 resection) and 0% in those with residual macroscopic tumour after resection (R2 resection) [33]. This indicates that complete removal of all microscopic or macroscopic tumour has to be the goal of any resection performed for oesophageal carcinoma.

Complete resection of the primary tumour is usually not a problem at the proximal and distal luminal borders of the resection, since a subtotal oesophagectomy can easily be performed either via the transhiatal or the transthoracic route. In our and others' experience, a transthoracic en bloc resection is, however, clearly superior to the transhiatal approach to achieve complete tumour removal in the mediastinum [12,41,44]. Whether an extensive transthoracic resection also improves the long-term prognosis as compared to a transhiatal resection is, however, debated [11,12,29,44].

In patients undergoing resection of oesophageal carcinoma, an adequate safety margin should not only be achieved in the area of the primary tumour, but also along its lymphatic drainage. This concept is supported by the independent prognostic effect which has been shown for the so-called lymph node ratio, i.e. the ratio of invaded and removed lymph nodes [33]. A significant drop in the survival rate occurs when more than 20% of the removed lymph nodes are involved. This ratio can be favourably influenced by a radical lymphadenectomy, which increases the number of removed lymph nodes. Theoretically, this implies that in a patient with oesophageal cancer the prognosis can be improved by extending the lymph node dissection [33,41]. It is, however, important to realize that lymph node metastases in patients with oesophageal carcinoma are usually further advanced than is detected with routine macroscopic and microscopic diagnostic techniques. This explains why the prognostic gain that can be achieved with lymph node dissection is highest in patients with apparently tumour free lymph nodes (N0 category) or patients with early and few lymph node metastases (N1 category) [33].

Based on these assumptions, an extension of the lymph node dissection to the so-called three-field lymphadenectomy, as proposed by several Japanese groups, appears reasonable [1,18]. Since three-field lymphadenectomy primarily provides an oral extension of the lymph node dissection, patients with tumours that metastasize orally, i.e., tumours with a close connection to the tracheobronchial tree, should benefit from this approach. These hypotheses, however, need to be confirmed by randomized prospective trials with a detailed subgroup analysis and a careful assessment of postoperative morbidity, which may increase substantially with the extension of the resection.

Combined Modality Therapy

Despite en bloc resection and extended lymph node dissection, a R0 resection is only possible in a minority of the patients presenting with oesophageal carcinoma. This is because at the time of presentation the tumour has frequently grown beyond the oesophageal wall, the tumour metastasizes early during the course of the disease and the proximity of the oesophagus to vital organs prohibits extensive resection in many patients with oesophageal tumours at unfavourable locations, i.e. tumours located at or above the level of the tracheal bifurcation. A variety of adjuvant, neoadjuvant and combined modality approaches have consequently been investigated in an effort to induce a down-staging of the primary tumour, to eliminate potential systemic micrometastasis, to treat residual tumour after surgical resection and ultimately to prolong survival in patients with oesophageal carcinoma [6].

Postoperative therapy has been applied in patients who have had a palliative or curative resection. Two recent randomized prospective trials, however, do not show an increase in survival time with postoperative radiation in patients with or without residual tumour after surgical resection [7,49]. Similarly, the use of adjuvant chemotherapy cannot currently be supported by controlled trials [6].

Due to the lack of effect of postoperative therapy, preoperative radiation, chemotherapy or radiochemotherapy followed by surgical resection has recently received increasing attention in patients with oesophageal carcinoma. While several prospective randomized trials showed no benefit of preoperative therapy in patients with potentially resectable tumours [20,34,36], combined modality treatment appears to increase the resection rate, rate of complete tumour resections and survival time in patients with locally advanced tumours [5,40,45]. However, most available studies show that a prognostic benefit from multimodal therapy can be expected only in patients who have an objective response to preoperative therapy with subsequent R0 resection or a complete histopathological response to preoperative treatment, i.e. no viable tumour in the resected specimen [4,6,10,36]. Neoadjuvant therapy for oesophageal carcinoma should therefore only be considered in patients who are fit for subsequent surgical resection. This requires adequate pulmonary, cardiac, renal and hepatic function as well as sufficient co-operation from the patient to withstand aggressive neoadjuvant therapy and a potentially prolonged postoperative course. In addition, parameters that would allow to predict the response to neoadjuvant therapy based on pretherapeutic data are clearly needed to avoid the excessive morbidity and mortality associated with combined modality treatment in patients who may not receive any benefit from this approach.

Other Treatment-Related Prognostic Factors

In a study by Sugimachi et al. [46], multivariate analysis identified postoperative complications, e.g. respiratory tract infections, anastomotic leakage and bleeding, as an independent predictor of survival in patients with squamous cell carcinoma of the oesophagus who had preoperative radio/chemotherapy. Of particular interest is the fact that the rate of postoperative complications and thus the perioperative mortality appears to be related to the experience of the surgeon [22]. Consequently, oesophageal resection should only be performed by surgeons who have sufficient experience with the technical details of oesophageal resection, reconstruction and the perioperative management. This appears to be particularly important in patients who have had preoperative neoadjuvant therapy.

Transfusions of packed red blood cells showed an independent effect on long-term survival after transhiatal oesophagectomy in one study from Switzerland [9]. This interesting observation has, however, so far not been confirmed by other groups.

Conclusion

The presence of haematogenous distant metastases, complete macroscopic and microscopic tumour removal and the nodal status are the only undisputed independent prognostic factors in patients with localized oesophageal carcinoma. With the use of modern imaging techniques, i.e. endoscopic ultrasonography and surgical laparoscopy, prediction of a R0 resection in the area of the primary tumour and the lymphatic drainage has become possible with a high degree of certainty. This will result in a more selective surgical approach to patients with oesophageal carcinoma and will help to identify those patients who may benefit from combined modality therapy.

References

1. Baba M, Aikou T, Yoshinaka H, Natsugoe S, Fukomoto T, Shimazu H, Akazawa K (1994) Long-term results of subtotal esophagectomy with three-field lymphadenectomy for carcinoma of the thoracic esophagus. Ann Surg 219: 310–316
2. Böttger T, Störkel S, Stöckle M, Wahl W, Jugenheimer M, Effenberger Kim O, Vinh T, Junginger T (1991) DNA image cytometry. A prognostic tool in squamous cell carcinoma of the esophagus? Cancer 67: 2290–2294
3. Brandmair W, Lehr L, Siewert J R (1989) Nutritional status in esophageal cancer: assessment and significance for preoperative risk assessment. Langenbecks Arch Chir 374: 25–31
4. Elias D, Lasser P, Mankarios H, Cabanes PA, Escudier B, Kac J, Rougier P (1992) Esophageal squamous cell carcinoma: the specific limited place of surgery defined by a prospective multivariate study of prognostic factors after surgical approach. Eur J Surg Oncol 18: 563–571
5. Fink U, Stein HJ, Lukas P, Gossmann A, Schiffner R, Dittler HJ, Roder JD, Siewert JR (1993) Combined modality treatment for locally advanced squamous cell esophageal carcinoma located at or above the level of the tracheal bifurcation. In: Nabeya K, Hanaoka T, Nogami H (eds) Recent advances in diseases of the esophagus. Springer, Berlin Heidelberg New York, pp 877–883
6. Fink U, Stein HJ, Bochtler H, Roder JD, Wilke HJ, Siewert JR (1994) Neoadjuvant therapy for squamous cell esophageal carcinoma. Ann Oncol 5: S17–S26
7. Fok M, Sham JST, Choy D, Cheng SWK, Wong J (1993) Postoperative radiotherapy for carcinoma of the esophagus: a prospective, randomized controlled study. Surgery 113: 138

8. Furihata M, Ohtsuki Y, Ogoshi S, Takahashi A, Tamiya T, Ogata T (1993) Prognostic significance of human papillomavirus genomes (type-16, -18) and aberrant expression of p53 protein in human esophageal cancer. Int J Cancer 54: 226–230

9. Gertsch P, Vauthey J-N, Lustenberger AA, Friedlander-Klar H (1993) Long-term results of transhiatal esophagectomy for esophageal carcinoma: a multivariate analysis of prognostic factors. Cancer 72: 2312–2319

10. Gill PG, Denham JW, Jamieson GG, Devitt PG, Yeoh E, Olweny C (1992) Patterns of treatment failure and prognostic factors associated with the treatment of esophageal carcinoma with chemotherapy and radiotherapy either as sole treatment or followed by surgery. J Clin Oncol 10: 1037–1043

11. Goldminc M, Maddern G, Le Prise E, Meunier B, Campion JP, Launois BTI (1993) Oesophagectomy by a transhiatal approach or thoracotomy: a prospective randomized trial. Br J Surg 80: 367–370

12. Hagen JA, Peters JH, DeMeester TR (1994) Superiority of extended en bloc esophagogastrectomy for carcinoma of the lower esophagus and cardia. J Thorac Cardiovasc Surg 106: 850–859

13. Hermanek P, Sobin LH (1987) UICC TNM classification of malignant tumours, 4th rev edn. Springer, Berlin Heidelberg New York

14. Hollstein MC, Smits AM, Galiana C et al (1988) Amplification of epidermal growth factor receptor gene but no evidence of ras mutations in primary human esophageal cancers. Cancer Res 48: 5119–5123

15. Iihara K, Shiozaki H, Tahara H, Kobayashi K, Inoue M, Tamura S, Miyata M, Oka H, Doki Y, Mori T (1993) Prognostic significance of transforming growth factor-alpha in human esophageal carcinoma. Implication for the autocrine proliferation. Cancer 71: 2902–2909

16. Iizuka T, Isono K, Kakegawa T, Watanabe H (1989) The Japanese Committee for registration of esophageal carcinoma cases: parameters linked to 10-year survival of resected esophageal carcinoma in Japan. Chest 96: 1005–1011

17. Kato H, Tachimori Y, Watanabe H, Iizuka T (1993) Evaluation of the new (1987) TNM classification for thoracic esophageal tumors. Int J Cancer 53: 220–223

18. Kato H, Watanabe H, Tachimori Y, Iizuka T (1991) Evaluation of neck lymph node dissection for thoracic esophageal cancer. Ann Thorac Surg 51: 931–935

19. Kitagawa Y, Ueda M, Ando N et al (1991) Significance of int2/hst-1 co-amplification as a prognostic factor in patients with esophageal squamous carcinoma. Cancer Res 51: 1504–1508

20. Le Prise E, Etienne P L, Meunier B, Maddern G, Hassel MB, Gedouin D et al (1993) A randomized study of chemotherapy, radiation therapy, and surgery versus surgery for localized squamous cell carcinoma of the esophagus. Cancer 73: 1779–1784

21. Lund O, Hasenkam JM, Aagaard MT, Kimose HH (1989) Time-related changes in characteristics of prognostic significance in carcinomas of the oesophagus and cardia. Br J Surg 76: 1301–1307

22. Mathews HR, Powell DJ, McCarley CL (1986) Effect of surgical experience on results of resection for oesophageal carcinoma. Br J Surg 73: 621–623

23. Matsuura H, Sugimachi K, Ueo H, Kuwano H, Koga Y, Okamura T (1986) Malignant potential of squamous cell carcinoma of the esophagus predicatble by DNA analysis. Cancer 57: 1810–1814

24. Mori M, Tokino T, Yanagisawa A, Kanamori M, Kato Y, Nakamura Y (1992) Association between chromosome 11q13 amplification and prognosis of patients with oesophageal carcinomas. Eur J Cancer 28A: 755–757

25. Morita M, Kuwano H, Matsuda H, Moriguchi S, Sugimachi K (1991) Prognostic significance of argyrophilic nucleolar organizer regions in esophageal carcinoma. Cancer Res 51: 5339–5341

26. Mukaida H, Toi M, Hirai T, Yamashita Y, Toge T (1991) Clinical significance of the expression of epidermal growth factor and its receptor in esophageal cancer. Cancer 68: 142–148

27. Nakamura T, Nekarda H, Hoelscher A H, Bollschweiler E, Hrabec N, Becker K, Siewert JR (1994) Prognostic value of DNA ploidy and c-ErbB-2 oncoprotein over-expression in adenocarcinoma of Barrett's esophagus. Cancer 73: 1785–1794

28. Ohno S, Mori M, Tsutsui S et al (1991) Growth pattern and prognosis of submucosal carcinoma of the esophagus. Cancer 68: 335–340

29. Orringer MB (1984) Transthoracic versus transhiatal esophagectomy: what difference does it make? Ann Thor Surg 38: 128–132

46   J.D. Roder et al.: Oesophageal Carcinoma

30. Ozawa S, Ued M, Ando N, Shimizu N, Abe O (1989) Prognostic significance of epidermal growth factor receptor in esophageal squamous cell carcinomas. Cancer 63: 2169–2173
31. Patil P, Redkar A, Patel SG, Mistry RC, Deshpande RK, Mittra I, Desai PB (1993) Prognosis of operable squamous cell carcinoma of the esophagus. Relationship with clinico-pathologic features and DNA ploidy. Cancer 72: 20–24
32. Robey-Cafferty SS, el Naggar AK, Sahin AA, Bruner JM, Ro J Y, Cleary KR (1991) Prognostic factors in esophageal squamous carcinoma. A study of histologic features, blood group expression, and DNA ploidy. Am J Clin Pathol 95: 844–849
33. Roder JD, Busch R, Stein HJ, Fink U, Siewert JR (1994) Ratio of invaded and removed lymph nodes as a predictor of survival in squamous cell carcinoma of the oesophagus. Br J Surg 81: 410–413
34. Roth JA, Pass HI, Flanagan MM, Graeber GM, Rosenberg JC, Steinberg S (1988) Randomized clinical trial of preoperative and postoperative adjuvant chemotherapy with cisplatin, vindesine, and bleomycine for carcinoma of the esophagus. J Thorac Cardiovasc Surg 96: 242–248
35. Ruol A, Segalin A, Panozzo M, Stephens J K, Dalla Palma P, Skinner DB, Peracchia A, Little AG (1990) Flow cytometric DNA analysis of squamous cell carcinoma of the esophagus. Cancer 65, 1185–1188
36. Schlag P, for the Chirurgische Arbeitsgemeinschaft für Onkologie der Deutschen Gesellschaft für Chirurgie Study Group (1992) Randomized trial of preoperative chemotherapy for squamous cell cancer of the esophagus. Arch Surg 127: 1146–1450
37. Schneeberger AL, Finley RJ, Troster M, Lohmann R, Keeney M, Inculet RI (1990) The prognostic significance of tumor ploidy and pathology in adenocarcinoma of the esophagogastric junction. Cancer 65: 1206–1210
38. Shimada Y, Imamura M (1993) Prognostic significance of cell culture in carcinoma of the oesophagus. Br J Surg 80: 605–607
39. Shimaya K, Shiozaki H, Inuoe M et al (1993) Significance of p53 expression as a prognostic factor in oesophageal squamous cell carcinoma. Virchows Arch [A] 422: 271–276
40. Sielezneff I, Thomas P, Giovanni M, Giudicelli R, Seitz JF, Fuentes P (1993) Esophageal carcinoma with doubtful extirpability: value of preoperative chemotherapy plus radiotherapy. Eur J Cardiothorac Surg 7: 606–611
41. Siewert JR, Bartels H, Bollschweiler E et al (1992) Plattenepithelcarcinom des Ösophagus. Behandlungskonzept der Chirurgischen Klinik der Technischen Universität München. Chirurg 63: 693–700
42. Siewert JR, Dittler HJ (1993) Esophageal carcinoma: impact of staging on treatment. Endoscopy 25: 28–32
43. Siewert JR, Hölscher AH, Bollschweiler E, Stein HJ, Fink U (1994) Chirurgie des Barrett Carcinoms. Chirurg 66: 102–109
44. Skinner DB, Little AG, Ferguson MK et al (1986) Selection of operation for esophageal carcinoma based on staging. Ann Surg 204: 391–402
45. Stahl M, Wilke H, Meyer H J, Preusser P, Berns T, Fink U et al (1994) 5-Fluorouracil, folinic acid, etoposide and cisplatin chemotherapy for locally advanced or metastatic carcinoma of the oesophagus. Eur J Cancer 30: 325–328
46. Sugimachi K, Matsuoka H, Ohno S et al (1988) Multivariate approach for assessing the prognosis of clinical oesophageal carcinoma. Br J Surg 75: 1115–1118
47. Sugimachi K, Matsuura H, Kai H, Kanematsu T, Inokuchi K, Jingu K (1986) Prognostic factors of esophageal carcinoma: univariate and multivariate analyses. J Surg Oncol 31: 108–112
48. Takubo K, Sasajima K, Yamashita K, Tanaka Y, Fujita K (1990) Prognostic significance of intramural metastasis in patients with esophageal carcinoma. Cancer 65: 1816–1819
49. Teniere P, Hay J-M, Fingerhut A, Fagniez P-L (1991) Postoperative radiation therapy does not increase survival after curative resection for squamous cell carcinoma of the middle and lower esophagus as shown by a multicenter controlled trial. Surg Gynecol Obstet 173: 123
50. Theunissen PHMH, Borchardt F, Poortvliet DCJ (1991) Histopathological evaluation of oesophageal carcinoma: the significance of venous invasion. Br J Surg 78: 930–932
51. Tsutsui S, Kuwano H, Mori M, Matsuura H, Sugimachi K (1992) Flow cytometric analysis of DNA content in primary and metastatic lesions of esophageal squamous cell carcinoma. Cancer 70: 2586–2591

6 Stomach Carcinoma

P. Hermanek, K. Maruyama, and L.H. Sobin

The overall prognosis of patients with stomach carcinoma is different in Western countries and Japan: at present about 70% of stomach cancer patients survive in Japan [57], but only about 35% in Germany [103] and about 20% in the United States [109]. These differences are predominantly dependent on differerent proportions of early carcinomas and of resection for cure (R0).

Despite some advances in medical and radiation therapy, the prognosis of a patient with stomach carcinoma is determined above all by the possibility of complete surgical resection (Fig. 1). Few, if any, patients will survive 5 years unless the carcinoma has been completely removed. Of course, this depends considerably on the pTNM defined stage, but sometimes resection for cure (R0) is not possible in the absence of metastasis, e.g., because of the general condition of the patient or associated comorbidity. Therefore, prognostic factors have to be considered separately for two patient groups:

1. For patients without resection of tumor and those with noncurative resection (R1, R2)
2. For patients with resection for cure (R0)

An overview on older studies of prognostic factors was published by Craven [14] in 1987 in which only two multvariate analyses were considered [7, 16]. Since then about 75 multivariate studies have been reported. Many of these, however, include only a relatively small number of patients (200 or less) and give only limited information. Thus, this overview is predominantly based on multivariate studies on several hundreds [7, 8, 12, 15, 23–25, 31, 34, 67, 68, 83, 84, 87, 127] or thousands of patients [9, 16, 47, 53, 55, 73, 75, 85, 97, 100, 103, 110]. It has to be emphasized that comparisons between various studies are sometimes difficult because the selection criteria, the analyzed factors and their definitions, and the end points (observed, adjusted, relative survival, disease-free survival, with or without surgical deaths, etc.) vary between institutions. Furthermore, sometimes a differentiation between curative and noncurative treatment is not made (no residual tumor classification).

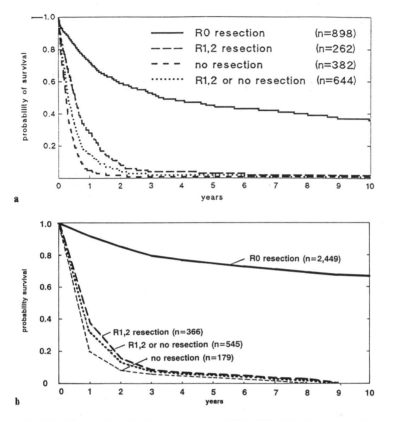

Fig. 1a,b. Observed survival in stomach cancer 1978–1989. Calculation according to Kaplan-Meier, surgical mortality not excluded. Unpublished data, see also Table 1. **a** Department of Surgery, University of Erlangen, Germany. **b** National Cancer Center Hospital, Oncological Surgery Division of the Stomach, Tokyo, Japan

Table 1. Observed survival in stomach cancer (1978–1989). Calculation according to Kaplan-Meier, surgical mortality not excluded. Unpublished data, see also Fig. 1

Patient group	Number of patients		Five-year survival rate (%)		Ten-year survival rate (%)		Median survival time (months)	
	Erlangen[a]	Tokyo[b]	Erlangen[a]	Tokyo[b]	Erlangen[a]	Tokyo[b]	Erlangen[a]	Tokyo[b]
R0	898	2449	44.7 ± 4.4	74.9 ± 1.9	36.2 ± 7.1	68.3 ± 2.6	39.2	n.d.
R1,2 resection	262	366	2.8 ± 2.3	5.7 ± 2.7	2.4 ± 2.3	0	6.4	10.2
No resection	382	179	0.5 ± 1.0	5.9 ± 4.0	0	0	2.8	6.9
No or R1,2 resection	644	545	1.5 ± 1.1	5.7 ± 2.2	1.3 ± 1.2	0	3.6	8.8

Survival rates with twofold standard deviation corresponding to the 95% confidence interval.
n.d., not defined.
[a] Department of Surgery, University of Erlangen, Germany.
[b] National Cancer Center Hospital, Oncological Surgery Division of the Stomach, Tokyo, Japan.

Patients Without Resection for Cure (R1,2)

For patients in whom resection for cure (R0) cannot be achieved, prognosis is very poor. A review of literature by Siewert et al. [111] showed a median survival time following exploratory laparotomy or gastroenterostomy between 3 and 5 months and following noncurative resection between 7 and 11 months. Only minor differences in survival can be observed, primarily depending on absence or presence of distant metastasis [7, 16, 23, 34, 123].

Multivariate studies in patients treated by chemotherapy demonstrated that peritoneal carcinomatosis is the most unfavorable form of metastasis [123]. Histologically confirmed response to chemotherapy is an indicator for longer survival time [58]. Additional adverse factors are weight loss [7, 36] and poor performance status [7, 63, 69]. In the study by Wilke et al. [123], women and patients with a diffuse-type carcinoma (Laurén) showed poor survival compared to men and those with intestinal-type carcinoma.

Patients with Resection for Cure (R0)

The most important prognostic factor is anatomic extent of tumor as described by the pTNM classification and stage grouping of UICC [36, 37] and AJCC [6]. In addition, there are some other tumor-related, patient-related, and treatment-related features which can be considered as proven or probable independent prognostic factors (Table 2).

Table 2. Prognostic factors in patients with stomach carcinoma resected for cure (R0)

Type of factors	Proven	Probable
Tumor-related factors	Anatomic extent – pTNM/stage – Number of involved nodes	Tumor site Small cell histology
Biological and molecular factors	Preoperative elevation of tumor marker serum level (CEA, CA 19–9)	Ploidy Proliferation markers: PCNA and BrdU c-*erbB*-2
Patient-related factors	–	–
Treatment-related factors	Hospital level/institution	Extent of lymph node dissection

CEA, carcinoembryonic antigen; PCNA, proliferating cell nuclear antigen; BrdU, bromodeoxyuridine.

Tumor-Related Factors

Anatomic Extent of Disease

All multivariate studies with larger number of patients showed a significant influence on prognosis for local spread (pT), regional lymph node metastasis (pN), and distant metastasis (M, pM). This applies to separate analysis of these features as well as for their condensation into stages (Table 3). In addition to the pN classification the number of involved nodes correlates with survival (review by Hermanek et al. [38]), e.g., according to Okusa et al. [98] the 5-year survival rates were 63% for one to three, 47% for four to six, and 29% for more than six nodes involved. Furthermore, the ratio of involved to examined lymph nodes correlates with survival [8, 103].

In one multivariate study [7] extension beyond the lymph node capsule was shown to be an additional independent adverse prognostic factor.

The independent prognostic influence of positive cytology on peritoneal lavage in patients without gross evidence of peritoneal involvement [74, 89, 93] remains to be proven. The same applies to the demonstration of isolated tumor cells in bone marrow by immunohistology (cytokeratin) [106].

Tumor Site

The long-term prognosis for patients with proximal carcinomas (upper third, cardiac, gastro-oesophageal junction) is poorer than for those with distal tumors [8, 57]. This may partly be explained by the higher surgical mortality [104] and the more advanced stage [86] of patients with proximal carcinoma; however, in some studies with larger numbers of patients proximal tumor site was an independent

Table 3. Relative 5-year survival rates (%) following resection for cure (R0); dependence on pTNM stage (UICC 1987)

Stage	Miwa [82] (1969–1973)	Maruyama 1992[a] (1978–1989)	Siewert 1992[a] (1982–1991)	Hermanek [35] (1978–1988)
IA	99.2 (n = 2376)	93.3 (n = 1146)	83.6 (n = 101)	91.5 (n = 157)
IB	88.4 (n = 1233)	87.2 (n = 316)	69.3 (n = 78)	83.0 (n = 138)
II	70.1 (n = 1548)	71.8 (n = 296)	45.5 (n = 81)	48.8 (n = 150)
IIIA	47.6 (n = 1611)	60.5 (n = 270)	29.3 (n = 93)	38.3 (n = 139)
IIIB	21.6 (n = 1431)	37.6 (n = 228)	24.1 (n = 63)	18.2 (n = 102)
IV	10.5 (n = 2375)	16.3 (n = 193)	17.9 (n = 89)	6.8 (n = 94)

[a] Unpublished data.

adverse prognostic factor [8, 9, 73, 87]. The stage-by-stage prognosis of gastric "stump" carcinoma is comparable to that of carcinomas in the nonoperated stomach [20] .

Histologic Type

In the second edition of the WHO International Histological Classification [122], the traditional typing (with papillary, tubular, mucinous adenocarcinoma, signet-ring cell, adenosquamous, squamous, small cell, and undifferentiated carcinoma) as well as the Laurén classification (intestinal and diffuse type) and the Ming classification (expanding and infiltrating type) are included.

As in other sites, the rare small cell carcinoma has an unfavorable prognosis [76, 114]. For the uncommon medullary carcinoma with lymphoid stroma a favorable prognosis was reported [91]. For the other types in the traditional classification most multivariate studies showed no independent prognostic influence. The same applies to the Laurén classification; the poorer prognosis of the diffuse type can be explained by the fact that diffuse-type carcinomas are, in general, more advanced than intestinal-type carcinomas [33].

There are only a few multivariate studies of curatively resected patients dealing with the histologic appearance of tumor margins – which is the basis of the Ming classification [5, 22, 25, 60, 102, 105, 108] – but the results are controversial.

Histologic Grade

The prognostic significance of histologic grade is unclear, and the results of large multivariate studies are controversial: a positive correlation was reported by Gabbert et al. [25] and Nakane et al. [87], while no influence of grade was observed by others [8, 34, 73, 84, 103].

Additional Pathologic Features

Controversial results from multivariate studies with more than 200 patients are listed in Table 4.

Peritumoral inflammatory reaction was a favorable factor only in univariate analyses (reviewed by Craven [14]) and in a single multivariate study on 75 patients [17], but could not be confirmed as independent in other multivariate studies [7, 102]. Hariguchi et al. [28] showed by univariate analysis that a morpho-volumetric classification gives useful prognostic information with relatively good prognosis for the funnel type and bad prognosis for the column and mountain type. The subdivision of carcinomas according to growth pattern into a superficially spreading (Super) type and penetrating (Pen) types A and B [41] may offer additional prognostic information, but needs proof by multivariate analysis.

Table 4. Pathological features whose prognostic significance in stomach carcinoma is controversial; only multivariate studies including more than 200 patients considered

Feature	Independent prognostic influence	
	Yes	No
Gross type (Borrmann)	Arveux et al. 1992 [3] ($n = 246$)	Kampschöer et al. 1989 [47] ($n = 1000$)
	Bedikian et al. 1984 [7] ($n = 246$)	Kim 1993 [53] ($n = 1488$)[a]
	Haugstvedt et al. 1983 [31] ($n = 513$)	Kim et al. 1992 [54] ($n = 2063$)[a]
	Korenaga et al. 1989 [60] ($n = 226$)	Maehara et al. 1992 [68] ($n = 916$)[a,c]
	Maruyama 1987 [73] ($n = 3994$)[a,b]	Maehara et al. 1994 [70] ($n = 221$)[a]
	Maruyama et al. 1993 [75] ($n = 2913$)[a]	Moriguchi et al. 1990 [83] ($n = 568$)
	Okajima et al. 1993 [97] ($n = 6540$)[a]	Moriguchi et al. 1992 [84] ($n = 648$)[c]
		Moriguchi et al. 1993 [85] ($n = 1019$)
		Nakane et al. 1994 [87] ($n = 865$)[a]
		Pacelli et al. 1993 [101] ($n = 238$)
		Roder et al. 1993 [103] ($n = 1182$)
		Tanaka et al. 1994 [118] ($n = 216$)[c]
Tumor site	Böttcher et al. 1992 [8] ($n = 702$)[a]	Arveux et al. 1992 [31] ($n = 246$)
	Maehara et al. 1992 [68] ($n = 916$)[a,c]	Bollschweiler et al. 1993 [9] ($n = 1928$)
	Maruyama et al. 1993 [75] ($n = 2913$)[a]	Bozzetti et al. 1986 [12] ($n = 361$)[d]
	Moriguchi et al. 1990 [83] ($n = 568$)	Gabbert et al. 1992 [25] ($n = 445$)
	Moriguchi et al. 1992 [84] ($n = 648$)[c]	Haugstvedt et al. 1993 [31] ($n = 512$)
	Moriguchi et al. 1993 [85] ($n = 1019$)	Hermanek 1989 [34] ($n = 533$)
	Nakane et al. 1994 [87] ($n = 865$)[a]	Kampschöer et al. 1989 [47] ($n = 1000$)
	Roder et al. 1993 [103] ($n = 1182$)	Korenaga et al. 1989 [60] ($n = 226$)
		Maehara et al. 1994 [70] ($n = 221$)[a]
		Maruyama 1987 [73] ($n = 3994$)[a,b]
		Okajima et al. 1993 [97] ($n = 6540$)[a]
		Shiu et al. 1987 [107] ($n = 210$)[a]
		Shiu et al. 1989 [108] ($n = 246$)
		Yonemura et al. 1990 [127] ($n = 442$)

Table 4 (*Contd.*)

Feature	Independent prognostic influence	
	Yes	No
Venous invasion	Gabbert et al. 1991 [24] (*n* = 529) Gabbert et al. 1992 [25] (*n* = 445) Korenaga et al. 1989 [60] (*n* = 226) Ribeiro et al. 1988 [102] (*n* = 227)	Bedikian et al. 1984 [7] (*n* = 246) Maehara et al. 1994 [70] (*n* = 221)[a] Maruyama 1987 [73] (*n* = 3994)[a,b]
Lymphatic invasion	Gabbert et al. 1991 [24] (*n* = 529) Gabbert et al. 1992 [25] (*n* = 445)	Bedikian et al. 1984 [7] (*n* = 246) Korenaga et al. 1989 [60] (*n* = 226) Maruyama 1987 [73] (*n* = 3994)[a,b] Tanaka et al. 1994 [118] (*n* = 216)[c]
Perineural invasion	Tanaka et al. 1994 [118] (*n* = 216)[c]	Bedikian et al. 1984 [7] (*n* = 246)
Desmoplasia	Ribeiro et al. 1988 [102] (*n* = 227)	Maruyama 1987 [73] (*n* = 3994)[a,b]
Sinus histocytosis of regional lymph node	Bedikian et al. 1984 [7] (*n* = 246)	Ribeiro et al. 1988 [102] (*n* = 227)

[a] Any R (all others R0 only).
[b] M0.
[c] pT2-4 only.
[d] Only tumors of middle and lower third of stomach.

Biological and Molecular Factors

Patients with higher preoperative tumor marker levels in serum of carcino-embryonic antigen (CEA), CA 19–9, CA125, Sialyl Tn antigen, ST-439, or alpha fetoprotein (AFP) have a worse prognosis than those without elevated levels [117]. This can be partly explained by the more advanced stage and the lower proportion of curative resections. However, in addition an independent prognostic influence was demonstrated by multivariate analysis for CEA [70, 87] and CA 19–9 [100].

CEA in peritoneal washings also may indicate poor prognosis [4]. After total gastrectomy, urinary pepsinogen I may be a marker predicting recurrences [126].

Table 5 shows biological and molecular markers which are assessed in tumor tissue and may be considered as probable independent indicators of prognosis.

Table 6 lists possible biological and molecular prognostic factors assessed in tumor tissue for which the independent prognostic significance remains to be proven.

Patient-Related Factors

The results of multivariate studies on the independent influence of age are controversial (Table 7).

Female gender was described as an independent favorable factor for R0 resected patients of all stages only in the study by Korenaga et al. [60] and

Table 5. Biological and molecular factors of probable prognostic significance in stomach carcinoma; results of multivariate analysis

Feature	Significant independent prognostic influence	
	Yes	No
Ploidy	Farley et al. 1992 [21] ($n = 48$)[a,c]	Böttcher et al. 1992 [8] ($n = 103$)
	Kimura et al. 1991 [56] ($n = 105$)[a,d]	Filipe et al. 1989 [22] ($n = 116$)
	Korenaga et al. 1989 [60] ($n = 226$)	Ohyama et al. 1992 [95] ($n = 171$)[a]
	Ohyama et al. 1990 [94] ($n = 117$)[a]	
	Rugge et al. 1994 [105] ($n = 76$)[b]	
	Yonemura et al. 1990 [127] ($n = 442$)	
PCNA	Maeda et al. 1994 [66] ($n = 152$)	
	Kakeji et al. 1994 [46] ($n = 181$)[e]	
	Yonemura et al. 1993 [130] ($n = 121$)[a]	
Bromodeoxyuridine	Tonemura et al. 1990 [119] ($n = 167$)[a]	Ohyama et al. 1992 [95] ($n = 172$)[a]
	Yonemura et al. 1990 [127] ($n = 442$)	
C-erbB-2	Jaehne et al. 1994 [43] ($n = 58$)[f]	
	Yonemura et al. 1991 [128] ($n = 189$)[a]	

For critical reviews see also Hattori [30], Katoh and Terada [49], Tahara [116], Wright et al. [124].
[a] Any R (all others R0 only).
[b] M0.
[c] pT1 only.
[d] pT2–4 only.
[e] Borrmann type IV only.
[f] Only for R0 stages III and IV.

Table 6. Biological and molecular factors (assessed in tumor tissue) of possible prognostic significance in stomach carcinoma

Marker	Selected references
A. Differentiation markers, receptors	
CA 19–9	Ikeda et al. 1991 [40]
Sialyl-Tn	Ma et al. 1993 [65]
Sialosyl-Tn	Yamada et al. 1993 [125]
Alpha fetoprotein (AFP)	Chang et al. 1991 [13]
E-cadherin*	Matsui et al. 1993 [78]
	Mayer et al. 1993 [80]*
	Oka et al. 1992 [96]
Alpha catenin	Matsui et al. 1993 [78]
Laminin	David et al. 1994 [18]
	Grigioni et al. 1994 [27]
Type IV collagen and collagenase	David et al. 1994 [18]
	Grigioni et al. 1994 [27]
Fibronectin	David et al. 1994 [18]
Helix pomatia agglutinin- binding activity	Kakeji et al. 1993 [45]
Alpha-2 macroglobulin	Grigioni et al. 1994 [27]
Epidermal growth factor (EGF)	Yonemura et al. 1992 [129]
Epidermal growth factor receptor (EGFR)	Lee et al. 1994 [64] Yonemura et al. 1992 [129]
Transforming growth factor (TGF-α)	Yonemura et al. 1992 [129]
Estrogen and progesterone receptors	Matsui et al. 1992 [77]
D5 (estrogen receptor-related protein)*	Harrison et al. 1991 [29]*
B. Proliferation markers	
S-phase fraction*	Filipe et al. 1991 [22]
	Johnson et al. 1993 [44]
	Ohyama et al. 1990 [94]*
Ki-67	Kakeji et al. 1993 [45]
AgNORs*	Kakeji et al. 1994 [46]*
Thymidine-labeling index	Amadori et al. 1993 [2]
p 105*	Kimura et al. 1991 [56]*
Ratio of bromodeoxyuridine- labeling index to DNA index*	Ohyama et al. 1992 [95]*
C. Molecular markers	
ras mutations	Deng et al. 1991 [19]
CD44*	Maruiwa et al. 1993 [72]
	Mayer et al. 1993 [79]*
nm23	Kodera et al. 1994 [59]
	Nakayama et al. 1993 [92]
p53	Kakeji et al. 1993 [45]
	Martin et al. 1992 [71]
c-*met* gene	Kuniyasa et al. 1992 [61]
MDR 1 gene	Wallner et al. 1993 [120]

* Factors for which independent prognostic significance was demonstrated by a single multivariate study and the respective reference are marked by an asterisk. For nonmarked factors multivariate studies have not yet been reported.
AgNOR, silver-staining nucleolar organizer region.

Table 7. Prognostic significance of age in stomach carcinoma; results of multivariate studies with more than 200 patients

Independent prognostic influence	
Yes	No
Arveux et al. 1992 [3]	Hermanek 1989 [34]
(n = 246)	(n = 533)
Bollschweiler et al. 1993 [9]	Kampschöer et al. 1989 [47]
(n = 1928)	(n = 1000)
Bozetti et al. 1980 [12]	Kim 1989 [52]
(n = 361)[a]	(n = 249)
Fujimoto et al. 1991 [23]	Kim 1993 [53]
(n = 264)	(n = 1488)[b]
Haugstvedt et al. 1993 [31]	Kim et al. 1992 [55]
(n = 513)	(n = 6589)[b]
Maruyama et al. 1993 [75]	Korenaga et al. 1989 [60]
(n = 2913)[b]	(n = 226)
Okajima et al. 1994 [97]	Maehara et al. 1992 [68]
(n = 6540)[b]	(n = 916)[b,c]
Omejc et al. 1994 [99]	Maehara et al. 1994 [70]
(n = 218)	(n = 221)[b]
Roder et al. 1993 [103]	Maruyama 1987 [73]
(n = 1139)	(n = 3994)[d]
Soreide et al. 1982 [113]	Meyers et al. 1987 [81]
(n = 274)[b]	(n = 255)[b]
	Moriguchi et al. 1990 [83]
	(n = 568)
	Moriguchi et al. 1992 [84]
	(n = 648)
	Moriguchi et al. 1993 [85]
	(n = 1019)
	Ribeiro et al. 1988 [102]
	(n = 227)
	Shiu et al. 1989 [108]
	(n = 246)[c]
	Yonemura et al. 1990 [127]
	(n = 493)[b]

[a] Only tumors of middle and lower third of stomach.
[b] Any R (all others R0 only).
[c] pT2-4 only.
[d] M0.

for subgroups by Bozzetti et al. [12] (pN0 only) and Hermanek [34] (stage IIIB only).

Performance status and comorbidity seem to influence prognosis independently only in patients with stage I [34] or pT1 [21].

The study by Cunningham et al. [15] showed that patients with a long history of symptoms (more than 6 months) survive longer than patients with a short history, and this finding persisted in multivariate analysis.

All other possible patient-related prognostic factors reported in univariate studies (e.g., place of residence, symptoms in general, weight loss, epigastric pain, hemoglobin level, immunoglobulin G, complement components in serum) have not yet been proven by multivariate analyses.

Treatment-Related Factors

In univariate analysis, Slisow et al. [112] demonstrated that for each stage of stomach carcinoma in different institutions both different rates of surgical mortality and different long-term results are observed. For "early" carcinoma data from 23 European centers [32] showed 5-year survival rates ranging between 40% and over 90% with a median value of 82.5%. Similar differences according to the hospital level were also reported in the United States by Wanebo et al. [121].

According to a multivariate analysis, the hospital level in Norway independently influenced survival [31], and Bollschweiler et al. [9], comparing the long-term results at the Technical University of Munich, Germany, and the National Cancer Center Hospital, Tokyo, Japan, showed that although there were differences in pT, pN, M, tumor site, and age, the center itself remained an independent prognostic factor. A multivariate analysis by Maruyama [73] failed to show an independent prognostic influence of the individual surgeon within a high-level institution.

Differences in survival between Western countries and Japanese reports on patients with advanced gastric carcinoma are generally explained by the different extent of lymph node dissection [11, 121]. The fact that extended node dissection can be performed without increased surgical mortality and major morbidity and that it results in better long-term survival was demonstrated by comparisons with historical controls in Japan [75, 90] as well as in some nonrandomized studies in Europe [10, 26, 50, 110, 115]. The value of extended node dissection was also shown by multivariate studies in Japan [60, 75, 87, 97, 100] and in Western countries [101, 107, 110]. However, there are also multivariate studies on large numbers of patients that do not show positive results, e.g., Hermanek [34], Kampschöer et al. [47], Maruyama [73], and Moriguchi et al. [85]. Prospective, randomized studies comparing extensive and limited node dissection are underway in the United Kingdom and the Netherlands.

An independent prognostic influence of the type of surgery (total or partial gastrectomy) has never been shown in multivariate analysis where the operation was performed with curative intention. Of course, adequate margins of clearance have to be observed.

An adverse influence of blood transfusion on the survival of gastric carcinoma patients was reported by Kaneda et al. [48]. However, their study was performed only by a univariate method. Multivariate analyses from two different Japanese institutions (National Cancer Center Tokyo, Kampschöer et al. [47], 1000 patients; Kyushu University Fukuoka, Moriguchi et al. [83], 568 patients) failed to demonstrate an independent influence of blood transfusions.

The data on the long-term influence of postoperative complications are controversial [42, 103, 113].

A meta-analysis of the results of postoperative adjuvant chemotherapy [39] showed that postoperative chemotherapy, although effective in some phase II studies, in general offers no additional survival benefit and, thus, at present cannot be considered as standard treatment. The same applies to neoadjuvant

chemotherapy, intraoperative radiotherapy [1], postoperative adjuvant immuno-
therapy [62], and immunochemotherapy [51, 53]. In particular, the subgroups
which may benefit from adjuvant and neoadjuvant treatment have yet to be
defined (for critical review see Nakajima [88]).

References

1. Abe M, Takahashi M (1981) Intraoperative radiotherapy: the Japanese experience. Int J Radiat Oncol Phys 13: 1821–1827
2. Amadori D, Bonagure C, Volpi A, Nanni O, Zoli W, Lundi N, Amadori A, Magni E, Saragoni A (1993) Cell kinetics and prognosis in gastric cancer. Cancer 71: 1–4
3. Arveux P, Faivre J, Boutron M-C, Piard F, Dusserre-Guion L, Monnet E, Hillon P (1992) Prognosis of gastric carcinoma after curative surgery. A population-based study using multivariate crude and relative survival analysis. Dig Dis Sci 37: 757–763
4. Asao T, Fukuda T, Yazawa S, Nagamachi Y (1991) Carcinoembryonic antigen levels in peritoneal washings can predict peritoneal recurrence after curative resection of gastric cancer. Cancer 68: 44–47
5. Baba H, Korenaga D, Okamura T, Saito A, Sugimachi K (1989) Prognostic factors in gastric cancer with serosal invasion, univariate and multivariate analysis. Arch Surg 124: 1061–1064
6. Beahrs OH, Henson DE, Hutter RVP, Kennedy BJ (eds) (1992) Manual for staging of cancer, 4th edn. Lippincott, Philadelphia
7. Bedikian AY, Chen TT, Khankhanian N, Heilbrun LK, McBride CM, McMurtrey MJ, Bodey GP (1984) The natural history of gastric cancer and prognostic factors influencing survival. J Clin Oncol 2: 305–310
8. Böttcher K, Becker K, Busch R, Roder JD, Siewert JR (1992) Prognosefaktoren beim Magencarcinom. Ergebnisse einer uni- und multivariaten Analyse. Chirurg 63: 656–661
9. Bollschweiler E, Boettcher K, Hoelscher AH, Sasako M, Kinoshita T, Maruyama K, Siewert JR (1993) Is the prognosis for Japanese and German patients with gastric cancer really different? Cancer 71: 2918–2925
10. Bonenkamp JJ, van de Velde CJH, Sasako M, Hermans J and cooperating investigators (1992) R2 compared with R1 resection for gastric cancer: morbidity and mortality in a prospective, randomised trial. Eur J Surg 158: 413–418
11. Bonenkamp JJ, van de Velde CJH, Kampschöer GHM, Hermans J, Hermanek P, Bemelmans M, Gouma DJ, Sasako M, Maruyama K (1993) Comparison of factors influencing the prognosis of Japanese, German, and Dutch gastric cancer patients. World J Surg 17: 410–415
12. Bozzetti F, Bonfanti G, Morabito A, Bufalino R, Menotti V, Andreola S, Doci R, Gennari L (1986) A multifactorial approach for the prognosis of patients with carcinoma of the stomach after curative resection. Surg Gynecol Obstet 162: 229–234
13. Chang Y-C, Nagasue N, Abe S, Taniura H, Kumar DD, Nakamura T (1992) Comparison between the clinicopathologic features of AFP-positive and AFP-negative gastric cancers. Am J Gastroenterol 87: 321–325
14. Craven JL (1987) Prognostic indices in stomach cancer. In: Stoll BA (ed) Pointers to cancer prognosis. Nijhoff, Dordrecht
15. Cunningham D, Hole D, Taggart DJ, Soukop M, Carter DC, McArdle CS (1987) Evaluation of the prognostic factors in gastric cancer: the effect of chemotherapy on survival. Br J Surg 74: 715–720
16. Curtis RE, Kennedy BJ, Myers MH, Hankey BF (1985) Evaluation of AJC stomach cancer staging using SEER population. Semin Oncol 12: 21–31
17. Davessar K, Pezzullo JC, Kessimian N, Hale JH, Jauregui HO (1990) Gastric adenocarcinoma: prognostic significance of several pathologic parameters and histologic classifications. Hum Pathol 21: 325–332
18. David L, Nesland JM, Holm R, Sobrinho-Simoes M (1994) Expression of laminin, collagen IV, fibronectin, and type IV collagenase in gastric carcinoma. Cancer 73: 518–527
19. Deng GR, Liu XH, Wang JR (1991) Correlation of mutations of oncogene c-Ha-ras at codon 12 with metastasis and survival of gastric cancer patients. Oncogene Res 6: 33–38

20. Domellöf L (1993) Remnant stomach and gastric cancer. In: Nishi M, Ichikawa H, Nakajima T, Maruyama K, Tahara E (eds) Gastric cancer. Springer, Berlin Heidelberg New York

21. Farley DR, Donohue JH, Nagorney DM, Carpenter HA, Katzmann JA, Ilstrup DM (1992) Early gastric cancer. Br J Surg 79: 539–542

22. Filipe MI, Rosa J, Sandey A, Imrie PR, Ormerod MG, Morris RW (1991) Is DNA ploidy and proliferative activity of prognostic value in advanced gastric carcinoma? Hum Pathol 22: 373–378

23. Fujimoto S, Furue H, Kimura T, Kondo T, Orita K, Taguchi T, Yoshida K, Ogawa N (1991) Clinical outcome of postoperative adjuvant immunochemotherapy with sizofiran for patients with resectable gastric cancer: a randomised controlled study. Eur J Cancer 27: 1114–1118

24. Gabbert HE, Meier S, Gerharz CD, Hommel G (1991) Incidence and prognostic significance of vascular invasion in 529 gastric-cancer patients. Int J Cancer 49: 203–207

25. Gabbert HE, Meier S, Gerharz CD, Hommel G (1992) Tumor-cell dissociation at the invasive front: a new prognostic parameter in gastric cancer patients. Int J Cancer 50: 202–207

26. Gall FP, Hermanek P (1993) Die systematische erweiterte Lymphknotendissektion in der kurativen Therapie des Magencarcinoms. Chirurg 64: 1024–1031

27. Grigioni WF, d'Errico A, Fortunato C, Fiorentino M, Mancini AM, Stetler-Stevenson G, Sobel ME, Liotta LA, Onisto M, Garbisa S (1994) Prognosis of gastric carcinoma revealed by interactions between tumor-cells and basement membrane. Modern Pathol 7: 220–225

28. Haraguchi M, Okamura T, Sugimachi K (1987) Accurate prognostic value of morpho-volumetric analysis of advanced carcinoma of the stomach. Surg Gynecol Obstet 164: 335–339

29. Harrison JD, Jones JA, Ellis IO, Morris DL (1991) Oestrogen receptor D5 antibody is an independent negative prognostic factor in gastric cancer. Br J Surg 78: 334–336

30. Hattori T (1993) DNA ploidy pattern and cell kinetics. In: Nishi M, Ichikawa H, Nakajima T, Maruyama K, Tahara E (eds) Gastric cancer. Springer, Berlin Heidelberg New York

31. Haugstvedt TK, Visto A, Eide GE, Soreide O and members of the Norwegian Stomach Cancer Trial (1993) Norwegian multicentre study of survival and prognostic factors in patients undergoing curative resection for gastric carcinoma. Br J Surg 80: 475–478

32. Heberer G, Teichmann RK, Krämling H-J, Günther B (1988) Results of gastric resection for carcinoma of the stomach: the European experience. World J Surg 12: 374–381

33. Hermanek P (1986) Prognostic factors in stomach cancer surgery. Eur J Surg Oncol 12: 241–246

34. Hermanek P (1989) Gastric carcinoma – precancerous conditions and lesions, classification, and prognosis. In: Hotz J, Meyer HJ, Schmoll HJ (eds) Gastric carcinoma. Springer, Berlin Heidelberg New York

35. Hermanek P (1991) Die Bedeutung der TNM-Klassifikation für die Beurteilung operierter Magenkarzinompatienten. In: Delbrück H (ed) Magenkarzinom. Zuckschwerdt, Munich

36. Hermanek P, Sobin LH (eds) (1987) UICC TNM classification of malignant tumours, 4th edn. Springer, Berlin Heidelberg New York

37. Hermanek P, Sobin LH (eds) (1992) UICC TNM classification of malignant tumours, 4th edn, 2nd rev. Springer, Berlin Heidelberg New York

38. Hermanek P, Henson DE, Hutter RVP, Sobin LH (eds) (1993) TNM Supplement 1993. A commentary on uniform use. Springer, Berlin Heidelberg New York

39. Hermans J, Bonenkamp JJ, Boon MC, Bunt AMG, Ohyama S, Sasako M, van de Velde CJH (1993) Adjuvant therapy after curative resection for gastric cancer: meta-analysis of random-ized trials. J Clin Oncol 11: 1441–1447

40. Ikeda Y, Mori M, Kido A, Shimono R, Matsushima T, Sugimachi K, Saku M (1991) Immunohistochemical expression of carbohydrate antigen 19–9 in gastric carcinoma. Am J Gastroenterol 86: 1163–1166

41. Inokuchi K, Sugimachi K (1993) Growth patterns of gastric cancer. In: Nishi M, Ichikawa H, Nakajima T, Maruyama K, Tahara E (eds) Gastric cancer. Springer, Berlin Heidelberg New York

42. Jaehne J, Meyer H-J, Maschek H, Geerlings H, Bruns E, Pichlmayr R (1992) Lympha-denectomy in gastric carcinoma. A prospective and prognostic study. Arch Surg 127: 290–294

43. Jaehne J, Cordon-Cardo C, Albino A, Meyer HJ, Pichlmayr R (1994) Pathogenetic and prognostic relevance of Her2/neu in gastric carcinoma. Eur J Surg Oncol 20: 362

44. Johnson H Jr, Belluco C, Masood S, Abou-Azama AM, Kahn L, Wise L (1993) The value of flow cytometric analysis in patients with gastric cancer. Arch Surg 128: 314–317

45. Kakeji Y, Korenaga D, Tsujitani S, Baba H, Anai H, Maehara Y, Sugimachi K (1993) Gastric cancer with p53 overexpression has high potential for metastasising to lymph nodes. Br J Cancer 67: 589–593
46. Kakeji Y, Maehara Y, Adachi Y, Baba H, Mori M, Furusawa M, Sugimachi K (1994) Proliferative activity as a prognostic factor in Borrmann type 4 gastric carcinoma. Br J Cancer 69: 749–753
47. Kampschöer GH, Maruyama K, Sasako M, Kinoshita T, van de Velde CJH (1989) The effect of blood transfusion on the prognosis of patients with gastric cancer. World J Surg 13: 637–643
48. Kaneda M, Hiromi M, Nimomiya M, Nagae S, Mukai K, Takeda I, Shimoyama H, Chohno S, Okabayashi T, Kagawa S, Orita K (1987) Adverse effect of blood transfusion on survival of patients with gastric cancer. Transfusion 27: 375–377
49. Katoh M, Terada M (1993) Oncogenes and tumor suppressor genes. In: Nishi M, Ichikawa H, Nakajima T, Maruyama K, Tahara E (eds) Gastric cancer. Springer, Berlin Heidelberg New York
50. Keller E, Stützer H, Heitmann K, Bauer P, Gebbensleben B, Rohde H and the German Stomach Cancer TNM Study Group (1994) Lymph node staging in 872 patients with carcinoma of the stomach and the presumed benefit of lymphadenectomy. J Am Coll Surg 178: 38–46
51. Kim J-P (1987) The concept of immunochemosurgery in gastric cancer. World J Surg 11: 465–472
52. Kim J-P (1989) Invited commentary. World J Surg 113: 123
53. Kim J-P (1993) Results of surgery in 6589 gastric cancer patients indicating immunochemosurgery as being the best multimodality treatment for advanced gastric cancer. In: Nishi M, Ichikawa H, Nakajima T, Maruyama K, Tahara E (eds) Gastric cancer. Springer, Berlin Heidelberg New York
54. Kim J-P, Yang H-K, Oh S-T (1992) Is the new UICC staging system of gastric cancer reasonable? (Comparison of 5-year survival rate of gastric cancer by old and new UICC stage classification) Surg Oncol 1: 209–213
55. Kim J-P, Kwon J, Sung T, Yang HK (1992) Results of surgery on 6589 gastric cancer patients and immunochemosurgery as the best treatment of advanced gastric cancer. Ann Surg 216: 269–279
56. Kimura H, Yonemura Y, Epstein AL (1991) Flow cytometric quantitation of the proliferation-associated nuclear antigen p105 and DNA content in advanced gastric cancers. Cancer 68: 2175–2180
57. Kinoshita T, Maruyama K, Sasako M, Okajima K (1993) Treatment results of gastric cancer patients: Japanese experience. In: Nishi M, Ichikawa H, Nakajima T, Maruyama K, Tahara E (eds) Gastric cancer. Springer, Berlin Heidelberg New York
58. Kiyohashi A, Kurihara M, Yoshida S, Ohkubo T, Suga S (1993) Antitumor effect and survival benefit of chemotherapy for unresectable advanced gastric cancer. Jpn J Clin Oncol 23: 41–45
59. Kodera Y, Isobe K-I, Yamauchi M, Kondoh K, Kimura N, Akiyama S, Itoh K, Nakashima I, Takagi H (1994) Expression of nm23 H-1 RNA levels in human gastric cancer tissues. A negative correlation with nodal metastasis. Cancer 73: 259–265
60. Korenaga D, Haraguchi M, Okamura T, Baba H, Saito A, Sugimachi K (1989) DNA ploidy and tumor invasion in human gastric cancer. Arch Surg 14: 314–318
61. Kuniyasa H, Yasui W, Kitadai Y, Yokozaki H, Ito H, Tahara E (1992) Frequent amplification of the c-met gene in scirrhous type stomach cancer. Biochem Biophys Res Commun 189: 227–232
62. Kyoto Research Group for Digestive Organ Surgery (1992) A comprehensive multi-institutional study on postoperative adjuvant immonotherapy with oral streptococcal preparation OK-432 for patients after gastric cancer surgery. Ann Surg 216: 44–54
63. Lavin PT, Bruckner HW, Plaxe StC (1982) Studies in prognostic factors relating to chemotherapy for advanced gastric cancer. Cancer 50: 2016–2023
64. Lee EY, Cibull ML, Strodel WE, Haley JV (1994) Expression of HER-2/neu oncoprotein and epidermal growth factor receptor and prognosis in gastric carcinoma. Arch Path Labor Med 118: 235–239
65. Ma XC, Terata N, Kodama M, Hattori T (1993) Sialyl Tn antigen as a predictor of survival time for patients with gastric carcinoma. In: Takahashi T (ed) Recent advances in management of digestive cancers. Springer, Berlin Heidelberg New York
66. Maeda K, Chung Y, Naoyoshi O, Kato Y, Nitta A, Arimoto Y, Yamada N, Kondo Y, Sowa M (1994) Proliferating cell nuclear antigen labeling index of preoperative biopsy specimens in gastric carcinoma with special reference to prognosis. Cancer 73: 528–533

67. Maehara Y, Morriguchi S, Kakeji Y, Orita H, Haraguchi M, Korenaga D, Sugimachi K (1991) Prognostic factors in adenocarcinoma in the upper one-third of the stomach. Surg Gynecol Obstet 173: 223–226
68. Maehara Y, Emi Y, Moriguchi S, Takahashi I, Yoshida M, Kusomoto H, Sugimachi K (1992) Postoperative chemotherapy for patients with advanced gastric cancer. Am J Surg 163: 577–580
69. Maehara Y, Sugimachi K, Ogawa M, Kakegawa T, Shimazu H, Tomita M (1993) Influence of preoperative performance status on survival time of patients with advanced gastric cancer following noncurative resection. Anticancer Res 13: 201–203
70. Maehara Y, Kusumoto T, Takahashi I, Kakeji Y, Baba H, Akazawa K, Sugimachi K (1994) Predictive value of preoperative carcinoembryonic antigen levels for the prognosis of patients with well-differentiated gastric cancer. Oncology 51: 859–862
71. Martin HM, Filipe MI, Morris RW, Lane DP, Silvestre F (1992) p53 expression and prognosis in gastric carcinoma. Int J Cancer 50: 859–862
72. Maruiwa M, Kumegawa H, Suematsu T, Kawabata S, Ohta J, Kodama I, Konfuji K, Takeda J, Kakegawa T (1993) Expression of CD 44 molecule in gastric cancer. In: Takahashi T (ed) Recent advances in management of digestive cancers. Springer, Berlin Heidelberg New York
73. Maruyama K (1987) The most important prognostic factors for gastric cancer patients. A study using univariate and multivariate analyses. Scand J Gastroenterol 22 [Suppl 133]: 63–68
74. Maruyama K (1991) Diagnosis of invisible peritoneal metastasis: cytologic examination by peritoneal lavage. In: Cordiano C, de Manzoni G (eds) Staging and treatment of gastric cancer. Piccin Nuova Libraria, Padua
75. Maruyama K, Sasako M, Kinoshita T, Okajima K (1993) Effectiveness of systematic lymph node dissection in gastric cancer surgery. In: Nishi M, Ichikawa H, Nakajima T, Maruyama K, Tahara E (eds) Gastric cancer. Springer, Berlin Heidelberg New York
76. Matsui K, Kitagawa M, Miwa A, Kuroda Y, Tsuji M (1991) Small cell carcinoma of the stomach: a clinico-pathologic study of 17 cases. Am J Gastroenterol 86: 1167–1175
77. Matsui M, Kojima O, Kawakami S, Uehara Y, Takahashi T (1992) The prognosis of patients with gastric cancer possessing sex hormone receptors. Surg Today 22: 421–425
78. Matsui S, Shiozaki H, Inoue M, Tamura S, Oka H, Doki Y, Iihara K, Kadowaki T, Iwazawa T, Shimaya K, Nagafuchi A, Tsukita A, Mori T (1993) Immunohistochemical evaluation of alpha-catenin, cadherin-associated intercellular protein, expression in human gastric cancer In: Takahashi T (ed) Recent advances in management of digestive cancers. Springer, Berlin Heidelberg New York
79. Mayer B, Jauch KW, Günthert U, Figdor CG, Schildberg FW, Funke I, Johnson JP (1993) De-novo expression of CD 44 and survival in gastric cancer. Lancet 342: 1019–1022
80. Mayer B, Johnson JP, Leitl F, Jauch KW, Heiss MM, Schildberg FW, Birchmeier W, Funke I (1993) E-cadherin expression in primary and metastatic gastric cancer: downregulation correlates with cellular dedifferentiation and glandular disintegration. Cancer Res 53: 1690–1695
81. Meyers WC, Damiano RJ, Rotolo FS, Postlethwait RW (1987) Adenocarcinoma of the stomach – changing patterns over the last 4 decades. Ann Surg 205: 1–8
82. Miwa K, Japanese Research Society for Gastric Cancer (1984) Evaluation of the TNM classification of stomach cancer and proposal for its rational stage-grouping. Jpn J Clin Oncol 14: 385–410
83. Moriguchi S, Maehara Y, Akazawa K, Sugimachi K, Nose Y (1990) Lack of relationship between perioperative blood transfusion and survival time after curative resection for gastric cancer. Cancer 66: 2331–2335
84. Moriguchi S, Maehara Y, Korenaga D, Sugimachi K, Hayashi Y, Nose Y (1992) Prediction of survival time after curative surgery for advanced gastric cancer. Eur J Surg Oncol 18: 287–292
85. Moriguchi S, Hayashi Y, Nose Y, Maehara Y, Korenaga D, Sugimachi K (1993) A comparison of the logistic regression and the Cox proportional hazard models in retrospective studies on the prognosis of patients with gastric cancer. J Surg Oncol 52: 9–13
86. Nakane Y, Okamura S, Boku T, Okusa T, Tanaka K, Hioki K (1993) Prognostic differences of adenocarcinoma arising from the cardia and the upper third of the stomach. Am Surg 59: 423–429
87. Nakane Y, Okamura S, Akehira K, Boku T, Okusa T, Tanaka K, Hioki K (1994) Correlation of preoperative carcinoembryonic antigen levels and prognosis of gastric cancer patients. Cancer 73: 2703–2708

88. Nakajima T (1993) Adjuvant and neoadjuvant chemotherapy in gastric cancer: a review. In: Nishi M, Ichikawa H, Nakajima T, Maruyama K, Tahara E (eds) Gastric cancer. Springer, Berlin Heidelberg New York

89. Nakajima T, Harashima S, Hirate M, Kajitani T (1978) Prognostic and therapeutic value of peritoneal cytology in gastric cancer. Acta Cytol 22: 225–229

90. Nakajima T, Nishi M (1989) Surgery and adjuvant chemotherapy for gastric cancer. Hepatogastroenterology 36: 79–85

91. Nakamura S, Ueki T, Yao T, Ueyama T, Tsuneyoshi M (1994) Epstein-Barr virus in gastric carcinoma with lymphoid stroma. Cancer 73: 2239–2249

92. Nakayama H, Yasui M, Yokozaki H, Tahara E (1993) Reduced expression of nm 23 is associated with metastasis of human gastric carcinomas. Jpn J Cancer Res 84: 184–190

93. Nekarda H, Schenck U, Luswig C, Stark M, Becker K, Fink U, Siewert JR (1994) Prognosis of free abdominal cancer cells in totally resected gastric cancer. Eur J Surg Oncol 20: 361

94. Ohyama S, Yonemura Y, Miyazaki I (1990) Prognostic value of S-phase fraction and DNA ploidy studied with in vivo administration of bromodeoxyuridine on human gastric cancers. Cancer 65: 116–121

95. Ohyama S, Yonemura Y, Miyazaki I (1992) Proliferative activity and malignancy in human gastric cancers. Significance of the proliferation rate and its clinical application. Cancer 69: 314–321

96. Oka H, Shiozaki H, Kobayashi K, Tahara H, Tamura S, Miyata M, Doki Y, Iihara K, Matsuyoshi N, Hirano S, Takeichi M, Mori T (1992) Immunohistochemical evaluation of E-cadherin adhesion molecule expression in human gastric cancer. Virchows Arch A 421: 149–156

97. Okajima K. Sasako M, Kinoshita T, Maruyama K (1993) Prognostic factors for gastric cancer patients – alternation of the significance in 6,540 patients treated over a 30-year period. In: Takahashi T (ed) Recent advances in management of digestive cancers. Springer, Berlin Heidelberg New York

98. Okusa T, Nakane Y, Boku T, Takada H, Yamamura M, Hioki K, Yomemato M (1990) Quantitative analysis of nodal involvement with respect to survival rate after gastrectomy for carcinoma. Surg Gynecol Obstet 170: 488–494

99. Omejc M, Repse S, Jelenc F, Cimerman M, Bitenc M, Jerman J, Lamovec J, Jutersek A, Herbst F (1994) Einfluß des Magenkarzinomtyps nach Laurén auf die Prognose nach potentiell kurativer Resektion. Acta Chir Austriaca 26: 155–159

100. Onorato A, Ohkura H, Okajima K, Sasako M, Kinoshita T, Maruyama K (1993) Non-anatomic prognostic factors for gastric cancer patients: significance of tumor markers. In: Takahashi T (ed) Recent advances in management of digestive cancers. Springer, Berlin Heidelberg New York

101. Pacelli F, Doglietto GB, Bellantone R, Alfieri S, Sgadari A, Crucitti F (1993) Extensive versus limited lymph node dissection for gastric cancer: a comparative study of 320 patients. Br J Surg 80: 1153–1156

102. Ribeiro MM, Seoxas M, Sobrinho-Simoes M (1988) Prognosis in gastric carcinoma. The preeminence of staging and futility of histological classification. Dig Dis Pathol 1: 51–68

103. Roder JD, Böttcher K, Siewert JR, Busch R, Hermanek P, Meyer H-J and the German Gastric Carcinoma Study Group (1993) Prognostic factors in gastric carcinoma. Results of the German Gastric Carcinoma Study 1992. Cancer 72: 2089–2097

104. Rohde H, Bauer P, Stützer H, Heitmann K, Gebbersieben B and the German Gastric Cancer TNM Study Group (1991) Proximal compared with distal adenocarcinoma of the stomach: differences and consequences. Br J Surg 78: 1242–1248

105. Rugge M, Sonego F, Panozzo M, Baffa R, Rubio J Jr, Farinati F, Nitto D, Ninfo V, Ming S-C (1993) Pathology and ploidy in the prognosis of gastric cancer with no extranodal metastasis. Cancer 73: 1127–1133

106. Schlimok G, Funke I, Pantel K, Strobel F, Lindemann F, Witte J, Riethmüller G (1991) Micrometastatic tumor cells in bone marrow of patients with gastric cancer. Methodological aspects of detection and prognostic significance. Eur J Cancer 27: 1461–1465

107. Shiu MH, Moore E, Sanders M, Huvos A, Freedman B, Goodbold J, Chaiyahruk S, Wesdorp R, Brennan MF (1987) Influence of the extent of resection on survival after curative treatment of gastric carcinoma – a retrospective multivariate analysis. Arch Surg 122: 1347–1351

108. Shiu MH, Perrotti M, Brennan MF (1989) Adenocarcinoma of the stomach: a multivariate analysis of clinical, pathologic and treatment factors. Hepatogastroenterology 36: 7–12

109. Shiu MH, Karpeh M, Brennan MF (1989) End results of surgical treatment of gastric adenocarcinoma: American experience. In: Nishi M, Ichikawa H, Nakajima T, Maruyama K, Tahara E (eds) Gastric cancer. Springer, Berlin Heidelberg New York

110. Siewert JR, Böttcher K, Roder JD, Busch R, Hermanek P, Meyer HJ, and the German Gastric Carcinoma Study Group (1993) Prognostic relevance of systematic lymph node dissection in gastric carcinoma. Br J Surg 80: 1015–1018

111. Siewert JR, Böttcher K, Roder JD, Fink U (1993) Palliative treatment from the surgical point of view. In: Nishi M, Ichikawa H, Nakajima T, Maruyama K, Tahara E (eds) Gastric cancer. Springer, Berlin Heidelberg New York

112. Slisów W, Marx G, Staneczek W, Seifart W, Greiner P (1985) Die therapeutische Situation beim Magenkarzinom in der DDR 1976 aus chirurgischer Sicht. Zbl Chir 110: 1361–1373

113. Soreide O, Lillestol J, Viste A, Bjerkeset T (1982) Factors influencing survival in patients with cancer of the stomach. Acta Chir Scand 148: 367–372

114. Staren ED, Lott S, Saavedra VM, Jansson DS, Deziel DJ, Saclarides TJ, Manderino GL, Gould VE (1992) Neuroendocrine carcinomas of the stomach: a clinicopathologic evaluation. Surgery 112: 1039–1047

115. Sue-Ling H, Johnston D (1993) Gastric cancer is curable in the West. Eur J Cancer Prev 2: 13–16

116. Tahara E (1993) Molecular mechanism of stomach carcinogenesis. J Cancer Res Clin Oncol 119: 265–272

117. Takahashi I, Maehara Y, Kusumoto T, Yoshida M, Kakeji Y, Kusumoto H, Furusawa M, Sugimachi K (1993) Predictive value of preoperative serum sialyl Tn antigen levels in prognosis of patients with gastric cancer. Cancer 72: 1836–1840

118. Tanaka A, Watanabe T, Okuno K, Yasutomi M (1994) Perineural invasion as a predictor of recurrence of gastric cancer. Cancer 73: 550–553

119. Tonemura Y, Kamata T, Ooyama S, Sugiyama K, Kimura H, Kosaka T, Yamaguchi A, Miyazaki I (1990) Relation of proliferative activity to survival in patients with gastric carcinoma. J Surg Oncol 43: 3–7

120. Wallner J, Depisch D, Gsur A, Götzl M, Haider K, Pirker R (1993) MDR 1 gene expression and its clinical relevance in primary gastric carcinomas. Cancer 71: 667–671

121. Wanebo HJ, Kennedy BJ, Chmiel J, Steele G, Winchester D, Osteen R (1993) Cancer of the stomach. A patient care study by the American College of Surgeons. Ann Surg 218: 583–592

122. Watanabe H, Jass JR, Sobin LH (1990) Histological typing of oesophageal and gastric tumours, 2nd edn. WHO International Histological Classification of Tumours. Springer, Berlin Heidelberg New York

123. Wilke H, Preusser P, Fink U, Achterrath W, Meyer HJ, Stahl M, Lenaz L, Meyer J, Siewert JR, Geerlings H, Köhne-Wömpner CH, Harstrick A, Schmoll H-J (1990) New developments in the treatment of gastric carcinoma. Semin Oncol 17 [Suppl 1]: 61–70

124. Wright PA, Quirke P, Attanoos R, Williams GT (1992) Molecular pathology of gastric carcinoma: progress and prospects. Hum Pathol 23: 848–859

125. Yamada T, Watanabe A, Sawada H, Yamada Y, Yano T, Ueyama N, Shino Y, Tanase M, Nakano H (1993) Expression of sialosyl Tn antigen in gastric cancer. In: Takahashi T (ed) Recent advances in management of digestive cancers. Springer, Berlin Heidelberg New York

126. Yamaguchi T, Takahashi T, Yokota T, Kitamura K, Noguchi A, Kamiguchi M, Doi M, Ahn T, Sawai K, Yamane T (1991) Urinary pepsinogen I as a tumor marker of stomach cancer after total gastrectomy. Cancer 68: 906–909

127. Yonemura Y, Ooyama S, Sugiyama K, Kamata T, de Aretxabala X, Kimura H, Kosaka T, Yamaguchi A, Miwa K, Miyazaki I (1990) Retrospective analysis of the prognostic significance of DNA ploidy patterns and S-phase fraction in gastric carcinoma. Cancer Res 50: 509–514

128. Yonemura Y, Nimomiya U, Ohoyama S, Kimura H, Yamaguchi A, Fushida S, Kosaka T, Miwa K, Miyazaki I, Endou Y (1991) Expression of c-erbB-2 oncoprotein in gastric carcinoma. Immunoreactivity for c-erbB-2 protein is an independent indicator of poor short-term prognosis in patients with gastric carcinoma. Cancer 67: 2914–2918

129. Yonemura Y, Takamura H, Ninomiya I, Fushida S, Tsugawa K, Kaji M, Nakai Y, Ohoyama S, Yamaguchi A, Miyazaki I (1992) Interrelationship between transforming growth factor-alpha and epidermal growth factor receptor in advanced gastric cancer. Oncology 49: 157–161

130. Yonemura Y, Kimura H, Fushida S, Tugawa K, Nakai Y, Kaji M, Fonseca L, Yamaguchi A, Miyazaki I (1993) Analysis of proliferative activity using anti-proliferating cell nuclear antigen antibody in gastric cancer tissue specimens obtained by endoscopic biopsy. Cancer 71: 2448–2453

7 Colorectal Carcinoma

P. Hermanek and L.H. Sobin

In 1991, an "International Documentation System for Colorectal Cancer (IDS for CRC)" was published by an international working party chaired by L.P. Fielding [32]. It includes a comprehensive overview on prognostic factors in colorectal carcinoma. Since then only a limited number of relevant papers have appeared, mainly confirming known factors or presenting preliminary data on possible new biological or molecular markers. Thus, this chapter is necessarily a condensed and updated version of the detailed description of prognostic factors by the IDS for CRC. Correspondingly, aside from key references only publications from the last 5 years are cited; for older literature see surveys [1, 22, 32]. In examining prognostic factors for most cancer types in general and colorectal carcinoma in particular, three special aspects have to be considered:

1. Surgical resection remains the most effective therapy for colorectal carcinoma [28]. Therefore, in the great majority of patients with colorectal carcinomas the primary tumor is removed by surgery, including endoscopic procedures. Thus, for most patients an estimation of prognosis includes the pathologic findings on the resection specimen.
2. In multi-institutional data sets, e.g., the SEER (Surveillance, Epidemiology, and End Results) Program 1983–1987, the overall observed 5-year survival rate (all races, males and females, all ages, colon and rectum) is about 40% and the relative rate 50% [50]. While the observed 5-year survival rates following complete tumor removal (residual tumor classification R0) today are between 50% and 60%, the prognosis for patients with residual tumor (R1, R2) is very poor (Fig. 1). Cure and long-term survival can be expected in general only in patients with resection for cure (R0). Exceptions are the uncommon patients with early-stage carcinomas in whom complete tumor destruction is achieved by radiotherapy or radiochemotherapy alone.
3. In patients with known residual tumor (R1, R2) the prognosis is relatively uniform and influenced by a limited number of prognostic factors; further-more, knowledge of these factors has only minor therapeutic implications. In contrast, patients with complete tumor resection (R0) have a wide spectrum of outcome. In this patient group, several factors determine outcome, and it is important to define high-risk patients for whom adjuvant and neoadjuvant treatment regimens may be considered. Thus, in the following, patients with (R1, R2) and those without residual tumor (R0) will be discussed separately.

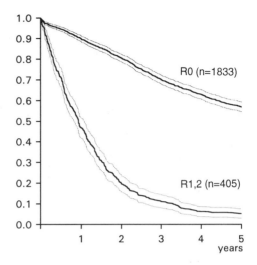

Fig. 1. Survival following tumor resection (any type) in relation to the residual tumor (R) classification. Data from the German Multicenter Study on Colorectal Carcinoma (SGCRC). Observed overall survival, calculated according to Kaplan-Meier, surgical mortality not excluded. Five-year survival rates with 95% confidence interval (%): R0, 56.9 (54.5–59.3); R1,2: 5.4 (2.9–7.9); $p < 0.001$. (From [57])

Prognostic Factors for Patients with Residual Tumor (R1, R2)

The prognosis of patients with known residual tumor (R1, R2) is poor. Median survival times of 10–11 months are reported [57, 105]. The 5-year survival rates are 6.9% [103] or 5.4% [57].

Multivariate analysis of patients with residual tumor shows that the presence or absence of distant metastases and the localization of residual tumor are the significant prognostic factors, while the extent of local spread and lymph node metastasis (T and N) have no influence on prognosis in these patients [105]. The median survival time was 13.8 months for locoregional residual tumor, 11.9 for distant residual tumor, and 7.6 months for residual tumor at both sites [105]. Similar figures are reported by Hermanek and Wittekind [57] (17.4, 9.8, and 6.7 months, respectively).

The residual tumor classification of the UICC (International Union Against Cancer) [55] and AJCC (American Joint Committee on Cancer) [10] differentiates between R1, microscopic residual tumor, and R2, macroscopic residual tumor. For R2 patients the prognosis is worse than for R1 (median survival times, 10.0 versus 18.7 months) [57]; however, most R2 patients have distant metastases, while most R1 patients have only locoregional residual tumor. For patients with multiple distant metastasis (at presentation or during follow-up) the performance status influences survival time; other possible factors such as number of symptoms, gender, hemoglobin level, lactate dehydrogenase (LDH) level, white blood count, blood sedimentation rate, albumin, carcinoembryonic antigen (CEA); and CA 19–9 serum levels have been considered, but not proven [25, 37, 76].

Prognostic Factors for Patients With Complete Resection of Tumor (No Residual Tumor, R0)

The prognosis of patients after tumor resection for cure (R0) is predominantly influenced by the anatomic extent of cancer as described by TNM [10, 55] and histologic grade. Table 1 presents an overview of proven and probable prognostic factors.

Tumor-Related Factors

Anatomic Extent of Disease

The anatomic extent is by far the most important prognostic factor. This is demonstrated in all multivariate analyses [17, 19, 58, 93, 94, 112, 139, 140]. The prognostic impact can be observed whether stage grouping or the components of

Table 1. Independent prognostic factors for colorectal carcinoma resected for cure (R0)

	Proven prognostic factors	Probable prognostic factors
Tumor related	Anatomic extent: pTNM and stage grouping (higher category) Histologic grade (high grade) Venous invasion (present, predominantly extramural)	Anatomic site of primary (lower rectum) Tumor perforation/obstruction (present) Lymphatic and perineural invasion (present) Histologic pattern of tumor margin (infiltrative) Peritumoral lymphoid cells/lymphoid aggregates (conspicious/present)
Patient related	–	Gender (male) CEA serum level (>5 mg/l)
Treatment related	Surgeon	Technique of tumor mobilization (other than "no-touch") Local spillage of tumor cells (iatrogeneous perforation of/incision into tumor)

Unfavorable level of covariates is shown in parentheses
CEA, carcinoembryonic antigen.

the stage grouping are included in the analysis. TNM stage grouping includes three components: (1) local spread of the primary tumor, i.e., depth of invasion (T); (2) regional lymph node status (N); and (3) absence or presence of distant metastasis (M). Although correlations between these three components exist, their independent influence on prognosis has been demonstrated by several multivariate analyses [14, 19, 36, 95, 106]. Futhermore, within the T3 category the extent of perimuscular invasion seems to influence prognosis, expecially in rectum carcinoma. Proposals to study this are presented in the TNM Supplement 1993 [56]. Tumor size has no independent influence on prognosis; the same applies to the gross tumor type, with the possible exception of the uncommon scirrhous or linitis plastica type [102, 123].

Concerning regional lymph node spread, the number of involved nodes as well as their localization (perirectal/pericolic or along the named vascular trunks) influence outcome [53, 105, 112, 113, 121].

The influence of pT, pN, and (p)M on prognosis is shown in Table 2 by the results of a prospective German multicenter study [52, 58]. Figure 2 shows survival in relation to stage grouping. It should be emphasized that stage III is prognostically nonhomogeneous, as shown in Table 3. Thus, whenever possible treatment results should be subdivided according to the individual pN categories. This is especially important in clinical trials on adjuvant treatment [51].

Table 2. Prognosis of colorectal carcinoma in relation to pTNM; patients with resection for cure (R0)

Patient groups		Patients (n)	Five-year survival rates with 95% confidence interval (%)	
pT	1	164	77	(70–84)
	2	349	72	(67–77)
	3	1119	54	(51–57)
	4	201	32	(25–39)
pN	0	1016	69	(66–72)
	1	356	48	(43–53)
	2	169	33	(26–40)
	3	219	32	(25–39)
(p)M	0	1772	58	(56–60)
	1	61	18	(6–26)

For patients and methods, see legend to Fig. 1.

Table 3. Prognostic inhomogeneity of stage III colorectal carcinoma; patients with resection for cure (R0)

Patient groups	Patients (n)	Five-year survival rates with 95% confidence interval (%)	
Any pT pN1 M0	344	46	(43–55)
Any pT pN2 M0	159	34	(26–42)
Any pT pN3 M0	197	34	(27–41)

For patients and methods, see legend to Fig. 1.

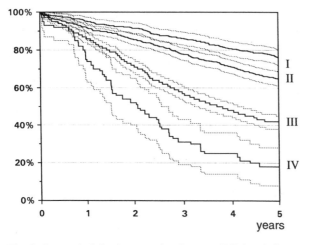

Fig. 2. Prognosis following resection for cure (R0) in relation to stage grouping. Data from the German Multicenter Study on Colorectal Carcinoma (SGCRC). Observed overall survival, calculated according to Kaplan-Meier, surgical mortality not excluded. Five-year survival rates with 95% confidence interval (%): stage I (n = 424), 76.2 (71.9–80.5); stage II (n = 646), 64.8 (60.9–68.7); stage III (n = 702), 41.5 (37.7–45.3); stage IV (n = 61), 16.4 (6.9–25.9)

Recently, histochemical methods have been used to identify isolated tumor cells in the bone marrow or in lymph nodes [39, 67, 85]. Larger studies are needed, however, to evaluate the prognostic significance of such findings. The same applies to the detection of malignant cells in peritoneal washings in patients without gross evidence of peritoneal involvement [83] and the immunohisto-chemical detection and enumeration of tumor cells in mesenteric venous blood samples [82].

Histologic Grade

Prognosis is also influenced by the histologic grade. For grading systems differentiating between low grade (G1, G2) and high grade (G3, G4), the independent prognostic value has been demonstrated by multivariate analyses [14, 17, 54, 64, 139, 140]. There are also a few multivariate analyses with negative results. These may be explained by limited numbers of patients, subjectivity of assessment, and interobserver variability. The additional prognostic information provided by morphometric analysis [4, 97] remains to be proven.

Histologic Type

The histologic type could not be demonstrated as an independent prognostic factor [54, 58, 65, 79, 93, 94]. Uncommon types such as signet ring cell, small cell, and undifferentiated carcinoma are always considered high grade and show an unfavorable prognosis. Mucinous adenocarcinomas in general present at a more advanced stage than nonmucinous adenocarcinomas, but stage-for-stage survival is not different [38].

Immunohistochemically, cells with endocrine differentiation (chromogranin A-positive cells) can sometimes be demonstrated in typical adenocarcinomas. The finding of a number of such cells (e.g., more than one per mm^2) seems to indicate poor prognosis [23, 44].

Additional Pathological Factors

Venous invasion was shown by multivariate analysis to be an independent adverse prognostic factor, at least in some substages [17, 54, 75, 93, 94]. Invasion of extramural veins especially can be considered an independent indicator of unfavorable outcome and the occurrence of hepatic metastases [47, 127].

Lymphatic invasion and perineural invasion have been shown in several multivariate studies to be independent indicators of poor prognosis [36, 54, 75, 79, 93–96]. Lymphatic invasion demonstrated in biopsies, polypectomy, or local excision specimens is – in addition to histologic grade and depth of invasion – an independent indicator of increased risk of lymph node metastases already present and thus of clinical significance in further treatment decisions [41].

The influence of tumor site on prognosis is not clear. Emergency cases (need for surgery within 48 h of admission [32]), e.g., due to obstruction, are more frequently observed in colon than rectum carcinoma and worsen prognosis. In elective surgery, rectum carcinoma seems to have a worse prognosis than colon carcinoma [13, 14]. This applies predominantly to carcinomas of the lower rectum; with decreasing distance from the anal verge both overall and disease-free survival worsen. However, with the introduction of new surgical methods and multimodal treatment the influence of tumor site has to be further studied.

Tumor obstruction and perforation occur predominantly in advanced colon carcinomas and require emergency surgery with increased surgical mortality. However, these tumor complications probably independently influence long-term outcome [17, 19, 31, 36, 58, 119].

The histologic pattern of tumor margins can be described as pushing (expansive) or infiltrating. Pushing borders seem to be an independent marker of favorable prognosis [65].

A conspicuous peritumoral lymphoid reaction at the deepest point of invasion and the presence of lymphoid aggregates in the surrounding tissues were reported as independent favorable prognostic factors [42, 47, 64]. The influence of the immunohistochemically detected phenotype of macrophages at the tumor–host interface [48] is unclear. The reports on the prognostic significance of follicular and paracortical hyperplasia of the regional lymph nodes are controversial [24, 98, 113].

Biological and Molecular Markers

With progress in laboratory methods, in recent years many new biological and molecular markers have been studied (Table 4). In most studies the number of patients was limited and mostly only univariate analyses of the prognostic influence were performed. Controversial results may, at least partly, be explained by the lack of standardization of methods. In summary, all the factors listed in Table 4 need further investigation before they can be accepted as probable or proven prognostic factors in colorectal carcinoma.

Patient-Related Factors

Reports on the prognostic influence of gender are controversial, although according to most larger studies women show better prognosis than men [17, 140].

General surveys on survival in relation to age show poorer survival for patients at the age of 40 years or younger and for patients over 70 or 80 years. In young patients a higher frequency of high-grade and advanced carcinomas is observed; within tumors of the same stage and grade, young age does not worsen prognosis [59, 72, 84, 88]. In the Swedish Cancer Registry, the prognosis for all cancers was better for patients below 40 years of age than for older patients; however, for adenocarcinomas there was no difference. This was explained by the inclusion of carcinoid tumors and their higher proportion in the younger patients [26]. With increasing age a higher surgical mortality in elective and especially in emergency surgery is observed; in addition, older age is associated with a significantly higher frequency of emergency cases. For patients surviving surgery, the observed overall survival is poorer in older patients (over 70 or 80 years); however, relative and adjusted (cancer-related) survival rates are not different for the various age-groups [6, 139].

Only in very large studies can minor differences in survival related to age be observed. The data of the SEER Program [71] show a decrease in relative survival rates with increasing age in women ($n = 11\ 809$) (but not in 11 777 men): the 5-year survival rate for all stages was 57.8% for ages less than 65 years, 55.4% for 65–74 years, and 53.9% for 75 years or more ($p < 0.01$); when stratified according to stage, there were significant differences only for localized tumors (86.5 versus 82.7 versus 81.3%, $p < 0.05$). A significant variation in stage distribution could not be observed between these three age-groups [143].

The adverse influence of low socioeconomic status on prognosis has been reported from several countries (Finland [7], France [100], the United States [124]). There are several reasons for this, e.g., diagnosis in more advanced stage, differences in treatment practice, different nutritional and immune status. Similar reasons may explain why in a study from France [80] rural patients, in particular women, had a worse prognosis than urban patients. Differences in prognosis between races as reported from the United States [2, 71, 114, 134] probably reflect differences in socioeconomic status.

Table 4. Possible biological and molecular prognostic factors in colorectal carcinoma for which the independent prognostic significance remains to be proven

Marker	Selected references
A. Differentiation markers, receptors	
Carcinoembryonic antigen (CEA)	Wiggers et al. 1988 [139]
CA 19–9 (Sialyl Le^a)	Shimono et al. 1984 [122]
Sialyl Le^x	Nakagoe et al. 1993 [101]
Sialosyl-Tn	Itzkowitz et al. 1990 [63]
Glycoproteins (glycoprotein 72, P-glycoprotein)	Guadagni et al. 1994 [40]
	Mayer et al. 1993 [90]
MUC 1-mucin	Nakamori et al. 1994 [104]
HLA (A,B,C;Dr)	Moeller et al. 1991 [99]
	Andersen et al. 1993 [5]
E-cadherin	von Aken et al. 1993 [133]
Integrins	Lindmark et al. 1993 [86]
Type IV collagen	Jeziorska et al. 1994 [68]
Gelatinase B (MMP-9)	Jeziorska et al. 1994 [68]
Laminin	Mafune et al. 1990 [89]
Tenascin	Riedl et al. 1991 [115]
Autocrine mobility factor (AMF) receptor (gp78)	Nakamori et al. 1994 [103]
Phospholipase C	Noh et al. 1994 [107]
Secretory component (SC) of immunoglobulin A (IgA)	Koretz et al. 1994 [77]
Metallothionein	Oefner et al. 1994 [109]
Urokinase-type plasminogen activator (uPA)	Vogelsang et al. 1994 [135]
Plasminogen inhibitor (PAI-1)	Vogelsang et al. 1994 [135]
EGFR (epidermal growth factor receptor)	Mayer et al. 1992 [90]
Gastrin receptor	Kameyama et al. 1993 [70]
Somatostatin receptors	Iftikhar et al. 1992 [61]
B. Ploidy and proliferation markers	
Ploidy/DNA index	Dean and Vernava 1992 [21]
	Kimura et al. 1992 [74]
	Bauer et al. 1993 [9]
	Böttger et al. 1993 [14]
S-phase fraction	Harlow et al. 1991 [46]
	Witzig et al. 1991 [141]
	Wahlström et al. 1992 [136]
PCNA (proliferating cell nuclear antigen)	Al-Sheneber et al.1993 [3]
	Mayer et al. 1993 [90]
Ki-67	Kubota et al. 1992 [78]^a
	Sahin et al. 1994 [120]
DNA polymerase alpha	Yamaguchi et al. 1992 [142]
Silver-staining nucleolar organizer regions (AgNORs)	Oefner et al. 1990 [108]
	Rüschoff et al. 1990 [118]
	Joyce et al. 1992 [69]
C. Molecular markers	
c-*myc*	Rowley et al. 1991 [116]
k-*ras*	Benhattar et al. 1993 [12]
	Bell et al. 1993 [11]
	Finkelstein et al. 1993 [33, 34]
pan *ras* 21	Sun et al. 1991 [125]
CD44	Tanabe et al. 1993 [128]
	Wielenga et al. 1993 [138]
nm23	Wang et al. 1993 [137]
	Campo et al. 1994 [16]
	Royds et al. 1994 [117]
	Tannapfel et al. 1995 [130]

Table 4 (*Contd.*)

Marker	Selected references
p53	Remvikos et al. 1992 [114]
	Sun et al. 1993 [126]
	Campo et al. 1994 [16]
	Hamelin et al. 1994 [43]
mdr	Mayer et al. 1993 [90]
Multiple molecular abnormalities	Hamilton 1992 [45]
	Laurent-Puig et al. 1992 [81]
	Iino et al. 1994 [62]
	Khine et al. 1994 [73]
D. Cytogenetics	
Cytogenetic abnormalities on short-term cultures	Bardi et al. 1993 [8]

[a] Indicator of chemosensitivity.

The different forms of clinical presentation reflect anatomic extent of carcinoma. Screen-detected asymptomatic carcinomas are in lower stages than symptomatic ones; patients presenting as an emergency are in advanced stages (see above under "Tumor-Related Factors").

Elevated serum levels of tumor markers, in particular CEA, indicate advanced tumor stage. The primary role that CEA has is for postoperative surveillance of those patients resected for cure who are at risk for recurrence. However, recent reports suggest that preoperative CEA levels may be independent prognostic factors with regard to recurrence rate and cancer-related survival [18, 139]. According to Meling et al. [92], stage II patients with preoperative CEA elevation (>5 mg/l) showed a significantly poorer prognosis than those with normal CEA levels.

The significance of other laboratory examinations such as serum levels of immunoglobulins (IgG, IgM) [132], soluble tumor necrosis factor receptors [74], or plasma prolactin [110] has still to be confirmed.

Treatment-Related Factors

It is now well documented that the surgeon influences not only short-term prognosis, i.e., surgical mortality, but also the frequency of locoregional recurrences and thus survival [30, 52, 58, 91, 111]. The wide variation in locoregional recurrence rates between and within institutions may be caused by inadequate resection of the primary tumor or the draining lymph nodes or both. Inadequate resection of a rectal primary tumor relates predominantly to incomplete excision of the mesorectum with remaining discontinuous satellites [49, 87]. Incomplete resection of the lymphatic drainage area may be the cause of a locoregional recurrence, as can be demonstrated by angiography of the remaining arterial supply [60].

Another cause of locoregional recurrence is intraoperative local tumor spillage [139, 144]. It can result from inadvertent perforation of the tumor, e.g., during the mobilization of a rectal carcinoma. It also occurs when a tumor attached to and invading an adjacent organ is not resected in an en bloc fashion [20, 35].

The "no touch" technique seems to reduce the frequency of hepatic metastasis [29], predominantly in carcinomas with venous invasion [64].

Several papers deal with the possible prognostic influence of blood products given perioperatively. The reported poorer prognosis after transfusions is probably caused by the circumstances (including surgical techniques) that necessitate them. It is not proven that in cancer surgery immunodepression after transfusions leads to a poorer survival [15, 27, 129, 131].

Multimodal treatment concepts are increasingly being used, and several clinical trials are currently open to participation. A discussion on the pros and cons and the indications is beyond the scope of this chapter.

Summary

In colorectal carcinoma patients, the anatomic extent of tumor is the strongest indicator of outcome. Prognosis following incomplete removal of the tumor is very poor; after resection for cure (no residual tumor, R0) the prognosis is determined at first by pTNM and stage grouping. Further proven prognostic factors are histologic grade, venous invasion, and the surgeon. Furthermore, other prognostic factors are probably significant and should be considered, e.g., anatomic site of the primary tumor, tumor perforation and obstruction, lymphatic and perineural invasion, histologic pattern of tumor margin, peritumoral lymphoid cells/aggregates, gender, CEA serum level, technique of tumor mobilization, and local spillage of tumor cells. A multitude of possible biological and molecular markers are under discussion; however, their prognostic significance remains to be established.

References

1. Abulafi AM, Williams NS (1994) Local recurrence of colorectal cancer: the problem, mechanisms, management and adjuvant therapy. Br J Surg 81: 7–19
2. Akerley WL, Moritz TE, Ryan LS, Henderson WG, Zacharski LR (1993) Racial comparison of outcome of male Department of Veterans Affairs patients with lung and colon cancer. Arch Intern Med 153: 1681–1688
3. Al-Sheneber IF, Shibata HR, Sampalis J, Jothy S (1993) Prognostic significance of proliferating cell antigen expression in colorectal cancer. Cancer 71: 1954–1959
4. Ambros PA, Pawel BB, Meshcheryakov I, Kotrotsios J, Lambert WC, Trost RC (1990) Nuclear morphometry as a prognostic indicator in colorectal carcinoma resected for cure. Anal Quant Cytol Histol 12: 172–176
5. Anderson SN, Rognum TO, Lund E, Meling GI, Hauge S (1993) Strong HLA-DR expression in large bowel carcinomas is associated with good prognosis. Br J Cancer 68: 80–85
6. Arnaud JP, Schloegel M, Ollier JC, Adloff M (1991) Colorectal cancer in patients over 80 years of age. Dis Colon Rectum 34: 896–898

7. Auvinen A (1992) Social class and colon cancer survival in Finland. Cancer 70: 402–409
8. Bardi G, Johansson B, Pandis N, Bak-Jensen E, Orndel C, Heim S, Mandahl N, Andren-Sandberg A, Mitelman F (1993) Cytogenetic aberrations in colorectal adenocarcinomas and their correlation with clinico-pathologic features. Cancer 71: 306–314
9. Bauer K, Bagwell C, Giaretti W, Melamed M, Zarbo R, Witzig T, Rabinovitch P (1993) Consensus review of the clinical utility of DNA flow cytometry in colorectal cancer. Cytometry 14: 486–491
10. Beahrs OH, Henson DE, Hutter RVP, Kennedy BJ (eds) (1992) American Joint Committee on Cancer (AJCC) manual for staging of cancer, 4th edn. Lippincott, Philadelphia
11. Bell SM, Scott N, Cross D, Sagar P, Lewis FA, Blair GE, Taylor GR, Dixon MF, Quirke P (1993) Prognostic value of p53 overexpression and c-Ki-ras gene mutations in colorectal cancer. Gastroenterology 104: 57–64
12. Benhattar J, Losi L, Chaubert P, Givel JC, Costa J (1993) Prognostic significance of K-ras mutations in colorectal carcinoma. Gastroenterology 104: 1044–1048
13. Bentzen SM, Balslev I, Pedersen M, Teglbjaerg PS, Hanberg-Srensen F, Bone J, Jacobsen NO, Sell A, Overgaard J, Bertelsen K (1992) Time to loco-regional recurrence after resection of Dukes'B and C colorectal cancer with or without adjuvant postoperative radiotherapy. A multivariate regression analysis. Br J Cancer 65: 102–107
14. Böttger TC, Potratz D, Stöckle M, Wellek S, Klupp J, Junginger T (1993) Prognostic value of DNA analysis in colorectal carcinoma. Cancer 72: 3579–3587
15. Busch OR, Hop WC, Hoynck van Papendrecht MA, Marquet RL, Jeekel J (1993) Blood transfusions and prognosis in colorectal cancer. New Engl J Med 328: 1372–1376
16. Campo E, Miquel R, Jares P, Bosch F, Juan M, Leone A, Vives J, Cardesa A, Yague J (1994) Prognostic significance of the loss of heterozygosity of nm23-H1 and p53 genes in human colorectal carcinomas. Cancer 73: 2913–2921
17. Chapuis PH, Dent OF, Fisher R, Newland RC, Pheils MT, Smyth E, Colquhoun KA (1985) A multivariate analysis of clinical and pathological variables in prognosis after resection of large bowel cancer. Br J Surg 72: 698–702
18. Chu D, Erickson C, Russell P, Lang N, Broadwater R, Westbrook K (1989) Elevated carcinoembryonic antigen (CEA) in colorectal carcinoma (CRC) predicts residual or recurrent disease but not survival. Proc Annu Meet Am Soc Clin Oncol 8: A474
19. Crucitti F, Sofo L, Doglietto GB, Bellantone R, Ratto C, Bossola M, Crucitti A (1991) Prognostic factors in colorectal cancer: current status and new trends. J Surg Oncol Suppl 2: 76–82
20. Curley StA, Carlson GW, Shumate CR, Wishnow KI, Ames FC (1992) Extended resection for locally advanced colorectal carcinoma. Am J Surg 163: 553–559
21. Dean PA, Vernava AM III (1992) Flow cytometric analysis of DNA content in colorectal carcinoma. Dis Colon Rectum 35: 95–102
22. Deans GT, Parks TG, Rowland BJ, Spence RAJ (1992) Prognostic factors in colorectal cancer. Br J Surg 79: 608–613
23. de Bruine AP, Wiggers T, Beek C, Volovics A, von Meyenfeldt M, Arends JW, Bosmann FT (1993) Endocrine cells in colorectal adenocarcinoma: incidence, hormone profile and prognostic relevance. Int J Cancer 54: 765–771
24. Dworak O, Altendorf-Hofmann A, Mansmann U (1993) Prognostic significance of lymph nodes in rectal carcinoma. Cancer Detect Prevent 17: 198
25. Edler L, Heim ME, Quintero C, Brummer T, Queisser W (1986) Prognostic factors of advanced colorectal cancer patients. Eur J Cancer Clin Oncol 22: 1231–1237
26. Enblad G, Enblad P, Adami H-O, Glimelius B, Krusemo U, Pahlman L (1990) Relationship between age and survival in cancer of the colon and rectum with special reference to patients less than 40 years of age. Br J Surg 77: 611–617
27. Faenza A, Cunsolo A, Selleri S, Lucarelli S, Farneti PA, Gozzetti G (1992) Correlation between plasma or blood transfusion and survival after curative surgery for colorectal cancer. Int Surg 77: 264–269
28. Fazio VW, Tjandra JJ (1991) Primary therapy of carcinoma of the large bowel. World J Surg 15: 586–575
29. Fielding LP (1988) The portal vein and colorectal cancer. Br J Surg 75: 402–403
30. Fielding LP, Stewart-Brown S, Dudley HA (1978) Surgeon-related variables and the clinical trial. Lancet ii: 778–779
31. Fielding LP, Phillips RKS, Fry JS, Hittinger R (1986) Prediction of outcome after curative resection for large bowel cancer. Lancet ii: 904–906

32. Fielding LP, Arsenault PA, Chapuis PH, Dent O, Gatright B, Hardcastle JD, Hermanek P, Jass JR, Newland RC (1991) Clinico-pathological staging for colorectal cancer: an International Documentation System (IDS) and an International Comprehensive Anatomical Terminology (ICAT). J Gastroenterol Hepatol 6: 325–344

33. Finkelstein SD, Sayegh R, Bakker A, Swalsky P (1993) Determination of tumor aggressiveness in colorectal cancer by K-ras-2 analysis. Arch Surg 128: 526–532

34. Finkelstein SD, Sayegh R, Christensen S, Swalsky PA (1993) Genotypic classification of colorectal adenocarcinomas. Biologic behaviour correlates with K-ras-2 mutation type. Cancer 71: 3827–3838

35. Gall FP, Tonak J, Altendorf A (1987) Multivisceral resections in colorectal cancer. Dis Colon Rectum 30: 337–341

36. Garcia-Peche P, Vazquez-Prado A, Fabra-Ramis R, Trullenque-Peris R (1991) Factors of prognostic value in long-term survival of colorectal cancer patients. Hepatogastroenterology 38: 438–443

37. Graf W, Glimelius B, Pahlman I, Bergstrom R (1991) Determinants of prognosis in advanced colorectal cancer. Eur J Cancer 27: 1119–1123

38. Green JB, Timmcke AE, Mitchell WT, Hicks TC, Gatright JB Jr, Ray JE (1993) Mucinous carcinoma: just another colon cancer? Dis Colon Rect 36: 49–54

39. Greenson JK, Isenhardt CE, Rice R, Mojzisik C, Houchens D, Martin EW Jr (1994) Identification of occult micrometastases in pericolic lymph nodes of Dukes' B colorectal cancer patients using monoclonal antibodies against cytokeratin and CC49. Cancer 73: 563–569

40. Guadagni F, Roselli M, Cosimelli M, Spila A, Cavaliere F, Arcuri R, Abbolito MR, Greiner JW, Schlom J (1994) Biologic evaluation of tumor-associated glycoprotein-72 and carcino-embryonic antigen expression in colorectal cancer, part I. Dis Colon Rectum 37 [Suppl]: S16-S23

41. Guggenmoos-Holzmann I, Hermanek P (1994) Einflußfaktoren für lymphgene Metastasierung bei frühen Formen des Rektumkarzinoms. In: Hermanek P, Marzoli GP (eds) Lokale Therapie des Rektumkarzinoms. Verfahren in kurativer Intention. Springer, Berlin Heidelberg New York

42. Halvorsen TB, Seim E (1989) Association between invasiveness, inflammatory reaction, desmoplasia and survival in colorectal cancer. J Clin Pathol 42: 162–166

43. Hamelin R, Laurent-Puig P, Olschwang S, Jego N. Asselaim B, Remvikos Y, Girodet J, Salmon RJ, Thomas G (1994) Association of p53 mutations with short survival in colorectal cancer. Gastroenterology 106: 42–48

44. Hamada Y, Oishi A, Shoji T, Tahada H, Yamamura M, Hioki K, Yamamoto M (1992) Endocrine cells and prognosis in patients with colorectal carcinoma. Cancer 69: 2641–2646

45. Hamilton SR (1992) Molecular genetic alterations as potential prognostic indicators in colorectal carcinoma. Cancer 69: 1589–1591

46. Harlow S, Eriksen B, Poggensee L, Chmiel J, Scarpelli D, Murad T, Bauer K (1991) Prognostic implications of proliferative activity and DNA aneuploidy in Astler-Coller-Dukes stage C colonic adenocarcinomas. Cancer Res 51: 2403–2409

47. Harrison JC, Dean PJ, El-Zeky F, Vander Zwaag R (1994) From Dukes through Jass: pathological prognostic indicators in rectal cancer. Hum Pathol 25: 498–505

48. Hauptmann S, Zwadlo-Kharwasser G, Hartung P, Klosterhalfen B, Kirkpatrick CJ, Mittermayer C (1994) Association of different macrophage phenotypes with infiltrating and non-infiltrating areas of tumor-host interface in colorectal carcinoma. Pathol Res Pract 190: 159–167

49. Heald RJ, Ryall RDH, Husband E (1982) The mesorectum in rectal cancer surgery: clue to pelvic recurrence. Br J Surg 69: 613–616

50. Henson DE, Gloeckler Ries LA (1994) On the estimation of survival. Semin Surg Oncol 10: 2–6

51. Hermanek P (1991) Data collection aspects for the design of adjuvant treatment protocols in colorectal carcinoma. Onkologie 14: 491–497

52. Hermanek P (1993) Long-term results of a German prospective multicenter study on colorectal cancer. In: Takahashi T (ed) Recent advances in management of digestive cancers. Springer, Berlin Heidelberg New York

53. Hermanek P, Altendorf A (1981) Classification of colorectal carcinoma with regional lymphatic metastases. Pathol Res Pract 173: 1–11

54. Hermanek P, Guggenmoos-Holzmann I, Gall FP (1989) Prognostic factors in rectal carcinoma. A contribution to the further development of tumor classification. Dis Colon Rectum 32: 593–599

55. Hermanek P, Sobin LH (eds) (1992) UICC TNM classification of malignant tumours, 4th edn 2nd rev. Springer, Berlin Heidelberg New York
56. Hermanek P, Henson DE, Hutter RVP, Sobin LH (eds) (1993) UICC TNM supplement 1993. A commentary on uniform use. Springer, Berlin Heidelberg New York
57. Hermanek P, Wittekind C (1994) Residual tumour (R) classification and prognosis. Semin Surg Oncol 10: 12–20
58. Hermanek P Jr, Wiebelt H, Riedl S, Staimmer D, Hermanek P und die Studiengruppe Kolorektales Karzinom (SGKRK) (1994) Langzeitergebnisse der chirurgischen Therapie des Coloncarcinoms. Ergebnisse der Studiengruppe Kolorektales Karzinom (SGKRK). Chirurg 65: 287–297
59. Heys SD, O'Hanrahan TJ, Brittenden J, Eremin O (1994) Colorectal cancer in young patients; a review of the literature. Eur J Surg Oncol 20: 225–231
60. Hohenberger P, Schlag P, Kretzschmar U, Herfarth C (1994) Regional mesenteric recurrence of colorectal cancer after anterior resection or left hemicolectomy: inadequate primary resection demonstrated by angiography of the remaining arterial supply. Int J Colorect Dis 6: 17–23
61. Iftikhar SY, Thomas WM, Rooney PS, Morris DL (1992) Somatostatin receptors in human colorectal cancer. Eur J Surg Oncol 18: 27–30
62. Iino H, Fukayama M, Maeda Y, Koike M, Mori T, Takahashi T, Kikuchi-Yanoshita R, Miyaki M, Mizuno S, Watanabe S (1994) Molecular genetics for clinical management of colorectal carcinoma. Cancer 73: 1324–1331
63. Itzkowitz SH, Bloom EJ, Kokal WA, Modin G, Hakomori S, Kim YS (1990) Sialosyl-Tn: a novel mucin antigen associated with prognosis in colorectal cancer patients. Cancer 66: 1960–1966
64. Jass JR, Atkin WS, Cuzick J, Bussey HJR, Morson BC, Northover JMA, Todd IP (1986) The grading of rectal cancer: historical perspectives and a multivariate analysis of 447 cases. Histopathology 10: 437–459
65. Jass JR, Love SB, Northover JMA (1987) A new prognostic classification of rectal cancer. Lancet i: 1303–1305
66. Jeekel J (1987) Can radical surgery improve survival in colorectal cancer? World J Surg 11: 412–417
67. Jeffers MD, O'Dowd GM, Mulcahy H, Stagg M, O'Donoghue DP, Toner M (1994) The prognostic significance of immunohistochemically detected lymph node micrometastases in colorectal carcinoma. J Pathol 172: 183–187
68. Jeziorska M, Haboubi NY, Schofield PF, Ogata Y, Nagase H, Wooley DE (1994) Distribution of gelatinase B (MMP-9) and type IV collagen in colorectal carcinoma. Int J Colorect Dis 9: 141–148
69. Joyce WP, Fynes M, Moran KT, Gough DB, Dervan P, Gorey TF, Fitzpatrick YM (1990) The prognostic value of nucleolar organiser regions in colorectal cancer: a 5-year follow-up study. Ann R Coll Surg Engl 74: 172–176
70. Kameyama M, Nakamori S, Imaoka S, Iwanaga T (1993) Relationship between gastrin receptor values in colorectal cancer tissue and clinical stage. In: Takahashi T (ed) Recent advances in management of digestive cancers. Springer, Berlin Heidelberg New York
71. Kant AK, Glover C, Horm J, Schatzkin A, Harris TB (1992) Does cancer survival differ for older patients? Cancer 70: 2734–2740
72. Kearney TJ, Price EA, Lee S, Silberman AW (1993) Tumor aneuploidy in young patients with colorectal cancer. Cancer 72: 42–45
73. Khine K, Smith DR, Goh H-S (1994) High frequency of allelic deletion in chromosome 17p in advanced colorectal cancer. Cancer 73: 28–35
74. Kimura K, Abe Y, Horiuchi A, Kimura S (1993) Elevated serum levels of soluble tumor necrosis factor receptors in patients with colorectal carcinoma. In: Takahashi T (ed) Recent advances in management of digestive cancers. Springer, Berlin Heidelberg New York
75. Knudsen JB, Nilsson T, Sprechler M, Johansen A, Christensen N (1983) Venous and nerve invasion as prognostic factors in postoperative survival of patients with resectable cancer of the rectum. Dis Colon Rectum 26: 613–617
76. Kouri M, Pyrhonen S, Kuusela P (1992) Elevated CA19-9 as the most significant prognostic factor in advanced colorectal carcinoma. J Surg Oncol 49: 78–85
77. Koretz K, Schlag P, Lehnert T, Quentmeier A, Möller P (1994) Evaluation of the secretory component (SC) as a prognostic variable in colorectal carcinoma. Eur J Surg Oncol 20: 294
78. Kubota Y, Petras RE, Easley KA, Bauer TW, Tubbs RR, Fazio VW (1992) Ki-67-determined growth fraction versus standard staging and grading parameters in colorectal carcinoma. Cancer 70: 2602–2609

79. Lasser P, Mankarios H, Elias D, Bognel C, Eschwege F, Wibault P, Kac J, Crespon B, Rougier P (1993) Etude pronostique uni- et multifactorielle de 400 adénocarcinomas rectaux réséqués. J Chir 130: 57–65

80. Launoy G, Le Coutour X, Gignoux M, Pottier D, Dugleux G (1992) Influence of rural environment on diagnosis, treatment, and prognosis of colorectal cancer. J Epidemiol Community Health 46: 365–367

81. Laurent-Puig P, Olschwang S, Delattre O, Remvikos Y, Asselain B, Melot T, Validire P, Muleris M, Girodet J, Salmon RJ, Thomas G (1992) Survival and acquired genetic alterations in colorectal cancer. Gastroenterology 102: 1136–1141

82. Leather AJM, Gallegos NC, Kocjan G, Savage F, Smales CS, Hu W, Boulos PB, Northover JMA, Phillips RKS (1993) Detection and enumeration of circulating tumour cells in colorectal cancer. Br J Surg 80: 777–780

83. Leather AJM, Kocjan G, Savage F, Hu W, Yiu C-Y, Boulos PB, Northover JMA, Phillips RKS (1994) Detection of free malignant cells in the peritoneal cavity before and after resection of colorectal cancer. Dis Colon Rectum 37: 8114–819

84. Li Destri G, Greco L, Craxi G, Rinzivillo C, Cordio S, Di Cataldo A, Puleo S (1994) Kolorektale Karzinome bei jungen Menschen: Eine schlechtere Prognose? Ist das wahr? Coloproctology 16: 56–61

85. Lindemann F, Schlimok G, Dirschedl P, Witte J, Riethmüller G (1992) Prognostic significance of micrometastatic tumour cells in bone marrow of colorectal cancer patients. Lancet 340: 685–689

86. Lindmark G, Gerdin B, Pahlman L, Glimelius B, Gehlsen K, Rubin K (1993) Interconnection of integrins α2 and α3 and structure of the basal membrane in colorectal cancer: relation to survival. Eur J Surg Oncol 19: 50–60

87. MacFarlane JK, Ryall RDH, Heald RJ (1993) Mesorectal excision for rectal cancer. Lancet 341: 457–460

88. Marble K, Banerjee S, Greenwald I (1992) Colorectal carcinoma in young patients. J Surg Oncol 51: 179–182

89. Mafune K, Ravikumar TS, Wong JM, Yow H, Chan LB, Steele GD (1990) Expression of a Mr 32,000 laminin-binding messenger RNA in human colon carcinoma correlates with disease progression. Cancer Res 50: 3888–3891

90. Mayer A, Takimoto M, Fritz E, Schellander G, Kofler K, Ludwig H (1993) The prognostic significance of proliferating cell nuclear antigen, epidermal growth factor receptor, and mdr gene expression in colorectal cancer. Cancer 71: 2454–2460

91. McArdle CS, Hole D (1991) Impact of variability among surgeons on postoperative morbidity and mortality and ultimate survival. Br Med J 302: 1501–1503

92. Meling GI, Rognum TO, Clausen OP, Brmer O, Lunde OC, Schlichting E, Havig O (1992) Serum carcinoembryonic antigen in relation to survival, DNA ploidy pattern, and recurrent disease in 406 colorectal carcinoma patients. Scand J Gastroenterol 27: 1061–1068

93. Michelassi F, Block GE, Vannucci L, Montag A, Chappell R (1988) A 5- to 21-year follow-up and analysis of 250 patients with rectal adenocarcinoma. Ann Surg 208: 379–387

94. Michelassi F, Ewing C, Montag A, Vannucci L, Segalin A, Panozzo M, Bibbo M, Dytch H, Chieco-Bianchi P (1992) Prognostic significance of ploidy determination in rectal cancer. Hepatogastroenterology 39: 222–225

95. Miholic J, End A, Loimer L, Möschl P, Wieselthaler G, Wolner E (1991) Multivariate Analyse von Risikofaktoren für Lokalrezidivierung beim Rektumkarzinom. Acta Chir Austriaca 23 [Suppl]: 129

96. Minsky BD, Mies C, Rich TA, Recht A (1989) Lymphatic vessel invasion is an independent prognostic factor for survival in colorectal cancer. Int J Rad Oncol Biol Phys 17: 311–318

97. Mitmaker B, Begin CR, Gordon PH (1991) Nuclear shape as a prognostic discriminant in colorectal carcinoma. Dis Colon Rectum 34: 249–259

98. Miura S, Tsuchiya H, Shikata J-i, Hosoda S, Shiina E (1989) Immunohistochemical analysis of mesocolic lymph node cells in human colorectal cancer. J Surg Oncol 40: 119–127

99. Möller P, Momburg F, Koretz K, Moldenhauer G, Herfarth C, Otto HF, Hämmerling GJ, Schlag P (1991) Influence of major histocompatibility complex class I and II antigens on survival in colorectal carcinoma. Cancer Res 51: 729–736

100. Monnet E, Boutron MC, Faivre J, Milan C (1993) Influence of socioeconomic status on prognosis of colorectal cancer. Cancer 72: 1165–1170

101. Nakagoe T, Fukushima K, Hirota M, Kusano H, Ayabe H, Tomita M, Kamihira S (1993) Immunohistochemical expression of sialyl Le antigen in relation to survival of patients with colorectal carcinoma. Cancer 72: 2323–2330

102. Nakahara H, Ishikawa T, Itabashi M, Hirota T (1992) Diffusely infiltrating primary colorectal carcinoma of linitis plastica and lymphangiosis types. Cancer 69: 901–906

103. Nakomori S, Watanabe H, Kameyama M, Imaoka S, Furukawa H, Ishikawa O, Sasaki Y, Kabuto T, Raz A (1994) Expression of autocrine motility factor receptor in colorectal cancer as a predictor for disease recurrence. Cancer 74: 1855–1862

104. Nakomori S, Ota DM, Cleary KR, Shirotani K, Irimura T (1994) MUC1 mucin expression as a marker of progression and metastasis of human colorectal carcinoma. Gastroenterology 106: 353–361

105. Newland RC, Dent OF, Chapuis PH, Bokey EC (1993) Clinicopathologically diagnosed residual tumor after resection for colorectal cancer. Cancer 72: 1536–1542

106. Newland RC, Dent OF, Lyttle MNB, Chapuis PH, Bokey EL (1994) Pathologic determinants of survival associated with colorectal cancer with lymph node metastases. Cancer 73: 2076–2082

107. Noh D-Y, Lee YH, Kim SS, Kim YI, Ryn S-H, Suh P-G, Park J-G (1994) Elevated content of phospholipase C-Gamma-1 in colorectal cancer tissues. Cancer 73: 36–41

108. Öfner D, Tötsch M, Sandbichler P, Hallbrucker C, Margreiter R, Mikuz G, Schmid KW (1990) Silver stained nucleolar organizer region proteins (AgNORs) as a predictor in prognosis in colonic cancer. J Pathol 162: 43–49

109. Oefner D, Naier H, Riedmann B, Bammer T, Rumer A, Winde G, Böcker W, Jasani B, Schmid KW (1995) Immunohistochemical metallothionein expression in colorectal adenocarcinoma. Correlation with tumor stage and patients survival. Virchows Arch A (in press)

110. Patel DD, Bhatavdekar JM, Ghosh N, Vora HH, Karelia NH, Shah NG, Suthar TP, Balar DB, Trivedi CR (1994) Plasma prolactin in patients with colorectal cancer. Value in follow-up and as a prognosticator. Cancer 73: 570–574

111. Phillips RKS, Hittinger R, Blesovsky L, Fry JS, Fielding LP (1984) Local recurrence following curative surgery for large bowel cancer; the overall picture. Br J Surg 71: 12–16

112. Phillips RKS, Hittinger R, Blesovsky L, Fry JS, Fielding LP (1984) Large bowel cancer. Survival, pathology and its relationship to survival. Br J Surg 71: 604–610

113. Pihl E, Nairn RC, Milne BJ, Cuthbertson AM, Hughes ESR, Rollo A (1980) Lymphoid hyperplasia. A major prognostic feature in 519 cases of colorectal carcinoma. Am J Pathol 100: 469–480

114. Remvikos Y, Tominaga O, Hammel P, Laurent-Puig P, Salmon RJ, Dutrillaux B, Thomas G (1992) Increased p53 protein content of colorectal tumours correlates with poor survival. Br J Cancer 66: 758–764

115. Riedl S, Möller P, Faissner A, Koretz K, Schlag P (1991) Tenascin – ein neuer immunhistologischer Marker für Tumorinvasion und Lymphknotenmetasierung beim colorectalen Carcinom. Langenbecks Arch Chir Suppl Chirurg Forum 1991, pp 161–164

116. Rowley S, Carpenter R, Newbold KM, Gearty J, Keighley MR, Donovan IA, Neoptolemos JP (1991) Use of the OM-11–906 monoclonal antibody for determining p62 c-myc expression by flow cytometry in relation to prognosis in colorectal cancer. Eur J Surg Oncol 17: 370–378

117. Royds JA, Alcock H, Sisley K, Silcocks PB, Cross SS, Rees RC, Scholefield JH, Shorthouse AJ, Stephenson TJ (1994) Nm 23 "antimetastatic" gene in colorectal cancer. Eur J Surg Oncol 20: 508

118. Rüschoff J, Bittinger A, Neumann K, Schmitz-Moormann P (1990) Prognostic significance of nucleolar organizing regions (NORs) in carcinomas of the sigmoid colon and rectum. Pathol Res Pract 186: 85–91

119. Runkel NS, Schlag P, Schwarz V, Herfarth C (1991) Outcome after emergency surgery for cancer of the large intestine. Br J Surg 78: 183–188

120. Sahin AA, Ro JY, Brown RW, Ordonez NG, Cleary KR, El-Naggar AK, Wilson P, Ayala AG (1994) Assessment of Ki-67-derived tumor proliferation activity in colorectal adenocarcinomas. Modern Pathol 7: 17–22

121. Shida H, Ban K, Matsumoto M, Masuda K, Imanari T, Machida T, Yamamoto T (1992) Prognostic significance of location of lymph node metastases in colorectal cancer. Dis Colon Rectum 35: 1046–1056

122. Shimono R, Mori M, Akazawa K, Adachi Y, Sugimachi K (1994) Immunohistochemical expression of carbohydrate antigen 19–9 in colorectal carcinomas. Am J Gastroenterol 89: 1010–1015

123. Shirouzu K, Isomoto H, Morodomi T, Ogato Y, Akagi Y, Kakegawa T (1994) Primary linitis plastica carcinoma of the colon and rectum. Cancer 74: 1863–1868

124. Steele GD Jr (1994) The National Cancer Data Base report on colorectal cancer. Cancer 74: 1979–1989
125. Sun XF, Hatschek T, Wingren S, Stal O, Carstensen JM, Zhang H, Boeryd B, Sjodahl R, Nordenskjold B (1991) Ras p21 expression in relation to histopathological variables and prognosis in colorectal adenocarcininoma. Acta Oncol 30: 933–939
126. Sun XF, Carstensen JM, Zhang H, Stal O, Wingren S, Hatschek T, Nordenskjold B (1992) Prognostic significance of cytoplasmic p53 oncoprotein in colorectal adenocarcinoma. Lancet 340: 1369–1373
127. Talbot IC, Ritchie S, Leighton M, Hughes A, Bussey H, Morson BC (1981) Invasion of veins by carcinoma of rectum: method of detection, histological features and significance. Histopathology 5: 141–163
128. Tanabe KK, Ellis LM, Saya H (1993) Expression of CD44R1 adhesion molecule in colon carcinomas and metastases. Lancet 341: 725–726
129. Tang R, Wang JY, Chang Chien Cr, Chen JS, Lin SE, Fan HA (1993) The association between perioperative blood transfusion and survival of patients with colorectal cancer. Cancer 72: 341–348
130. Tannapfel A, Köckerling F, Katalinic A, Wittekind C (1995) The expression of nm23-H1 predicts lymph node involvement in colorectal carcinoma. Dis Colon Rectum (in press)
131. Tartter PI (1992) The association of perioperative blood transfusion with colorectal cancer recurrence. Ann Surg 216: 633–638
132. Tsavaris N, Tsigalakis D, Bobota A, Tsoutsos E, Sarafidou M, Papazachariou M, Komitsopoulou P, Kosmidis P (1992) Prognostic value of serum levels of immunoglobulins (IgA, IgM, IgG, IgE) in patients with colorectal cancer. Eur J Surg Oncol 18: 31–36
133. Van Aken J, Cuvelier CA, De Wever N, Roels J, Gao Y, Mareel MM (1993) Immunohisto-chemical analysis of E-cadherin expression in human colorectal tumours. Pathol Res Pract 189: 975–978
134. Villar HV, Menck HR (1994) The National Cancer Data Base report on cancer in Hispanics. Cancer 74: 2386–2395
135. Vogelsang H, Nekarda H, Angermeier C, Huber F, Roder J, Fink U, Siewert JR (1994) Prognostic impact of uPA and PAI-1 on survival of patients with resected colorectal cancer. International Gastro-Surgical Club 1994. 5th Joint Meeting of Surgeons and Gastroenterologists, Munich, April 27–30, 1994 (abstract 10)
136. Wahlström B, Branchög I, Stierner U, Sunzel H, Holmberg E (1992) Association of ploidy and cell proliferation, Dukes' classification and histopathological differentiation in adenocarcinomas of colon and rectum. Eur J Surg 158: 237–243
137. Wang I, Patel U, Ghosh L, Chen HC, Banerjee S (1993) Mutation in the nm 23 gene is associated with metastasis in colorectal cancer. Cancer Res 53: 717–720
138. Wielenga VJ, Heider KH, Offerhaus GJ, Adolf GR, van der Berg FM, Ponta H, Herrlich P, Pals ST (1993) Expression of C44 variant proteins in human colorectal cancer is related to tumor progression. Cancer Res 53: 4754–4756
139. Wiggers T, Arends JW, Volovics A (1988) Regression analysis of prognostic factors in colorectal cancer after curative resections. Dis Colon Rectum 34: 33–41
140. Wiggers T, Arends JW, Schutte B, Volovics L, Bosman FT (1988) A multivariate analysis of pathologic prognostic indicators in large bowel cancer. Cancer 61: 386–395
141. Witzig T, Loprinzi C, Gonchoroff N, Reiman H, Cha S, Weiand H, Katzman J, Paulsen J, Moertel C (1991) DNA ploidy and cell kinetic measurements as predictors of recurrence and survival in stage B2 and C colorectal adenocarcinomas. Cancer 68: 879–888
142. Yamaguchi A, Hirono Y, Fushida S, Kurosaka J, Kanno M, Yonemura Y, Miyazaki I (1992) DNA polymerase alpha positive-cell rate in colorectal cancer and its relationship to prognosis. Br J Cancer 65: 421–424
143. Yancik R, Ries LA (1994) Cancer in older-persons, Magnitude of the problem – how do we apply what we know? Cancer 74: 1995–2003
144. Zirngibl H, Husemann B, Hermanek P (1990) Intra-operative spillage of tumor cells for rectal cancer. Dis Colon Rectum 33: 610–614

8 Anal Canal Carcinoma

B.J. Cummings

The principal prognostic factors for carcinomas which arise in the anal canal are similar to those of most other epithelial malignancies. The prognosis for survival deteriorates as the primary tumour enlarges and worsens as cancer metastasises to the regional lymph nodes and to extrapelvic sites. The relative rarity of anal canal carcinoma (incidence about 0.5–1 per 100 000) has meant that prognostic factors have, for the most part, been evaluated by univariate analysis in small groups of patients. Conflicting results have been common. More recently, larger series have been assembled and assessed by multivariate analysis or similar statistical techniques.

Major changes in treatment and classification over the past decade make intercomparison of studies more difficult.

(a) In treatment, there has been a shift from radical resection to primary radiation therapy, delivered alone or in combination with cytotoxic chemotherapy [4]. As a result, detailed gross and histopathological assessment of excised pelvic tissues, which formed the cornerstone of many earlier analyses, is no longer possible. It has not yet been established that all features of prognostic value in patients treated surgically are equally predictive of outcome following radiation with/without chemotherapy.

(b) The 1987 edition of the TNM Classification System introduced major changes in the staging of the primary tumour [21]. T category is now determined by the largest diameter of the primary carcinoma measured in centimetres. Formerly, it was necessary to estimate clinically the proportion of the length or circumference of the canal involved and whether the external sphincter was infiltrated [19].

(c) In 1987, it was recommended that the anal canal be defined as that part of the intestine which extends from the rectum to the perianal skin (to the junction with the hair-bearing skin) [21]. Prior to this, no definition of the canal was included in the UICC (International Union Against Cancer) manual, and many centres classified any cancer lying wholly or mostly below the pectinate (dentate) line as a carcinoma of the anal margin rather than of the canal.

The histological classification of malignancies of the anal canal did not change substantially between the 1976 [25] and 1989 [22] descriptions of the WHO Classification System. The 1989 edition identifies three major subtypes of squamous cell carcinoma, namely large cell keratinizing, large cell non-keratinizing (transitional) and basaloid. Many investigators, conceding that the prognostic value of histological subtyping is marginal, group all three subtypes as squamous cell or epidermoid carcinomas.

Patient-Related Factors

The unexplained female preponderance in the incidence of anal canal carcinoma is not generally considered a prognostic factor. Occasional multivariate analyses do suggest that women have a better prognosis than men [11, 14], but this is not a general finding [1]. The converse has not been reported.

Age at diagnosis has not been reported to be of independent prognostic significance [1, 5, 14]. However, since most analyses are of patients treated radically, those unfit for radical treatment by virtue of advanced age or poor performance status are often excluded.

The duration of symptoms is not generally thought to be significant, although in one series it was found that those treated within a month of onset of symptoms fared better [38]. Small cancers found incidentally at surgery for benign anal conditions also have a good prognosis [18].

Pre-existing or coincidental benign conditions affecting the anal canal or perianal skin do not appear to have any prognostic significance [17].

Although epidemiological studies indicate that a history of venereal disease, anoreceptive intercourse in males and current cigarette smoking are each associated with a higher risk of development of anal carcinoma [6], these factors are not known to be important prognostically. An association has been demonstrated between anal squamous cell carcinomas and human papilloma virus (HPV) types 16 and 18, and herpes simplex virus (HSV) [30, 35]. The finding of HPV type 16 DNA in anal tissues or tumours is associated with an increased risk of multicentric anogenital carcinoma, particularly in women. In analyses of serum, the immunoglobulin A (IgA) response to peptide E2:9 (derived from HPV type 16 E2 region) had a marginally significant association with poorer prognosis which was independent of tumour size [20]. No correlation was found with antibody responses to several other antigens derived from papilloma virus [20].

The risk of carcinoma of the anal canal is increased in immunosuppressed patients such as renal transplant recipients [32] and probably also in those with the acquired immunodeficiency syndrome (AIDS) [29]. The prognosis in such patients is unpredictable, reflecting factors related to both anal carcinoma and immunosuppression.

Tumour-Related Factors

Anatomic Extent of Disease

The size of the primary tumour and the depth to which the tumour penetrates into and through the anal wall are strongly prognostic for both survival and local tumour control [1, 2]. There is no agreement on the break-points for division by size. In series not subject to detailed examination of excised tissues, the prognostic value of the T category is a surrogate for a combination of tumour size, depth of invasion and likelihood of metastases to the pelvic lymph nodes. The risk of nodal metastases correlates reasonably well with the histological subtype, grade and size of the primary tumour [1].

In patients treated by radiation therapy and studied by multivariate analysis, the size of the primary tumour was generally predictive for both survival and local control [5, 14, 34]. Three-year local control rates of 89% for tumours up to 4 cm in size and 73% for larger tumours were reported for one large series treated by radiation alone [31]. In patients treated by radiation with 5-fluorouracil and mitomycin C, local control rates for primary tumours up to 2 cm in size were in the range of 95%–100%, for 2–5 cm 80%–95%, and for larger than 5 cm 65%–80% [5, 42]. Five-year survival rates, corrected for deaths from intercurrent disease, were typically about 95%–100% when the primary tumour was less than 2 cm in size, and in the range of 60%–70% for larger tumours, reflecting the relatively good surgical salvage rates for local relapse after treatment with radiation-based protocols [5,42]. In one large series of patients treated surgically and analyzed by multivariate analysis, it was found that, after adjustment for stage (determined by depth of invasion, presence of pelvic node metastases or of distant metastases, and resectability), tumour size was no longer a significant prognostic factor [1]. Some investigators consider that the depth of invasion is of greater prognostic significance than regional lymph node metastases [7]. However, most authors have concluded that when nodal metastases are present, the depth of invasion is of lesser prognostic significance [1, 11].

The current, and previous, UICC criteria for determining the T category create some confusion by not relying solely on the measured size of the primary tumour, tumour size being superseded by the presence or absence of invasion of adjacent organs to establish the T4 category [19, 21]. There is considerable disagreement, particularly in reports of patients treated by radiation with/without chemotherapy, as to whether invasion of adjacent organs such as the vagina or prostate is truly of major negative prognostic import for survival or for local control and preservation of anal function [3, 5, 8, 14, 31, 33, 39]. There is similar disagreement whether the extent of circumferential involvement of the anal canal reduces the likelihood of preservation of function [31, 33].

The negative prognostic influence of regional lymph node metastases on survival that has been established from series managed by surgery is not as clear since the emphasis changed to non-surgical treatment. In surgical series, histopathologically confirmed involvement of metastases in the perirectal, superior hemorrhoidal, pelvic or inguinal node groups was associated with 5-year survival rates of about 50%, some 25% worse than those of patients who did not have nodal metastases [12, 17, 37, 38]. The prognosis was somewhat better when inguinal node metastases were diagnosed several months after primary treatment, provided they were the only site of recurrence [12, 17].

While many series treated by radiation with/without chemotherapy have not found a statistically significant adverse prognosis for those with inguinal node metastases, the trend in survival rates for those patients was generally worse [5, 33, 34]. The widespread practice of including clinically normal inguinal nodes electively in the volume irradiated has greatly reduced the risk of late failure in those nodes, but the effect of such elective irradiation on survival rates has not been determined [4]. The presence of inguinal or pelvic lymph node metastases has not correlated with control of the primary tumour in patients managed with radiation [5, 31].

Extrapelvic metastases, to either lymph nodes or parenchymal organs, are associated with a very poor prognosis, median survival being in the range of 6–12 months [17, 42]. Solitary metastases are uncommon, but have occasionally been amenable to potentially curative treatment [40].

Results for composite TNM stage groups have been reported infrequently [15], it being much more common to classify patients by the separate tumour characteristics outlined above.

Pathological Features

Histological Type

The histological subtype of squamous cell carcinoma has generally not been found to carry independent prognostic significance for survival or local tumour control. Although the histological classification often appeared related to survival in univariate analysis, multivariate models for the most part showed that, when corrected for stage, this significance was lost. This was true whether stage was determined by the size of the primary tumour only in patients treated by radiation [5, 14, 34] or by surgico-histopathological systems which assessed tumour depth and the presence of node metastases [1, 14, 37]. A few rare variants, such as small cell carcinomas and microcystic squamous cell carcinomas, have a very poor prognosis and are characterised by early dissemination [1, 37].

Histological Grade

When independent significance for histopathological grade is found, poorly differentiated tumours carry a worse prognosis than moderately or well-differentiated cancers [1, 11, 13, 15, 17]. In a series of 235 patients, the 5-year survival rate was 95% for those patients with well-differentiated tumours, compared to 60% for those with moderately or poorly differentiated tumours [37]. Others have found that histological grade lost the prognostic significance apparent on univariate analysis when adjustment was made for stage [1].

Cytometric and Cytogenetic Analysis

In one large study of flow cytometric DNA analysis of paraffin-embedded tissue from anal carcinomas managed surgically, ploidy was found by multivariate analysis to be strongly predictive of outcome, patients with diploid tumours having a 5-year survival rate of 75% compared to 55% for non-diploid tumours [37]. A similar, but not statistically significant, trend was found in a smaller group of surgically treated patients [36]. However, in another retrospective study of patients managed by radiation and/or surgery, in which DNA was assessed by image cytophotometry, no correlation was found between ploidy and prognosis [13]. The prognostic significance of the recurrent deletions of chromosomes 11q and 3p in tumour cells from a small series of anal canal carcinomas is not known [26].

Associated Intraepithelial Neoplasia

The finding of dysplasia or intraepithelial neoplasia in the anal canal (ACIN) in addition to invasive carcinoma is of unknown prognostic significance when the patient is treated by radical surgery or by radiation with/without chemotherapy. Since ACIN is often multicentric and frequently exhibits foci of microinvasion [9], the presence of ACIN may account for the relatively high frequency of recurrence after apparently complete local excision of small carcinomas. It has been suggested that the demonstration by immunohistochemical techniques of the accumulation of mutant p53 protein [28] and/or overexpression of C-*myc* [27] may serve as a marker of likely disease progression from ACIN grade III to invasive carcinoma.

Biological and Molecular Factors

The marker of greatest interest currently is serum squamous cell carcinoma antigen (SCCAg), although it has not been studied widely and results have been conflicting. In one multivariate analysis, elevated SCCAg was the most significant determinator of risk for overall and tumour-specific death rates as well as for residual and recurrent carcinoma [16]. Elevated pretreatment SCCAg superseded tumour stage, size and histopathological grade as a prognostic factor. These findings were contrary to those in a smaller series, in which no prognostic value was identified for pretreatment SCCAg levels [10]. Serum carcinoembryonic antigen (CEA) or tumour CEA levels did not correlate with prognosis in patients managed by radiation combined with 5-fluorouracil and mitomycin C [41].

Treatment-Related Factors

There have been no major differences apparent in the 5-year survival rates in patients managed by surgery or by radiation with/without chemotherapy, the rates ranging from about 35%–80% with an average of about 55% [4]. The likelihood of retaining anorectal function was much greater after radiation-based treatment, when it was about 75% [4]. Some multivariate analyses have indicated that prognosis is better following higher doses of radiation [14, 34]. The overall time in which radiation was delivered by uninterrupted or split course was not significant [5, 34]. The presence of residual carcinoma in the canal at the completion of radical radiation was not predictive of eventual local control [34]. Carcinoma residual after radiation and chemotherapy was associated with poor outcome after attempted salvage surgery in some [23] but not all series [5, 24]. The extent of clinical response to chemotherapy and/or radiation in recurrent and metastatic carcinoma correlated with the duration of subsequent survival [40].

Summary

The most deleterious prognostic factor for survival is the presence of extrapelvic metastases. For carcinoma confined to the pelvis, the size of the primary tumour provides the most useful indicator for survival and local control and preservation of anorectal function. After tumour size and T category, the status of the regional lymph nodes correlates fairly well with survival, but not with control of the primary carcinoma. Poor histological grade is the most discriminatory histopathological prognostic feature, histological subtype being generally of little significance. Other tumour-related features such as DNA ploidy, serum and tissue markers and genetic markers are of potential value but have not yet been studied widely. Most patient-related factors such as gender, age at diagnosis and a history of co-morbid or associated conditions appear to be of little prognostic value, provided the patient is able to tolerate radical treatment of a cancer confined to the pelvis.

References

1. * Boman BM, Moertel CG, O'Connell MJ, Scott M, Weiland LH, Beart RW, Gunderson LL, Spencer RJ (1984) Carcinoma of the anal canal. A clinical and pathological study of 188 cases. Cancer 54: 114–125
2. Cummings BJ (1982) The place of radiation therapy in the treatment of carcinoma of the anal canal. Cancer Treat Rev 9: 124–147
3. Cummings BJ (1991) Preservation of anorectal function in advanced epidermoid anal cancer. Dis Colon Rectum 34: P4 (abstract)
4. Cummings BJ (1992) Epidermoid cancer of the anal canal. In: Horwich A (ed) Combined radiotherapy and chemotherapy in clinical oncology. Arnold, London, pp 127–137

Studies analyzed by multivariate analysis are marked*

5. * Cummings BJ, Keane TJ, O'Sullivan B, Wong CS, Catton CN (1991) Epidermoid anal cancer: treatment by radiation alone or by radiation and 5-fluorouracil with and without mitomycin C. Int J Radiat Oncol Biol Phys 21: 1115–1125
6. Daling JR, Weiss NS, Hislop TG, Maden C, Coates RJ, Sherman KJ, Ashley RL, Beagrie M, Ryan JA, Corey L (1987) Sexual practices, sexually transmitted diseases, and the incidence of anal cancer. N Engl J Med 317: 973–977
7. Dougherty BG, Evans HL (1985) Carcinoma of the anal canal: a study of 79 cases. Am J Clin Pathol 83: 159–164
8. Eschwege F, Lasser P, Chavy A, Wibault P, Kac J, Rougier P, Bognel C (1985) Squamous cell carcinoma of the anal canal: treatment by external beam irradiation. Radiother Oncol 3: 145–150
9. Fenger C, Nielsen VT (1986) Intraepithelial neoplasia in the anal canal. The appearance and relation to genital neoplasia. Acta Pathol Microbiol Immunol Section [A] 94: 343–349
10. Fontana X, Lagrange JL, Francois E, Bowry J, Chauvel P, Sordage M, Lapalus F, Namer M (1991) Assessment of squamous cell carcinoma antigen (SCC) as a marker of epidermoid carcinoma of the anal canal. Dis Colon Rectum 34: 126–131
11. Frost DB, Richards PX, Montague ED, Giacco GG, Martin RG (1984) Epidermoid cancer of the anorectum. Cancer 53: 1285–1293
12. Golden GT, Horsley JS (1976) Surgical management of epidermoid carcinoma of the anus. Am J Surg 131: 275–280
13. Goldman S, Auer G, Erhardt K, Seligson U (1987) Prognostic significance of clinical stage, histologic grade, and nuclear DNA content in squamous cell carcinoma of the anus. Dis Colon Rectum 30: 444–448
14. * Goldman S, Glimelius B, Glas U, Lundell G, Pahlman L, Stahle E (1989) Management of anal epidermoid carcinoma – an evaluation of treatment results in two population-based series. Int J Colorectal Dis 4: 234–243
15. * Goldman S, Glimelius B, Pahlman L, Stahle E, Wilander E (1988) Anal epidermoid carcinoma: a population-based clinico-pathological study of 164 patients. Int J Colorectal Dis 3: 109–118
16. * Goldman S, Svensson C, Bronnergard M, Glimelius B, Wallin G (1993) Prognostic significance of serum concentration of squamous cell carcinoma antigen in anal epidermoid carcinoma. Int J Colorectal Dis 8: 98–102
17. Greenall MJ, Quan SH, Decosse JJ (1985) Epidermoid cancer of the anus. Br J Surg 72 [Suppl]: S97-S103
18. Grodsky L (1967) Unsuspected anal cancer discovered after minor anorectal surgery. Dis Colon Rectum 10: 471–478
19. Harmer MH (ed) (1978) UICC TNM classification of malignant tumours, 3rd edn. International Union Against Cancer, Geneva
20. Heino P, Goldman S, Lagerstedt U, Dillber J (1993) Molecular and serological studies of human papillomavirus among patients with anal epidermoid carcinoma. Int J Cancer 53: 377–381
21. Hermanek P, Sobin LH (eds) (1987) UICC TNM classification of malignant tumours, 4th edn. Springer, Berlin Heidelberg New York
22. Jass JR, Sobin LH (1989) Histological typing of intestinal tumours, 2nd edn. Springer, Berlin Heidelberg New York, pp 41–44
23. Leichman L, Nigro N, Vaitkevicius VK, Considine B, Buroker T, Bradley G, Seydel HG, Olchowski S, Cummings G, Leichman C, Baker L (1985) Cancer of the anal canal. Model for preoperative adjuvant combined modality therapy. Am J Med 78: 211–215
24. * Miller EJ, Quan SH, Thalar HT (1991) Treatment of squamous cell carcinoma of the anal canal. Cancer 67: 2038–2041
25. Morson BC, Sobin LH (1976) Histological typing of intestinal tumors. World Health Organization, Geneva, pp 62–65
26. Muleris M, Salmon RJ, Girodet J, Zafrani B, Dutrillaux B (1987) Recurrent deletions of chromosomes 11q and 3p in anal canal carcinoma. Int J Cancer 39: 595–598
27. Ogunbiyi OA, Scholefield JH, Rogers K, Sharp F, Smith JHF, Polacarz SV (1993) C-myc oncogene expression in anal squamous neoplasia. J Clin Pathol 46: 23–27
28. Ogunbiyi OA, Scholefield JH, Smith JHF, Polacarz SV, Rogers K, Sharp F (1993) Immunohistochemical analysis of p53 expression in anal squamous neoplasia. J Clin Pathol 46: 507–512

Studies analyzed by multivariate analysis are marked*

29. * Palefsky JM, Gonzales J, Greenblatt RM, Ahn DK, Hollander H (1990) Anal intraepithelial neoplasia and anal papillomavirus infection among homosexual males with Group IV HIV disease. JAMA 263: 2911–2916
30. Palefsky JM, Holly EA, Gonzales J, Berline J, Ahn DK, Greenspan JS (1991) Detection of human papillomavirus DNA in anal intraepithelial neoplasia and anal cancer. Cancer Res 51: 1014–1019
31. Papillon J, Montbarbon JF (1987) Epidermoid carcinoma of the anal canal. A series of 276 cases. Dis Colon Rectum 30: 324–333
32. Penn I (1986) Cancer of the anogenital region in renal transplant recipients. Analysis of 65 cases. Cancer 58: 611–616
33. Salmon RJ, Fenton J, Asselain B, Mathieu G, Girodet J, Durand JC, Decroix YC, Pilleron JP, Rousseau J (1984) Treatment of epidermoid anal canal cancer. Am J Surg 147: 43–48
34. * Schlienger M, Touboul E, Mauban S, Ozsahin M, Pene F, Krzisch C, Marsiglia H, Laugier A, Parc R, Tiret E, Malajosse M, Gallot D, Sezeur A, Loygue J (1991) Resultats du traitement de 286 cas de cancers epidermoides du canal anal dont 236 par irradiation a visée conservatrice. Lyon Chir 87: 61–69
35. Scholefield JH, McIntyre P, Palmer JG, Coates PJ, Shepherd NA, Northover JMA (1990) DNA hybridization of routinely processed tissue for detecting HPV DNA in anal squamous cell carcinomas over 40 years. J Clin Pathol 43: 133–136
36. * Scott NA, Beart RW, Weiland LH, Cha SS, Lieber MM (1989) Carcinoma of the anal canal and flow cytometric DNA analysis. Br J Cancer 60: 56–58
37. * Shepherd NA, Scholefield JH, Love SB, England J, Northover JMA (1990) Prognostic factors in anal squamous carcinoma: a multivariate analysis of clinical, pathological and flow cytometric parameters in 235 cases. Histopathology 16: 545–555
38. Stearns MW, Urmacher C, Sternberg SS, Woodruff J, Attiyeh F (1980) Cancer of the anal canal. Curr Prob Cancer 4: 1–44
39. Svensson C, Goldman S, Friberg B (1993) Radiation treatment of epidermoid cancer of the anus. Int J Radiat Oncol Biol Phys 27: 67–73
40. Tanum G (1993) Treatment of relapsing anal carcinoma. Acta Oncol 32: 33–35
41. Tanum G, Stenwig AE, Bormer OP, Tveit KM (1992) Carcinoembryonic antigen in anal carcinoma. Acta Oncol 31: 333–335
42. Tanum G, Tveit K, Karlsen KO, Hauer-Jensen M (1991) Chemotherapy and radiation therapy for anal carcinoma. Survival and late morbidity. Cancer 67: 2462–2466

Studies analyzed by multivariate analysis are marked*

9 Hepatocellular Carcinoma

C. Wittekind

Introduction

Long-term survival and cure of patients with hepatocellular carcinoma (HCC) can be expected only after resection or hepatectomy followed by transplantation. Thus, prognosis primarily depends on the possibility of resective surgery, which is determined predominantly by the anatomic extent of disease but also by the general condition of the patient.

Since surgery has developed in this field, along with the introduction of early detection efforts, prognosis has significantly improved, particularly in Japan, as a number of studies have shown [1, 4, 6, 12, 13, 27, 28, 33, 34, 37, 39]. Most of these studies focused on the prognosis of HCC in relation to surgical and medical treatment [3, 10, 11, 22]. The prognosis of untreated patients is extremely poor. A recent Italian study evaluating 130 unselected patients showed an overall mean survival time of 23 weeks [8]. After 1 year, 11.5% of patients were alive. In a multivariate analysis only two variables (presenting symptoms and serum bilirubin levels) were independent prognostic factors [8].

The reported resectability rate of liver carcinomas varied from 7% to 36% [18, 22, 24, 32, 34]. Despite the success of surgery, the question of whether surgical resection improves survival in HCC patients was recently raised by a study by Cottone et al [9]. In this study only 37 asymptomatic patients (all Child A class) were included. Twelve of these 37 patients underwent resection, while 25 were not resected. In a later report, the same study group was able to show that survival became markedly better after 3 years for operated patients [10]. Bruix et al. [3], who doubted the observation made by Cottone et al. [9], also reported that surgical resection effectively improves prognosis in Western patients with HCC, particularly for patients with HCC less than 5 cm.

Since the resectability rate of HCC is lower than for colorectal cancer, many authors have described parameters with prognostic significance in patients with non-resectable HCC, although the prognosis for these patients is poor. Median survival time in untreated patients ranges from 2 to 12.4 months [3, 27]. On the other hand, there are only a few studies dealing with factors influencing prognosis after resection [23, 30, 34]. Because of the dismal prognosis of untreated HCC, it is inevitable that there is a multitude of different approaches to management under investigation. The different treatment modalities will not be covered in this review, especially because controlled prospective studies are not available.

The first part of this review deals with factors that become relevant after resection or transplantation and that have prognostic significance in univariate or multivariate analyses. The second part consists of an overview of factors that have prognostic relevance in patients at the time of first diagnosis who will not be resected or transplanted.

Prognostic Factors in Surgically Treated Patients: Resection or Transplantation

Multivariate analyses of prognosis after operation of HCC were performed by Iwatsuki et al. [24], Lai et al. [25], Nagorney et al. [30] and Ringe et al. [34]. In these studies it could be shown unequivocally that resection for cure [25, 30, 34] and anatomic extent of the tumours were the most important prognostic factors. The R (residual tumour) classification was not mentioned in the study by Iwatsuki et al. [24]; however, patients with "positive surgical margins" had a statistically shorter mean survival time in univariate analysis.

Prognostic factors other than TNM and R can be grouped into clinical findings and pathological features. As to clinical findings, performance status was an important prognostic parameter in a multivariate analysis by Nagorney et al. [30]. Prothrombin time and hypercalcaemia were evaluated only in the study by Nagorney et al. [30] and were found to be prognostically important. The effect of other factors on prognosis has been controversial (Table 1).

As might be expected, studies on pathological factors yielded different results. Histological grade had an influence in Nagorney's patients [30] but not in those of Ringe et al. [34] and was not evaluated in the study by Iwatsuki et al. [24]. The majority of factors were only investigated in univariate analyses (Table 1).

Prognostic Factors in Patients Not Treated by Resective Surgery

The prognostic importance of anatomic extent (as expressed by the TNM classification [16, 17] or related parameters) is emphasized in many studies. It is noteworthy that TNM classification itself is not used regularly by all authors. Certain parameters such as tumour size [1, 5, 21, 31] or presence of metastases are used as descriptors of tumour extension [1, 5, 7]. Variables other than anatomic extent found at diagnosis to be of value in predicting prognosis are shown in Table 2. In this second part, papers that deal with larger numbers of cases and that use multivariate analysis will be covered more extensively.

Calvet et al. [5] investigated prognostic factors in 206 patients with confirmed HCC, taking into account clinical and laboratory variables. The median survival time in the entire series of patients was 3.3 months. Twenty-three per cent of the patients lived longer than 1 year. In addition to factors included in the TNM

Table 1. Prognostic factors in surgically treated patients

Factor	Multivariate analysis		Univariate analysis	
	Significant	Not significant	Significant	Not significant
Anatomic extent				
TNM	24, 34		38,43	
R classification	25, 30, 34		40	
Other pathological features				
Co-existing cirrhosis	30[a]		38	15, 18
Histological type	30[a]		30, 40, 42[b]	
Grade	30	34	15,35	19, 20, 38
Capsule formation	25		14, 20, 29	
Satellites			14, 19, 35	
Dysplasia			19	
Inflammatory reaction			19	
Necrosis			35	
Bile production			35	
Mitotic activity			15, 35	
Clinical findings (pretherapeutic)				
Patient-related factors				
Age			40, 41, 43	15, 18
Sex		34	30	18, 26, 29, 35
Performance status	30			
Symptoms			22, 26	
Hepatitis B status		30, 34		
Tumour-related factors				
Tumour site		34		26
Hepatomegaly			35	
Preoperative AFP level	34		25, 29, 38	18
Prothrombin time	30			
Hypercalcaemia	30			

AFP, alpha-fetoprotein.
[a] Resection only.
[b] For tumours larger than 5 cm.

classification (tumour size and presence of metastases), ascites, toxic syndrome (defined by the presence of weight loss of more than 10% pre-morbid weight, malaise and anorexia) and laboratory variables such as bilirubin, blood urea nitrogen, gamma-glutamyltranspeptidase and serum sodium were independent predictors of survival [5].

In a study by Chlebowski et al. [7], multivariate analysis indicated that increased bilirubin or presence of pulmonary metastases adversely influenced outcome. Furthermore, North American patients younger than 45 years of age had a significantly ($p < 0.01$) longer survival (median, 40 versus 9 weeks) than older patients with the disease, although clinical and laboratory features were not different. Sutton et al. [36] found in a multivariate analysis that only cirrhosis was a risk factor for death.

Table 2. Prognostic factors (other than TNM) in patients not treated with resective surgery

Factor	Multivariate analysis		Univariate analysis (Significant)
	Significant	Not significant	
Patient-related factors			
Age	5, 7		11
Sex			11, 36
Performance status			11, 20
Cirrhosis	36		
Tumour-related factors			
Jaundice			5, 11, 21
Ascites	1, 5	2, 7	
Portal vein thrombosis			5
Toxic syndrome	5		
Encephalopathy	2		
Laboratory variables			
Bilirubin	2, 5, 7		1
Blood urea nitrogen	2, 5		
GGT	5		
Serum sodium	5		
Alkaline phosphatase			5
Alpha-fetoprotein			5, 31, 36
Serum creatinine			5
Haemoglobin level			5
Platelet count			5
Prothrombin time			5
Serum albumin			6

GGT, gamma-glutamyltranspeptidase.

In most of the studies the possible relevance of encephalopathy was not discussed, whereas Attali et al. [2] found that encephalopathy was the best variable for predicting 60-day survival of HCC patients. This fact may be explained by the very poor prognosis of the 127 patients in their study, encephalopathy possibly being less important in patients with better median survival times.

In a multivariate study by Akashi et al. [1], four variables had prognostic influence, namely gross appearance of HCC, encapsulation (assessed by US, abdominal computed tomography, CT, and celiac angiography), clinical stage (according to the scheme of the Liver Cancer Group of Japan) and treatment by transcatheter arterial embolization (TAE). These observations have not yet been confirmed by other institutions.

References

1. Akashi Y, Koreeda C, Enomoto S, Uchiyama S, Mizuno T, Shiozaki Y, Sameshima Y, Inoue K (1991) Prognosis of unresectable hepatocellular carcinoma: an evaluation based on multivariate analysis of 90 cases. Hepatology 14: 262–268

2. Attali P, Prod'Homme S, Pelletier G, Papoz L, Ink O, Buffet C, Etienne JP (1987) Prognostic factors in patients with hepatocellular carcinoma. Attempts for the selection of patients with prolonged survival. Cancer 59: 2108–2111

3. Bruix J, Cirera I, Calvet X, Fuster J, Bru C, Ayuso C, Vilana R, Boix L, Visa J, Rodés J (1992) Surgical resection and survival in western patients with hepatocellular carcinoma. J Hepatol 15: 350–355

4. Callea F (1988) Natural history of hepatocellular carcinoma as viewed by the pathologist. Appl Pathol 6: 105–116

5. Calvet X, Bruix J, Gines P, Bru C, Sole M, Vilana R, Rodes J (1990) Prognostic factors of hepatocellular carcinoma in the West: a multivariate analysis in 206 patients. Hepatology 12: 753–60

6. Chen DS, Sung JL, Sheu JC, Lai MY, How SW, Hsu HC, Lee CS, Wei TC (1984) Serum alpha-fetoprotein in the early stage of human hepatocellular carcinoma. Gastroenterology 86: 1404–1409

7. Chlebowski RT, Tong M, Weismann J, Block JB, Ramming KP, Weiner JM, Bateman JR, Chlebowski JS (1984) Hepatocellular carcinoma: diagnostic and prognostic features in North American patients. Cancer 53: 2701–2706

8. Colloredo Mels G, Leandro G, Scorpiniti A, Christini P, Angeli G (1993) Natural history of hepatocellular carcinoma in northern Italy. Multivaried analysis of prognostic factors. J Exp Cancer Res 12: 101–106

9. Cottone M, Virdona R, Fusco G, Orlando A, Turri M, Caltagirone M, Maringhini A, Sciarrino E, Demma I, Nicoli N, Tine F, Sammarco S, Pagliaroo L (1989) Asymptomatic hepatocellular carcinoma in Child's A cirrhosis. A comparison of natural history and surgical treatment. Gastroenterol 96: 1566–1571

10. Cottone M, Virdone R, Orlando A, Turri M, Caltagirone M (1990) Letter to the editor, reply. Gastroenterology 98: 1992–1996

11. Falkson G, Cnaan A, Schutt AJ, Ryan LM, Falkson HC (1988) Prognostic factors for survival in hepatocellular carcinoma. Cancer Res 48: 7314–7318

12. Fortner JG, Kim DK, Maclean BJ, Barrett MK, Iwatsuki S, Turnbull AD, Howland WS, Beattie EJ Jr (1978) Major hepatic resection for neoplasia. Personal experience in 108 patients. Ann Surg 188: 363–371

13. Fortner JG, Maclean BJ, Kim DK, Howland WS, Turnbull AD, Goldiner P, Carlon G, Beattie EJ Jr (1981) The seventies evolution in liver surgery for cancer. Cancer 47: 2161–2166

14. Franco D, Capusotti L, Smadja C, Bouzari H, Meakins J, Kemeny F, Grange D, Dellepiane M (1990) Resection of hepatocellular carcinomas. Results in 72 European patients with cirrhosis. Gastroenterology 98: 733–738

15. Haratake J, Takeda S, Kasai T, Nakano S, Tokui N (1993) Predictable factors for estimating prognosis of patients after resection of hepatocellular carcinoma. Cancer 72: 1178–1183

16. Hermanek P, Sobin LH (eds) (1987) UICC TNM classification of malignant tumours, 4th edn. Springer, Berlin Heidelberg New York

17. Hermanek P, Sobin LH (eds) (1992) UICC TNM classification of malignant tumours, 4th edn, 2nd rev. Springer, Berlin Heidelberg New York

18. Heuschen UA, Hofmann WJ, Otto HF, Schlag P, Herfarth C (1990) Clinico-pathological features and surgical management of primary epithelial hepatic malignancies. Eur J Surg Oncol 16 332–345

19. Hsu HC, Sheu JC, Lin YH, Chen DS, Lee CS, Hwang LY, Beasley RP (1985) Prognostic histologic parameters in resected small cell hepatocellular carcinoma (HCC) in Taiwan. A comparison with resected large HCC. Cancer 56: 672–680

20. Hsu HC, Wu TT, Wu MZ, Shen JC, Lee CS, Chen DS (1988) Tumor invasiveness and prognosis in resected hepatocellular carcinoma. Clinical and pathogenetic implications. Cancer 61: 2095–2099

21. Ihde DC, Matthews MJ, Makuch RW, McIntire KR, Eddy JL, Seeff LB (1985) Prognostic factors in patients with hepatocellular carcinoma receiving systemic chemotherapy. Identification of two groups of patients with prospects for prolonged survival. Am J Med 78: 399–406

22. Iwatsuki S, Shaw BW, Starzl TE (1983) Experience with 150 liver resections. Ann Surg 197: 247–253

23. Iwatsuki S, Gordon RD, Shaw BW, Starzl TE (1985) Role of liver transplantation in cancer therapy. Ann Surg 202: 401–407

24. Iwatsuki S, Starzl TE, Sheahan DG, Yokoyama I, Demetris AJ, Todo S, Tzakis AG, van Thiel DH, Carr B, Selby R, Madariaga J (1991) Hepatic resection versus transplantation for hepatocellular carcinoma. Ann Surg 214: 221–229

25. Lai EC-S, Ng IO-L, Lok AS-F, Tam P-C, Fan S-T, Choi T-K, Wong J (1990) Long-term results of resection for large hepatocellular carcinoma: a multivariate analysis of clinicopathological features. Hepatology 11: 815–818

26. Lee CS, Sung JL, Hwang LY, Cheu JC, Chen DS, Lin TY, Beasley RP (1986) Surgical treatment of 109 patients with symptomatic and asymptomatic hepatocellular carcinoma. Surgery 99: 481–490

27. Lin TY, Lee CS, Chen KM, Chen CC (1987) Role of surgery in the treatment of primary carcinoma of the liver: a 31-year experience. Br J Surg 74: 839–842

28. McDermott WV, Cady B, Georgi B, Steele G, Khettry U (1989) Primary cancer of the liver: evaluation, treatment and prognosis. Arch Surg 124: 552–555

29. Nagao T, Inoue S, Goto S, Mizuta T, Omori Y, Kawano N, Morioko Y (1987) Hepatic resection for hepatocellular carcinoma. Clinical features and long-term prognosis. Ann Surg 205: 33–40

30. Nagorney DM, van Heerden JA, Ilstrup DM, Adson MA (1989) Primary hepatic malignancy: surgical management and determinants of survival. Surgery 106: 740–749

31. Nomura F, Onishi K, Tanabe Y (1989) Clinical features and prognosis of hepatocellular carcinoma with reference to serum alpha-fetoprotein levels: analysis of 606 patients. Cancer 64: 1700–1707

32. O'Grady JG, Polson RJ, Rolles K, Calne RY, Williams R (1988) Liver transplantation for malignant disease: results in 93 consecutive patients. Ann Surg 207: 373–379

33. Okuda K, Ohtsuki T, Obata H, Tomimatsu M, Okazaki N, Hasegawa H, Nakajima Y, Onishi K (1985) Natural history of hepatocellular carcinoma and prognosis in relation to treatment: Study of 850 patients. Cancer 56: 918–928

34. Ringe B, Pichlmayr R, Wittekind C, Tusch G (1991) Surgical treatment of hepatocellular carcinoma: experience with liver resection and transplantation in 198 patients. World J Surg 15: 270–285

35. Smalley SR, Moertel CG, Hilton JF, Weiland LH, Weiand HS, Adson MA, Melton LJ, Batts K (1988) Hepatoma in the noncirrhotic liver. Cancer 62: 1414–1424

36. Sutton FM, Russell NC, Guinee VF, Alpert E (1988) Factors affecting the prognosis of primary liver carcinoma. J Clin Oncol 6: 321–328

37. Takayasu K, Muramatsu Y, Moriyama N, Hasegawa H, Makuuchi M, Okazaki N, Hirohashi S, Tsugane S (1989) Clinical and radiological assessments of the results of hepatectomy for small hepatocellular carcinoma and therapeutic arterial embolization for postoperative recurrence. Cancer 64: 1848–1852

38. Tang ZY, Yu YQ, Zhou XD, Ma ZC, Yang R, Lu JZ, Lin ZY, Yang BH (1989) Surgery of small hepatocellular carcinoma. Cancer 64: 536–541

39. Tsuzuki T, Sugioka A, Ueda M, Iida S, Kanai T, Yoshii H, Nakayasu K (1990) Hepatic resection for hepatocellular carcinoma. Surgery 107: 511–520

40. Wood WJ, Rawlings M, Evans H, Lim CNH (1988) Hepatocellular carcinoma: importance of histologic classification as a prognostic factor. Am J Surg 155: 663–666

41. Yamanaka N, Okamoto E, Toyosaka A, Mitunobu M, Fujihara S, Kato T, Fujimoto J, Oriyama T, Furukawa K, Kawamura E (1990) Prognostic factors after hepatectomy for hepatocellular carcinomas. A univariate and multivariate analysis. Cancer 65: 1104–1110

42. Yokoyama I, Todo S, Iwatsuki S, Starzl TE (1990) Liver transplantation in the treatment of primary liver cancer. Hepatogastroenterology 37: 188–193

43. Zhao G, Su S, Borek D, Friesen S, Holmes F (1990) Long survival and prognostic factors in hepatocellular carcinoma. J Surg Oncol 45: 257–60

10 Carcinoma of the Gallbladder

M.T. Carriaga and D.E. Henson

Introduction

Carcinoma of the gallbladder is an uncommon but highly lethal disease that often causes death in less than 1 year after diagnosis [2, 11]. In a collected series of more than 1700 patients, the 5-year survival rate after surgical resection was 2.6% [9]. At the Beth Israel Medical Center in New York, the 5-year survival rate was 11.3% [18]. In an analysis of 2354 cases from the Surveillance, Epidemiology, and End Results (SEER) Program of the National Cancer Institute, the overall 5-year survival rate was 12.1% [7]. Because carcinomas of the gallbladder are relatively rare and known to have a poor outcome, investigators have not systematically evaluated new prognostic factors. In this report, we describe the prognostic factors for carcinomas of the gallbladder based on our analysis of published data. There has been no multivariate analysis reported on combinations of the different prognostic factors.

Patient-Related Factors

Age

Age has no effect on survival. Carcinoma of the gallbladder predominantly affects the older population: in the SEER Program, the median age was 73 years and the average age was 72 years. Approximately 75% of patients were older than 65 years. In these older age groups, there are many competing causes of death.

Race

The SEER data for the years 1983–1987 showed a higher 5-year survival rate for whites (15.7%) than for blacks (7.6%), all stages combined [7]. This difference in survival was not associated with a shift in the stage distribution at diagnosis; racial differences were present within each stage. For example, the 5-year survival rate for localized-stage adenocarcinoma was 43% for whites and 21% for blacks. Since these differences may reflect variations in patient care, however, race should not be used as an independent prognostic factor in assessing outcome.

Clinical and Laboratory Findings

Early stage gallbladder carcinoma is often asymptomatic. In the SEER Program, fewer than 25% of cases were diagnosed, while the disease was still confined to the gallbladder [7]. Signs and symptoms, such as weight loss, anemia, jaundice, or right upper quadrant pain, usually indicate regional spread of the tumor to the liver or to the extrahepatic bile ducts. Jaundice is often a sign of unresectable liver involvement or bile duct obstruction. Laboratory abnormalities include hyperbilirubinemia, bilirubinuria, and increased levels of serum alkaline phosphatase and lactic dehydrogenase. Although these clinical findings are considered poor prognostic signs, they have not been integrated into a prognostic system, since they are found in nearly all patients. Seeding of the abdominal cavity can occur, and ascites secondary to intra-abdominal tumor spread also indicates a very poor prognosis. As with other cancer sites, assessment of performance status can also be used as a prognostic factor. Although tumor cells produce carcinoembryonic antigen (CEA), serum levels of CEA cannot be used to estimate tumor bulk, since they also increase with bile duct obstruction due to other causes [3, 21]. Elevated serum CA 19–9 levels have been demonstrated in patients with gallbladder carcinoma, but are also nonspecific.

Tumor-Related Factors

Anatomic Extent of Disease

The stage of disease is an important prognostic factor in gallbladder carcinoma. As expected, in situ carcinomas are associated with excellent patient outcome. The 5-year relative survival rate for patients with in situ carcinoma is 90%. Most in situ carcinomas are discovered fortuitously in specimens removed for cholelithiasis [1, 5, 20].

In the SEER Program, the stage of disease is reported as "localized", "regional", or "distant." Localized cancers, i.e., those confined to the gallbladder, have the most favorable prognosis. In SEER, the 5-year survival rate for localized invasive carcinomas was 42%. Localized cancers can be further subdivided by the depth of invasion into the wall of the gallbladder as assessed histologically. However, the size of the primary tumor does not appear to be a useful prognostic factor. For patients with regional disease, i.e., extension to the liver or regional lymph nodes, the 5-year survival rate was less than 5%. The 5-year rate was virtually zero for cases with distant metastases at diagnosis. Table 1 shows survival by stage of disease and histologic type.

Histologic Type

An important prognostic variable is the histologic type. Papillary carcinomas have the most favorable prognosis with a 5-year survival rate of 40.5% compared to less than 10% for other histologic types, all stages combined [7]. Unfortunately, papillary carcinomas are not common, comprising only 5.5% of all carcinomas of the gallbladder. Patients with undifferentiated, large cell, anaplastic, or pleomorphic carcinomas have a very poor prognosis. Small cell carcinomas are also associated with poor patient outcome: the 2-year survival rate is 0.0%. In summary, published data show a relationship between the histologic type and survival, although the differences at 5 years are only significant for papillary carcinomas. Tables 1 and 2 show the relative survival rates for the most common histologic types of gallbladder carcinoma recorded in the SEER Program [7].

Table 1. Five-year relative survival rates (%) by histologic type and stage of disease (1978–1986)

| | Stage | | | | | |
	Localized[a]	Regional[b]	Distant[c]	Unstaged	All[d]	Total (n)
All types	41.9	3.8	0.7	4.3	12.1	2354
Carcinoma (all)	42.1	3.9	0.7	4.6	12.3	2330
Adenocarcinoma	42.3	4.0	0.8	6.9	13.0	2138
Adenocarcinoma (NOS)	37.5	4.6	0.7	7.6	11.3	1774
Papillary	63.4[f]	–	–	–	40.5[f]	119
Mucinous	–	0.0	0.0	–	7.8	117
Other	44.9[f]	2.3	0.0	–	13.0	128
Squamous cell carcinoma	–	–	–	–	8.8	42
Carcinoma (NOS)[e]	–	0.0	0.0	–	2.0	138

From [7]. Where no value is given, there were fewer than 25 cases.
NOS, not otherwise specified.
[a] Confined to the gallbladder.
[b] Extension to the liver or regional lymph nodes.
[c] Distant metastases.
[d] All cases, staged and unstaged, combined.
[e] Includes undifferentiated, anaplastic, pleomorphic, etc.
[f] $0.05 < S.E. \leq 0.10$.

Table 2. Two-year relative survival rates and median survival times for the most common histologic types of gallbladder carcinoma recorded in the SEER program (1977–1986)

	Total (n)	Two-year survival rate (%)	Median survival (months)
Adenocarcinoma	1970	14	4
Carcinoma (NOS)	200	6	2
Papillary adenocarcinoma	151	47	20
Mucinous	125	12	4
Adenosquamous	95	8	3
Squamous cell carcinoma	45	9	4
Oat cell	13	0	2

From [11].
NOS, not otherwise specified; SEER, Surveillance, Epidemiology, and End Results.

Histologic Grade

As in other cancers, the histologic grade is associated with outcome (Table 3). There is an inverse correlation between increasing grade and survival rates [11]. The difference between grades 3 and 4 is not significant. Other investigators have also observed a relationship between grade and outcome in gallbladder carcinoma [10, 16, 24]. According to Yamaguchi and Enjoji, for example, the cumulative survival rate was 33.3% for poorly differentiated carcinomas at 1 year compared to 79.5% for well-differentiated carcinomas [24].

Vascular Invasion

The presence of vascular or lymphatic invasion is a significant prognostic factor, since it reduces survival time. For localized stage disease, the 5-year survival rate for patients with vascular invasion was 13%, compared with 31% for patients without known vessel invasion. The median survival time for patients with vascular invasion was 10 months; without vascular invasion, the median survival was 18 months [11].

Other Tumor-Related Factors

There is little information on the loss of suppressor genes, oncogene amplification, chromosome changes, or biochemical markers as potential prognostic factors for cancers of the gallbladder. Amplification of c-*erb*B-2 gene and increased production of c-*erb*B-2 protein was not found to be associated with outcome [23].

Evidence indicates that tumor acid mucopolysaccharide content may prove to be a useful prognostic factor. High mucopolysaccharide content has been associated with a better prognosis [15].

Table 3. Relation between histologic grade and survival for adenocarcinoma of the gallbladder

Grade	Total (*n*)	Median Survival (months)	Two-year relative survival rate (%)
1	265	7	30
2	443	6	14
3	594	4	8
4	38	3	7

From [11].

Treatment-Related Factors

Despite new surgical and chemotherapeutic approaches to treatment [4, 8, 17, 20], the 5-year survival rate for invasive carcinomas increased only slightly from 8% to 14% during the 15-year period covered in the SEER Program. The role of radiation therapy has been studied in small series; some investigators reported longer median survival times in patients receiving adjuvant postoperative radiotherapy compared to patients undergoing surgery alone [6, 13]. Further improvements in survival will most likely depend upon the earlier detection of in situ or localized stage tumors in patients at risk for gallbladder cancer.

Discussion

With current information, stage of disease, histologic type (papillary or nonpapillary), and histologic grade are the most reliable prognostic factors for carcinomas of the gallbladder. Vascular invasion can serve as an additional prognostic marker, but the presence or absence of vascular invasion is not reported in the vast majority of cases. Based on our estimation, vascular invasion reduces survival to the next lower stage of disease [11]. Numerous authors have commented on the correlation that exists between survival and the anatomic extent of disease at time of diagnosis: patients with regional or distant stage disease show much shorter survival times than patients in whom the disease is confined to the gallbladder. For practical purposes, the TNM stage is probably the most powerful predictor of outcome.

Of all the histologic types, papillary carcinomas have the most favorable prognosis [11, 12, 19, 22]. Papillary carcinomas are associated with localized disease more than any other histologic type. In the SEER Program, 64% of patients with papillary carcinoma had localized disease at diagnosis. This association is not surprising, since papillary carcinomas are usually exophytic in growth. Unfortunately, papillary carcinomas are found in fewer than 10% of patients.

Patients with carcinomas that exhibit metaplasia may have a better outcome than patients with carcinomas that do not demonstrate metaplastic changes [25], but this finding requires confirmation. Reports also suggest that predominant neuroendocrine differentiation is associated with a reduced survival time [14]. Although investigators are beginning to report genetic mutations in gallbladder cancer, there are no reports correlating these changes with survival.

This review has been based on the analysis of individual prognostic factors; no multivariate analyses have been reported. In practice, this may not be important, since short survival can be safely predicted if the tumor has invaded the liver or abdominal cavity. In summary, the major prognostic factors for carcinomas of the gallbladder include the extent of disease as defined by the TNM staging system, histologic type, and histologic grade.

References

1. Albores-Saavedra J, Angeles-Angeles A, Manrique JJ, Henson DE (1984) Carcinoma in situ of the gallbladder: a clinico-pathologic study of 18 cases. Am J Surg Pathol 8: 323–333
2. Albores-Saavedra J, Henson DE (1986) Tumors of the gallbladder and extrahepatic bile ducts. Armed Forces Institute of Pathology, Washington DC
3. Albores-Saavedra J, Nadji M, Morales AR, Henson DE (1983) Carcinoembryonic antigen in normal, preneoplastic, and neoplastic gallbladder epithelium. Cancer 52: 1069–1072
4. Andrews W, Smith F (1987) Chemotherapy for cholangiocarcinoma and gallbladder cancer. In: Wanebo HJ (ed) Hepatic and biliary cancer. Dekker, New York, pp 453–457
5. Bergdahl L (1980) Gallbladder carcinoma first diagnosed at microscopic examination of gallbladders removed for presumed benign disease. Ann Surg 191: 19–22
6. Bosset JF, Mantion G, Gillet M et al. (1989) Primary carcinoma of the gallbladder: adjuvant postoperative external irradiation. Cancer 64: 1843–1847
7. Carriaga MT, Henson DE (1995) Liver, gallbladder, extrahepatic bile ducts, and pancreas: incidence and prognosis by histologic type. SEER population-based data, 1973–1987. Cancer (in press)
8. Donohue JH, Nagorney DM, Grant CS, Tsushima K, Ilstrup DM, Adson MA (1990) Carcinoma of the gallbladder: does radical surgery improve outcome? Arch Surg 125: 234–241
9. Dowdy GS Jr (1969) The biliary tract. Lea and Febiger, Philadelphia
10. Guo KJ, Yamaguchi K, Enjoji M (1988) Undifferentiated carcinoma of the gallbladder: a clinicopathologic, histochemical, and immunohistochemical study of 21 patients with a poor prognosis. Cancer 61: 1872–1879
11. Henson DE, Albores-Saavedra J, Corle D (1992) Carcinoma of the gallbladder: histologic types, stage of disease, grade, and survival rates. Cancer 70: 1493–1497
12. Hisatomi K, Haratake J, Horie A, Ohsato K (1990) Relation of histopathological features to prognosis of gallbladder cancer. Am J Gastroenterol 85: 567–572
13. Houry S, Schlienger M, Huguier M, Lacaine F, Penne F, Laugier A (1989) Gallbladder carcinoma: role of radiation therapy. Br J Surg 76: 448–450
14. Hsu W, Deziel DJ, Gould VE, Warren WH, Gooch GT, Staren ED (1991) Neuroendocrine differentiation and prognosis of extrahepatic biliary tract carcinoma. Surgery 110: 604–610
15. Johnson LA, Lavin PT, Dayal YY, Geller SA, Doos WG, Cooper HS, Gerber JE, Masse ST, Weiland LH, Moertel CG , Engstrom PS (1986) Gallbladder adenocarcinoma: prognostic significance of tumor acid mucopolysaccharide content. J Surg Oncol 33: 243–245
16. Johnson LA, Lavin PT, Yogeshwar YD, Geller SA et al (1987) Gallbladder adenocarcinoma: the prognostic signficance of histologic grade. J Surg Oncol 34: 16–18
17. Matsumoto Y, Fujii H, Aoyama H, Yamamoto M, Sugahara K, Suda K (1992) Surgical treatment of primary carcinoma of the gallbladder based on the histologic analysis of 48 surgical specimens. Am J Surg 163: 239–245
18. Nadler LH, McSherry CK (1992) Carcinoma of the gallbladder: review of the literature and report on 56 cases at the Beth Israel Medical Center. Mt Sinai J Med 59: 47–52
19. Ouchi K, Owada Y, Matsumo S, Sato T (1987) Prognostic factors in the surgical treatment of gallbladder carcinoma. Surgery 101: 731–737
20. Shirai Y, Yoshida K, Tsukada K, Muto Y (1992) Inapparent carcinoma of the gallbladder: an appraisal of a radical second operation after simple cholecystectomy. Ann Surg 215: 326–331
21. Strom BL, Iliopoulos D, Atkinson B, Herlyn M, West SL, Maislin G, Saul S, Varello MA, Rodriguez-Martinez HA, Rios-Dalenz J, Soloway RD (1989) Pathophysiology of tumor progression in human gallbladder: flow cytometry, CEA, and CA 19–9 levels in bile and serum in different stages of gallbladder disease. J Natl Cancer Inst 81: 1575–1580
22. Sumiyoshi K, Nagai E, Chijiwa K, Nakayama F (1992) Pathology of carcinoma of the gallbladder. World J Surg 15: 315–321
23. Suzuki T, Takano Y, Kakita A, Okudaira M (1993) An immunohistochemical and molecular biological study of c-erb-B2 amplification and prognostic relevance in gallbladder cancer. Pathol Res Pract 189: 283–292
24. Yamaguchi K, Enjoji M (1988) Carcinoma of the gallbladder: a clinicopathology of 103 patients and newly proposed staging. Cancer 62: 1425–1432
25. Yamamoto M, Makajo S, Tahara E (1989) Carcinoma of the gallbladder: the correlation between histogenesis and prognosis. Virchows Arch [A] 414: 83–90

11 Carcinoma of the Extrahepatic Bile Ducts

M.T. Carriaga and D.E. Henson

Introduction

Compared to carcinomas of the gallbladder, carcinomas of the extrahepatic bile ducts are less common, occur more often in men than in women, are usually not associated with lithiasis, and have a different epidemiologic distribution [1–3, 7, 12]. The prognosis for extrahepatic bile duct carcinomas is very poor, with an overall 5-year survival rate of only about 12%. Herein we describe the results of our analysis of the prognostic factors for carcinomas of the extrahepatic bile ducts. This analysis is based primarily on published reports on the prognostic factors in cancers of the extrahepatic bile ducts, including data from the Surveillance, Epidemiology, and End Results (SEER) Program of the National Cancer Institute. No multivariate analysis has been reported on combinations of the different prognostic factors.

Patient-Related Factors

Clinical Findings

Obstructive jaundice is a presenting symptom in the majority of patients. Clinical findings such as abdominal pain, weight loss, pruritus, anemia, and abdominal mass are also common. Laboratory findings include hyperbilirubinemia and elevated serum alkaline phosphatase levels. Because these clinical observations are found in almost all patients, they have not been classified into a prognostic system.

Tumor-Related Factors

Anatomic Extent of Disease

The stage of disease is associated with survival. The relatively early appearance of obstructive symptoms in bile duct carcinoma often results in its detection before the development of distant metastases. In the SEER Program, the stage of disease is reported as "localized," i.e., confined to the extrahepatic bile ducts without nodal involvement, "regional," denoting regional lymph node involvement or direct extension of tumor to adjacent organs, or "distant," when distant metastases are present. Only 23.8% of cases were staged as distant at diagnosis. The overall 5-year survival rate, all histologic types combined, was 26.5% for localized disease, 12.4% for regional disease, and 1.3% for distant disease [4].

Published data also indicate that the depth of invasion into the wall of the extrahepatic bile duct is an important prognostic factor [7, 8, 10]. Most cases, however, are found after the carcinomas have penetrated the wall of the extrahepatic ducts.

Location Within the Biliary Tree

Another important factor in prognosis is the location of the tumor within the biliary tree. Tumors located in the lower third of the bile duct can be more successfully resected than those in the upper (proximal) portions [5, 6, 14, 16]. Unfortunately, the majority of tumors originate within the upper third of the bile ducts, i.e., above the junction of the cystic and hepatic ducts [1, 8, 11, 15]. Bile duct tumors can be diffusely infiltrative or multifocal; these are more difficult to resect and are thus associated with a less favorable prognosis.

Histologic Type

Histologic type has an influence on survival. Table 1 shows the most common histologic types recorded in the SEER Program and their corresponding 5-year relative survival rates. Papillary carcinomas, which comprise only 9.3% of all invasive cancers, have the highest 5-year survival rate (33.7%) of all histologic types reviewed, all stages combined. Papillary adenocarcinomas also show the highest proportion of localized disease (41%), and fewer than 10% are associated

Table 1. Five-year relative survival rates of the most common histologic types of carcinomas of the extrahepatic bile ducts (1978–1986, all stages combined)

	Total (n)	Five-year survival rate (%)
Adenocarcinoma	1762	12.9
Adenocarcinoma (NOS)	1403	10.9
Papillary	147	33.7
Mucinous	87	2.9
Other adenocarcinoma	1251	7.9
Carcinoma (NOS)[a]	106	9.8
Squamous cell carcinoma	8	_[b]

From [4].
NOS, not otherwise specified.
[a] Includes undifferentiated, anaplastic, pleomorphic, etc.
[b] Fewer than 25 cases.

with distant metastases. Ouchi et al. have also reported high survival rates for patients with papillary carcinoma and much shorter survival times for patients with poorly differentiated carcinomas [10]. In SEER, mucinous adenocarcinomas were associated with the lowest 5-year survival rates (2.9%, all stages combined).

Histologic Grade

As a group, the carcinomas of the extrahepatic bile ducts are better differentiated than carcinomas of the gallbladder. The 2-year survival rates by histologic grade are listed in Table 2. For all stages combined, there was a correlation between histologic grade and outcome. Median survival times also fell with advancing histologic grade.

Treatment-Related Factors

Surgical resection of bile duct tumors is complicated by their anatomic location. In recent years, ultrasonography, computed tomography, cholangiography, and cytologic examination of cholangiography specimens have led to the earlier diagnosis of bile duct tumors. This earlier detection has led to improvements in patient management and to reductions in operative mortality [15], but survival rates remain unchanged.

Discussion

Because carcinoma of the extrahepatic bile ducts is not common, there are only a small number of reports that deal specifically with its prognostic factors. Major prognostic factors include the anatomic extent of disease [7, 11, 15], histologic type [1, 2, 7, 9, 10], histologic grade [7], and the site of origin of the tumor within the biliary tree. Published data suggest that vascular invasion is also an important

Table 2. Relation between histologic grade and survival for adenocarcinomas (NOS) of the extrahepatic bile ducts

Grade	Total (n)	Median survival (months)	Two-year relative survival rate (%)
1	221	10	24
2	241	8	16
3	212	4	7
4	6	2	0

From [7].
NOS, not otherwise specified.

prognostic factor [10]. Other potential prognostic factors, especially tumor markers or molecular markers, have not been systematically investigated [17].

As a group, carcinomas of the extrahepatic bile ducts are detected at an earlier stage than gallbladder carcinomas. The early appearance of obstructive symptoms and improved diagnostic procedures contribute to the earlier detection of bile duct tumors. Although carcinomas of the bile ducts are often diagnosed before the occurrence of distant metastases, the overall 5-year survival rate remains poor; according to published data, the overall rate is 12%.

Of all histologic types, papillary carcinomas have been consistently associated with the best prognosis [7, 9, 13]. The relatively good prognosis is probably related to the stage of disease. In the SEER Program, 41% of patients with papillary carcinoma had localized disease, compared with only 13% of patients with mucinous carcinoma. Mucinous adenocarcinomas have the lowest proportion of localized stage disease and the lowest 5-year survival [4].

The location of the tumor within the biliary tree is an important prognostic factor. Carcinomas that arise in the hepatic hilus are associated with a very poor prognosis because of direct extension into adjacent vital organs, including the hepatic artery and portal vein. Proximal tumors are also more difficult to resect than those occurring in the lower portions of the biliary tree.

In summary, the stage of disease, histologic type, histologic grade, and location of tumor are dependable prognostic factors for carcinomas of the extrahepatic bile ducts. Other potential prognostic factors, such as performance status, clinical findings, ploidy and chromosomal changes have not been systematically classified into a prognostic system. Although the TNM stage is the most useful prognostic factor clinically, the 5-year survival rate for localized disease is only 25%, reflecting the difficulty in the surgical treatment and postoperative management of these tumors. The presence of residual disease represents another important prognostic factor, for which new treatment approaches, such as intraoperative radiation therapy, adjuvant radiation and chemotherapy, and liver transplantation are being investigated.

References

1. Albores-Saavedra J, Henson DE (1986) Tumors of the gallbladder and extrahepatic bile ducts. Armed Forces Institute of Pathology, Washington DC
2. Alexander F, Rossi RL, O'Bryan M, Khettry V, Braasch JW, Watkins E (1984) Biliary carcinoma: a review of 109 cases. Am J Surg 147: 503–509
3. Anderson JB, Cooper MJ, Williamson RCN (1985) Adenocarcinoma of the extrahepatic biliary tree. Ann Roy Coll Surg Engl 67: 139–143
4. Carriaga MT, Henson DE (1995) Liver, gallbladder, extrahepatic bile ducts, and pancreas: incidence and prognosis by histologic type. SEER population-based data, 1973–1987. Cancer (in press)
5. Chao TC, Greager JA (1991) Carcinoma of the extrahepatic bile ducts. J Surg Oncol 46: 145–150
6. Fortner JG, Vitelli CE, MacLean BJ (1989) Proximal extrahepatic bile duct tumors: analysis of a series of 52 consecutive patients treated over a period of 13 years. Arch Surg 124: 1275–1279
7. Henson DE, Albores-Saavedra J, Corle D (1992) Carcinoma of the extrahepatic bile ducts. Cancer 70: 1498–1501

8. Kozuka S, Tsuborne M, Hachisuka K (1984) Evolution of carcinoma in the extrahepatic bile ducts. Cancer 54: 65–72
9. Nakajima T, Kondo Y (1989) Well differentiated cholangiocarcinoma: diagnostic significance of morphologic and immunohistochemical parameters. Am J Surg Pathol 13: 569–573
10. Ouchi K, Suzuki M, Hashimoto L, Sato T (1989) Histologic findings and prognostic factors in carcinoma of the upper bile duct. Am J Surg 157: 552–556
11. Reding R, Buard JL, Lebeau G, Saunois B (1991) Surgical management of 552 carcinomas of the extrahepatic bile ducts (gallbladder and periampullary tumors excluded): results of the French Surgical Association Survey. Ann Surg 213: 236–241
12. Strom BL, Hibberd PL , Soper KA, Stolley PD, Nelson WL (1985) International variations in epidemiology of cancers of the extrahepatic biliary tract. Cancer Res 45: 5165–5168
13. Todoroki T, Okamura T, Fukao K et al (1980) Gross appearance of carcinoma of the main hepatic duct and its prognosis. Surg Gynecol Obstet 150: 33–40
14. Tompkins RK, Saunders K , Roslyn JJ, Longmire WP Jr (1990) Changing patterns in diagnosis and management of bile duct cancer. Ann Surg 211: 614–620
15. Tompkins RK, Thomas D, Wile A, Longmire WP (1981) Prognostic factors in bile duct carcinoma: analysis of 96 cases. Ann Surg 194: 447–457
16. Tsuzuki T, Ueda M, Kuramochi S, Iida S, Takahashi S, Iri H (1990) Carcinoma of the main hepatic duct junction: indications, operative morbidity and mortality, and long-term survival. Surg 108: 495–501
17. Yamaguchi K, Enjoji M, Nakayama F (1988) Cancer of the extrahepatic bile duct: a clinico-pathologic study of immunohistochemistry for CEA, CA 19–9, and p21. World J Surg 12: 11–17

12 Exocrine Pancreatic Carcinoma

M. Yamamoto, Y. Saitoh, and P. Hermanek

Introduction

More than 90%–95% of malignant tumours of the pancreas are exocrine carcinomas. Surgical resection remains the only potentially curative approach, although the resectability is still low and the prognosis is still poor compared with cancer in other digestive organs. The median survival time for all diagnosed patients with exocrine pancreatic carcinoma is reported to be between 4 and 7 months [18, 42, 66]; the overall 5-year survival rate is extremely low: in the older literature figures are under 1% [22]; recently, figures of 1%–3% [18, 48] have been reported.

The prognosis of a patient with exocrine pancreatic carcinoma is determined above all by the possibility of resection. This is dependent primarily on the anatomic extent of disease as defined by the TNM classification and stage grouping [6, 25], but sometimes resection is not possible even for localized stages, e.g. because of the general condition of patients or associated co-morbidity. In the literature the resection rate for exocrine pancreatic carcinoma lies between 15% and 30% [5, 18, 20, 27, 38, 66]. The outcome of patients after tumour resection is significantly better than that of patients who do not undergo resection. While long-term survival without resection is practically never observed, the 5-year survival rate following resection in specialized centres is between 20% and 25% [11, 20, 61, 65]. The median survival time is 3–9 months without resection [10, 20, 27, 38, 49] compared to 10–20 months with resection [5, 18, 20, 55]. Therefore, prognostic factors will be considered separately for patients without and with tumour resection.

In the following, the relevant international literature as well as the results of a national survey by the Pancreatic Cancer Registry of the Japan Pancreas Society [51] will be considered. There are difficulties in reviewing the literature because carcinomas of the head of the pancreas are often not separated from those of the ampulla of Vater and those of the distal common bile duct. Futhermore, the recent reduction of surgical mortality to less than 5% [13, 21, 60] has to be considered, particulary for pre-1980 data.

Prognostic Factors for Patients Without Tumour Resection

Because of the very poor prognosis for patients without resection, only a limited influence of prognostic factors can be expected.

In a recent Norwegian prospective study [4] multivariate analysis revealed jaundice on presentation as the only unfavourable independent prognostic factor for patients who did not receive surgical treatment. In patients who received bypass surgery or laparotomy only, invasion of the superior mesenteric vein, regional lymph node metastasis and weight loss on presentation were independent unfavourable prognostic factors, whereas the surgical procedure (laparotomy, biliary bypass or double bypass) did not influence survival.

In a retrospective study on 3741 patients operated on between 1982 and 1988 at 148 French institutions [29], the median survival times for different nonresective surgical procedures were as follows: 2.6 months for surgically placed biliary stents, 3.2 months for cholecysto-enteric bypass and between 5.0 and 5.5 months for the various types of choledocho-enteric bypass with or without gastrojejunostomy.

A retrospective study of 1180 patients who underwent palliative surgery in 158 hospitals of the USA Department of Veterans Affairs from 1987 to 1991 showed that survival after biliary or combined biliary and gastric bypass was significantly longer than after gastric bypass alone (8.6 and 9.3 versus 6.9 months) [49].

Prognostic Factors for Patients with Tumour Resection

Because the prognosis of pancreatic carcinoma is so poor and the number of resected cases at individual institutions is limited, the influence of various possible prognostic factors is unclear. Most reports are based on univariate analysis. Only one published multivariate study [20] includes more than 100 resected patients, while the other multivariate studies [2, 4, 8, 9, 16, 17, 41, 52, 57, 63, 70] are not conclusive because of their small number of patients. Further difficulties arise from inaccuracies of topographical and histopathological diagnosis (inclusion of prognostically more favourable ampullary and/or endocrine carcinomas) and the absence of residual tumour classification in several reports.

Tumour-Related Factors

The most important and generally accepted tumour-related factors are listed in Table 1.

The most frequent histological type (over 90%) of exocrine pancreatic carcinoma is the ductal adenocarcinoma, including such variants as mucinous

Table 1. Prognostic factors for patients with exocrine pancreas carcinoma treated by resection

Factor	Favourable variant
Histological type	Mucinous cystadenocarcinoma
	Intraductal papillary mucinous carcinoma
Histological grade	G1 (G2)
Anatomic extent	
Local spread	Limited to pancreas (T1/pT1)
Tumour size	≤ 2 cm (≤ 2.5 cm, < 4 cm)
Regional lymph node	N0/pN0
metastasis (N/pN)	
Distant metastasis	M0/pM0
Stage grouping	Stage I

non-cystic, adenosquamous, anaplastic and osteoblast-like giant cell carcinoma. The mucinous cystadenocarcinoma (about 1% of all cases or 5% of resected cases) has a relatively good prognosis [12, 14], e.g. in Japanese patients, a 5-year survival rate of 54.3%. Similarly, the uncommon intraductal papillary mucinous carcinoma [54] has a better prognosis than the common ductal adenocarcinoma. Therefore, it is important to separate cystadenocarcinomas and intraductal papillary mucinous carcinomas from ductal adenocarcinomas. In the following discussion these two tumour types will be excluded, as will in situ carcinomas.

There are conflicting reports on the prognostic significance of histological grade. In the Japanese Registry [51], the 5-year survival rates were similar (11.7%, 9.1% and 9.1%) for G1, G2 and G3, respectively. On the other hand, Klöppel et al. [35] and Boettger et al. [8] found a correlation between grade and survival. Grade was an independent prognostic factor in the multivariate analysis published by Geer and Brennan [20]. These authors found a 5-year survival rate for poorly differentiated carcinomas of about 10% compared to nearly 50% for well-differentiated carcinomas.

Tumour size has been recognized as a significant prognostic factor. In multivariate analysis [2, 20] patients with tumours larger than 2.5 cm (greatest dimension) had a lower survival rate than those with smaller tumours (20% versus 40%); the hazard ratio for death was 2.77 for tumours of more than 2.5 cm [20]. Baumel et al. [5] found in the retrospective French multicentre study a worsening of prognosis for tumours of 4 cm or more. In the Japanese series, tumours of 2 cm or less accounted for only 5% of the total. Despite recent advances in diagnostic modalities, an obvious increase over time in the frequency of these small tumours could not be found. The resectability rate for small tumours was over 90%, and the postoperative survival rates were relatively favourable as compared with tumours greater than 2 cm in size. The 5-year survival rate was 40.5% for 407 patients with tumours of 2.0 cm or less; 14.4% for 1559 patients with tumours of 2.1–4.0 cm, 10.9% for 938 patients with tumours of 4.1–6.0 cm and 19.2% for 583 patients with tumours greater than 6.0 cm.

According to the TNM classification [6, 25] local tumour spread is described by T. It is divided into three categories: T1, tumour limited to the pancreas; T2, tumour extends directly to any of the following: duodenum, bile duct or peripancreatic tissues; T3, tumour involves one or more of the following; stomach, spleen, colon or adjacent large vessels. The importance of invasion beyond the pancreas was demonstrated by several authors in univariate analysis [5, 24, 45]. In the Japanese series, the prognosis of patients with tumours limited to the pancreas was significantly better than those with tumours extending directly to adjacent organs or large vessels. According to the Japanese Cancer Registry the postoperative survival rates of pT1 patients reached 58.6% at 5 years, whereas pT2 patients had 19.7% and pT3 patients only 7.1% 5-year survival rates (Fig. 1).

pT1 is subdivided into pT1a (tumour size of 2.0 cm or less) and pT1b (tumour greater than 2.0 cm in size). In the Japanese Registry no difference in prognosis between pT1a and pT1b tumours could be found.

The presence and extent of peripancreatic invasion was the most important prognostic factor, but it has been suggested that the frequency of tumour invasion is strongly correlated with tumour size. A retroperitoneal invasion was found in 19.3% of the tumours 2 cm or less in size, 53% of those 2.1–4.0 cm in size, 77.2% of those 4.1–6 cm in size, and 89.5% in the tumours greater than 6 cm in size. However, small tumours were not necessarily early-stage tumours. Even in patients in whom tumour size was 2 cm or less, the invasion of retroperitoneal tissue or the portal vein was found in 19.3% and 17.3%, respectively. Therefore, tumour size was not a major determinant of prognosis per se, but correlated with

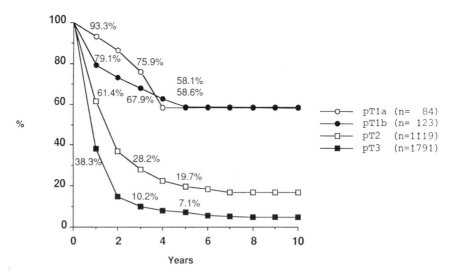

Fig. 1. Observed postoperative survival following resection in relation to pT [6, 25]

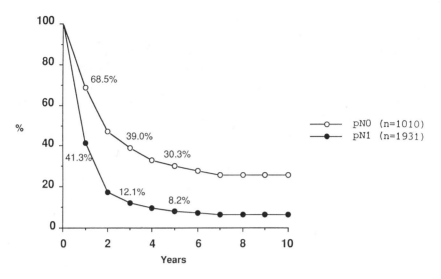

Fig. 2. Observed postoperative survival following resection in relation to pN [6, 25]

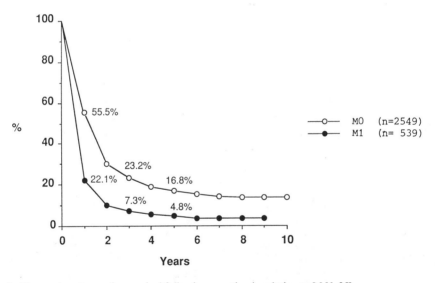

Fig. 3. Observed postoperative survival following resection in relation to M [6, 25]

the presence and extent of peripancreatic invasion, which determined the post-operative prognosis.

Lymph node metastases and distant metastases were of definite influence on the prognosis following resection. Figures 2 and 3 show the postoperative survival according to pN and M/pM categories of TNM. The relation of survival to N and M was demonstrated by most authors reporting larger number of patients [5, 8, 20, 53, 55].

According to the Japanese classification system [32], the lymph nodes are divided into three groups including 18 stations (Table 2). The location of involved nodes influences prognosis. In the Japanese Registry [51], the cumulative survival rates were 30.2% at 5 years in 1151 patients when no nodes were involved, 7.2% in 1250 patients within group 1, 3.2% in 350 patients within group 2, and no 3-year survivors in 147 patients within group 3. A similar influence of node metastasis location on prognosis could also be demonstrated by Nagakawa et al. [45] in a group of 43 patients who underwent extended radical pancreatectomy by the translateral retroperitoneal approach including complete excision of the lymph nodes and nerve plexus of both the celiac axis and the

Table 2. Subdivision of lymph nodes according to the Japanese Pancreas Society [32]

Node stations		Group classification	
		Head of the pancreas	Body or tail of the pancreas
5:	Suprapyloric	3	3[a]
6:	Infrapyloric	1	3[a]
7:	Along the left gastric artery	3	2[a]
8:	Along the common hepatic artery	1	1[a]
9:	Celiac	2	1[a]
10:	At the hilus of the spleen	3[a]	1
11:	Along the splenic artery	2[a]	1
12:	In the hepatoduodenal ligament		
12 h:	At the porta hepatis	3	3
12a1:	Along the upper portion of the proper hepatic artery	2	3
12a2:	Along the lower portion of the proper hepatic artery	1	2
12p1:	Along the upper portion of the portal vein	2	3
12p2:	Along the lower portion of the portal vein	1	2
12b1:	Along the proximal bile duct	2	3
12b2:	Along the distal bile duct	1	2
12c:	Along the cystic duct	2	3
13:	Posterior pancreaticoduodenal	1	2
14:	Along the superior mesenteric artery		
14a:	At the origin of the superior mesenteric artery	2	2
14b:	At the origin of the inferior pancreaticoduodenal artery	1	2
14c:	At the origin of the middle colic artery	1	2
14d:	At the origin of the jejunal artery	1	2
14v:	Along the superior mesenteric vein	1	2
15:	Along the middle colic artery	2[a]	2[a]
16:	Para-aortic	2[a]	2[a]
17:	Anterior pancreaticoduodenal	1	2
18:	Inferior body and tail	2	1

[a] According to the UICC TNM classification [25] these nodes are considered as non-regional; involvement is classified as distant metastasis.

superior mesenteric artery. The 5-year survival for pN0 was 67% and 21% for pN1 with group 1 involvement; however, no patient with group 2 metastasis survived 2 years.

Hermanek [23] pointed out that if two or more lymph nodes were involved, a dramatic worsening of prognosis following resection for cure was observed, so that the number of involved lymph nodes should be stated in the histological report of tumour resection specimens.

On the other hand, Mannell et al. [41] looked at the Mayo Clinic experience and found that, of the patients who lived for 3 years or longer, 71% had had negative nodes, but of the patients who had died within the first year, 76% had had negative nodes. They concluded that nodal involvement was not a significant prognosis factor.

Pancreatic carcinoma may penetrate the peritoneum and result in peritoneal metastasis. Sometimes peritoneal spread can be detected only by peritoneal washings [64]. This indicates a very poor prognosis.

The anatomic extent of carcinoma can be described by condensing T, N and M or pT, pN and pM into stage groups [6, 25]. The prognosis after resection depending on stage grouping is shown for Japanese patients in Fig. 4. In the Western literature, lower survival rates are reported; nevertheless stage grouping indicates prognosis [4, 8, 15, 24].

In the multivariate analysis carried out by Geer and Brennan [20], tumour site had no independent influence on prognosis. According to most reports, the prognosis for patients with carcinomas of the head is more favourable than for other sites [5, 18]. A survey compiling data from the literature [19] shows that tumours treatable by left-sided resection have a 5-year survival rate of 0% versus

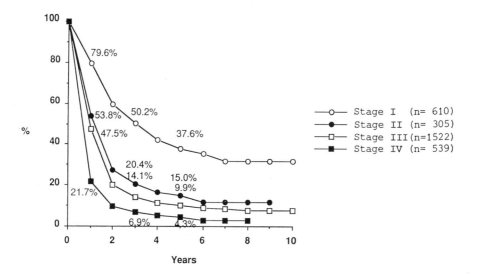

Fig. 4. Observed postoperative survival following resection in relation to stage grouping [6,25]

5.1% for tumours of the pancreatic head treated by partial duodenopancreatectomy; the average survival time was 11.4 versus 13.7 months. In general, carcinomas of the body and tail of the pancreas are diagnosed at a more advanced stage. However, after resection for cure (R0) the same results are achieved as for carcinomas of the pancreatic head [20].

During recent years, DNA ploidy and cell cycle analysis have been extensively studied by flow [1, 3, 9, 17, 26, 52, 57, 67, 73] and image (absorption) cytometry [2, 8, 9]. According to most, but not all reports, aneuploid carcinomas seem to behave poorer than diploid tumours; however, diploid carcinomas may be rapidly fatal. Perhaps this may be explained by the heterogeneity of pancreas carcinomas resulting in a relatively low reliability of detecting aneuploidy [17]. According to Alanen et al. [1], DNA ploidy is correlated with histological grade; however, this could not be confirmed by other authors [8, 17]. Reports on the prognostic importance of the S-phase fraction and the G2 fraction are contradictory [1, 3, 9, 17, 57]. At present, cytometry needs further investigation, especially in prospective studies, predominantly for stratifying patients [65].

Additional possible tumour-related prognostic factors have been reported either in single studies only or in limited numbers of patients, sometimes with conflicting results. They are listed in Table 3. The clinical significance of these factors requires further investigation.

Table 3. Possible tumour-related prognostic factors which need further confirmation

Factor	Selected references
Multicentricity	63
Round cell infiltrate at the tumour margin	41
Lymphatic, venous and perineural invasion	11, 20, 46
Extent of involvement of portal or superior mesenteric vein	31
Epithelial atypia in the uninvolved pancreatic ducts	41
Histoquantitative finding: nuclear morphometry, M/V index (volume-corrected mitotic index)	16, 37
Proliferation markers	39, 50
Growth factors and growth factor receptors (EGF, TGF-α, EGFR)	28, 71, 72
Oncogenes and oncogene products:	
erbB2	28, 71
erbB3	36
Ki-ras	28, 43
p53	28
nm23	47

EGF, epidermal growth factor; TGF, transforming growth factor; EGFR, EGF receptor.

Patient-Related Factors

In patients for whom tumour resection is possible, there are no proven patient-related prognostic factors. In the data of Bakkevold and Kambestad [4], neither age, gender or presenting symptoms demonstrated an independent influence on prognosis. In contrast, some authors reported a more favourable prognosis in patients with a short history of symptoms (not more than 8 weeks) [7], with good performance status [34], without backache [5, 7] and with low preoperative CA 19–9 serum levels (less than 400 IU/ml) [7]. However, CA 19–9 reflects the tumour burden (except in patients with negative Lewis blood type and some of those with poorly differentiated carcinomas), and an independent prognostic influence has not been proven [59].

Baumel et al. [5] observed a better prognosis in patients with jaundice than in those without. Preoperative alpha 1-antitrypsin serum levels of more than 100 mg/100 ml seem to signify a poor prognosis [62].

Treatment-Related Factors

The prognosis is definitely related to the radicality of resection. According to the UICC, tumour status following tumour resection is described by the residual tumour (R) classification. In R1 resections (microscopic residual tumour) the majority of cases show tumour transsection on the dorsal (retroperitoneal) resection margins (73% [68] and 88% [69]). In the Japanese Cancer Registry [51], R0 resection (no residual tumour) was performed on 1018 patients, corresponding to 36% of the resected cases. The 1-, 3- and 5-year survival rates were 70%, 38% and 28%, respectively. These results were significantly better than for R1 and R2 resections. The prognosis of patients with remaining macroscopic residual tumour (R2) was not more favourable than for patients who were treated without resection.

In the Western literature, the proportion of R0 resection varies between 47% [55], 49% [68] and 66% [18]. The 2- and 5- year relative survival rates for R0 resections are 35% and 16% and for R1 and R2 resections 10% and 0%, respectively. The median survival time in non-curative resections was 7.2 months compared to 3.4 months for patients with bypass surgery only [18]. The highly significant worsening of prognosis in cases of remaining loco-regional residual tumour was recently confirmed by Willet et al. [68]: no survivors beyond 41 months versus a 22% 5-year survival rate for R0 resection.

It is generally accepted that radical resection to cure pancreatic carcinoma (partial, subtotal or total duodenopancreatectomy, subtotal left pancreatectomy) includes en bloc dissection of the regional lymph nodes and the surrounding connective tissue with its lymphatic and perineural spaces. An extension of the dissection to non-regional lymph nodes, especially to the para-aortic nodes down to the aortic bifurcation, has been recommended by some Japanese authors [31, 40, 44, 45]. This is supported by the demonstration of lymphatic spread to superior mesenteric and para-aortic lymph nodes even in patients with small carcinomas [33]. The published reports on a relatively limited number of patients (22 [31] and 74 [40]) and unpublished recent data of the Japanese Cancer Registry suggest that such extended dissection may prolong survival in patients with less-advanced carcinomas, namely those with tumours of 4 cm or less, metastasis to peripancreatic nodes only and absent or slight portal vein involvement [30]. In the Western literature, opinions on the usefulness of such extended resection are contradictory [20, 53].

With regard to the recently proposed pylorus-preserving resections, Sharp et al. [58] reported an increased frequency of local recurrences. The superiority of conventional radical surgery in terms of frequency of R0 resections and survival was shown by Roder et al. [56].

The prognostic influence of blood transfusions is unclear [2, 11, 20] and the results of multimodal treatment are not uniform [10, 20, 74].

Summary

In comparison with other digestive tract carcinomas, exocrine pancreatic carcinoma has a very poor prognosis. To date, cure is possible only by complete surgical resection. For patients with curatively resected tumours (R0 resection) anatomic extent, histological type and grade are accepted prognostic factors. Other factors need further investigation.

Acknowledgements. This publication has been supported by the Japan Pancreas Society, in co-operation with a large number of surgeons in Japan, and partly supported by a grant from the Japanese TNM Committee.

References

1. Alanen KA, Joensuu H, Klemi PJ, Nevalainen TJ (1990) Clinical significance of nuclear DNA content in pancreatic carcinoma. J Pathol 160: 313–320
2. Allison DC, Bose KK, Hruban RH, Piantadosi S, Dooley WC, Boitnott K, Cameron JL (1991) Pancreatic cancer cell DNA content correlates with long-term survival after pancreatoduodenectomy. Ann Surg 214: 648–656
3. Baisch DC, Klöppel G, Reinke B (1990) DNA ploidy and cell-cycle analysis in pancreatic and ampullary carcinoma: flow cytometric study on formalin-fixed paraffin-embedded tissue. Virchows Arch [A] 417: 145–150
4. Bakkevold KE, Kambestad B (1993) Long-term survival following radical and palliative treatment of patients with carcinoma of the pancreas and papilla of Vater – the prognostic factors influencing the long-term results. Eur J Surg Oncol 19: 147–161
5. Baumel H, Huguier M, Manderscheid JC, Fabre JM, Houry S, Fagot H (1994) Results of resection for cancer of the exocrine pancreas: a study from the French Association of Surgery. Br J Surg 81: 102–107
6. Beahrs OH, Henson DE, Hutter RVP, Kennedy BJ (eds) (1992) AJCC: manual for staging of cancer, 4th edn. Lippincott, Philadelphia
7. Boettger T, Zech W, Sorger K, Junginger T (1990) Relevant factors in the prognosis of ductal pancreatic carcinoma. Acta Chir Scand 156: 781–788

8. Böttger TC, Störkel S, Wellek S, Stöckle M, Junginger T (1994) Factors influencing survival after resection of pancreatic cancer. Cancer 73: 63–73

9. Bose KK, Allison DC, Hruban RH, Piantadosi S, Zahurak M, Dooley WC, Lin P, Cameron JL (1993) A comparison of flow cytometric and absorption cytometric DNA values as prognostic indicators for pancreatic carcinoma. Cancer 71: 691–700

10. Brennan MF, Kinsella TJ, Casper ES (1993) Cancer of the pancreas. In: de Vita VT Jr, Hellman S, Rosenberg SA (eds) Cancer. Principles and practice of oncology, 4th edn. Lippincott, Philadelphia

11. Cameron JL, Crist DW, Sitzmann JV, Hruban RH, Brittnot JK, Seidlerr AJ, Coleman J (1991) Factors influencing survival after pancreaticoduodenectomy for pancreatic cancer. Am J Surg 161: 120–124

12. Connolly MM, Dawson PJ, Michelassi F, Moossa AR, Lowenstein F (1987) Survival in 1,001 patients with carcinoma of the pancreas. Ann Surg 206: 366–370

13. Christ DW, Sitzmann JV, Cameron JL (1987) Improved hospital morbidity, mortality, and survival after the Whipple procedure. Ann Surg 206: 358–365

14. Eskelinen M, Lipponen P (1992) A review of prognostic factors in human pancreatic adenocarcinoma. Cancer Detect Prev 16: 287–295

15. Eskelinen M, Lipponen P, Collan Y, Vainio O, Marin S, Alhava E (1991) Cancer of the pancreas: clinical stage, histological grade, surgical therapy and survival. Surg Res Commun 10: 9–14

16. Eskelinen M, Lipponen P, Marin S, Haapasalo H, Mäkinen K, Ahtola H, Puittinen J, Nuntinen P,Alhava E (1991) Prognostic factors in human pancreatic cancer, with special reference to quantitatve histology. Scand J Gastroenterol 26: 483–490

17. Eskelinen M, Lipponen P, Marin S, Haapasalo H, Mäkinen K, Puittinen J, Alhava E, Nordling S (1992) DNA ploidy, S-phase fraction, and G2 fraction as prognostic determinants in human pancreatic cancer. Scand J Gastroenterol 27: 39–43

18. Gall FP, Kessler H, Hermanek P (1991) Surgical treatment of ductal pancreatic carcinoma. Eur J Surg Oncol 17: 173–181

19. Gall FP, Zirngibl H (1984) Chirurgische Therapie der Pankreastumoren. In: Gebhardt C (ed) Chirurgie des exokrinen Pankreas. Thieme, Stuttgart

20. Geer RJ, Brennan MF (1993) Prognostic indicators for survival after resection of pancreatic adenocarcinoma. Am J Surg 165: 68–73

21. Grace PA, Pitt HA, Tompkins RK, Den Besten L, Longmire WP Jr (1986) Decreased morbidity and mortality after pancreaticoduodenectomy. Am J Surg 151: 141–149

22. Gudjonsson B (1987) Cancer of the pancreas. 50 years of surgery. Cancer 60: 2284–2303

23. Hermanek P (1991) Staging of exocrine pancreas carcinoma. Eur J Surg Oncol 17: 167–172

24. Hermanek P (1995) UICC TNM classification and stage grouping. In: Beger HG, Büchler MW, Schoenberg MH (eds) Cancer of the pancreas. Universitätsverlag, Ulm

25. Hermanek P, Sobin LH (eds) (1992) UICC TNM classification of malignant tumours, 4th edn, 2nd rev. Universitatsverlag, Ulm

26. Herrera MF, van Heerden JA, Katzmann JA, Weiland LH, Nagorney DM, Ilstrup D (1992) Evaluation of DNA nuclear pattern as a prognostic determinant in resected pancreatic ductal adenocarcinoma. Ann Surg 215: 120–124

27. Hohenberger W, Zirngibl H, Gall FP (1989) Pancreatic and periampullary carcinoma, In: Veronesi U, Arnesjo B, Burn I, Denis L, Mazzeo F (eds) Surgical oncology. A European handbook. Springer, Berlin Heidelberg New York

28. Hoorens A, Lemoine NR, McLellan E, Morohoshi T, Kamisawa T, Heitz PhU, Stamm B, Rüschoff J, Wiedenmann B, Klöppel G (1993) Pancreatic acinar cell carcinoma. An analysis of cell lineage markers, p53 expression, and Ki-ras mutation. Am J Surg Pathol 143: 685–698

29. Huguier M, Baumel H, Manderscheid J-C, Houry S, Fabre JM (1993) Surgical palliation for unresected cancer of the exocrine pancreas. Eur J Surg Oncol 19: 342–347

30. Ishikawa O (1993) What constitutes curative pancreatectomy for adenocarcinoma of the pancreas? Hepatogastroenterology 40: 414–417

31. Ishikawa O, Ohigashi H, Imaoka S, Furukawa H, Sasaki Y, Fujita M, Kurada C, Iwanaga T (1992) Preoperative indications for extended pancreatectomy for locally advanced pancreas cancer involving the portal vein. Ann Surg 215: 231–236

32. Japan Pancreas Society (1993) General rules for the study of the pancreatic cancer, 4rd edn. Kanehara, Tokyo

33. Kayahara M, Nagakawa T, Kobayashi H, Mori K, Nakano T, Kadoya N, Ohta T, Ueno K, Miyazaki I (1992) Lymphatic flow in carcinoma of the head of the pancreas. Cancer 70: 2061–2066
34. Kalser MH, Barkin J, MacIntyre JM (1985) Pancreatic cancer: assessment of prognosis by clinical presentation. Cancer 56: 397–402
35. Klöppel G, Lindenthal G, von Bülow M, Kern HF (1985) Histological and fine structural feature of pancreatic ductal adenocarcinomas in relation to growth and prognosis. Histopathology 9: 841–856
36. Lemoine NR, Lobresco M, Leung H, Barton C, Hughes CM, Prigent SA, Gullick WJ, Klöppel G (1993) The erb-B-3 gene in human pancreatic cancer. J Pathol 168: 269–273
37. Lipponen PK, Eskelinen MJ, Collan Y, Marin S, Alhava E (1990) Volume-corrected mitotic index in human pancreatic cancer. Scand J Gastroenterol 25: 548–554
38. Livingston EH, Welton ML, Reber HA (1991) Surgical treatment of pancreatic cancer. Int J Pancreatol 9: 153–157
39. Maekinen K, Eskelinen M, Lipponen P, Nuntinen P, Marin S, Alhava E (1993) Ag-Nors related to flow cytometry, morphometry and prognosis in patients with pancreatic cancer. Anticancer Res 13: 157–160
40. Manabe T, Ohsio G, Baba N, Miyashita T, Asano N, Tamura K, Yamaki K, Nonaka A, Tobe T (1989) Radical pancreatectomy for ductal cell carcinoma of the head of the pancreas. Cancer 64: 1132–1137
41. Mannell A, Weiland LH, van Heerden JA, Ilstrup DM (1986) Factors influencing survival after resection for ductal adenocarcinoma of the pancreas. Ann Surg 203: 403–407
42. Mohinddin M, Rosato F, Schuricht A, Barbot D, Biermann W, Cantor R (1994) Carcinoma of the pancreas – the Jefferson experience 1975–1988. Eur J Surg Oncol 20: 13–20
43. Motojima K, Urano T, Nagata Y, Shiku H, Tsurifune T, Kanemitsu T (1993) Detection of point mutations in the Kirsten-ras oncogene provides evidence for the multicentricity of pancreatic carcinoma. Ann Surg 217: 138–143
44. Nagakawa T, Kurachi M, Konishi K, Miyazaki I (1982) Translateral retroperitoneal approach in radical surgery for pancreatic carcinoma. Jpn J Surg 12: 229–233
45. Nagakawa T, Konishi I,Ueno K, Ohta T, Akiyama T, Kanno M, Kayahara M, Miyazaki I (1991) The results and problems of extensive radical surgery for carcinoma of the head of the pancreas. Jpn J Surg 21: 262–267
46. Nagakawa T, Kayahara M, Ueno K, Konishi I, Ueda N, Miyazaki I (1992) A clinicopathologic study on neural invasion in cancer of the pancreatic head. Cancer 69: 930–935
47. Nakamori S, Ishikawa O,Ohhigashi H, Kameyama M, Furukawa H, Sasaki Y, Inaji H, Higashiyama M, Imaoka S, Iwanaga T (1993) Expression of nucleoside diphosphate kinase /nm 23 gene product in human pancreatic cancer: an association with lymph node metastasis and tumor invasion. Clin Exp Metastasis 11: 151–158
48. National Cancer Institute (1990) Annual cancer statistics review: 1973–1988. National Institutes of Health Publ 90–2789, Bethesda
49. Neuberger TJ, Wade TP, Swope JT, Virgo KS, Johnson FE (1993) Palliative operations for pancreatic cancer in the hospitals of the U.S.Department of Veterans Affairs from 1987 to 1991. Am J Surg 166: 632–637
50. Ohta T, Nagakawa T, Tsukioka Y, Mori K, Takeda T, Kayahara M, Ueno K, Fonseca L, Miyazaki I, Terada T (1993) Expression of argyrophilic nucleolar organizer regions in ductal adenocarcinoma of the pancreas and its relationship to prognosis. Int J Pancreatol 13: 193–200
51. Pancreatic Cancer Registration Committee of the Japan Pancreas Society (1993) Annual report of registered cases of pancreatic cancer in Japan (in Japanese). Japan Pancreas Society, Tokyo
52. Porschen R, Remy U, Bevers G, Schauseil S, Hengels K-J, Borchard F (1993) Prognostic significance of DNA ploidy in adenocarcinoma of the pancreas. Cancer 71: 3846–3850
53. Reber HA (1990) Lymph node involvement as a prognostic factor in pancreatic cancer. Int J Pancreatol 7: 125–127
54. Rickaert F, Cremer M, Devière J, Tavares L, Lambilliotte JP, Schröder S, Wurbs D, Klöppel G (1991) Intraductal mucin-hypersecreting neoplasms of the pancreas. Gastroenterology 101: 512–519
55. Roder JD, Siewert JR (1992) Analyse prognose-assoziierter Faktoren beim Pankreaskopf- und periampullären Carcinom. Chirurg 63: 410–415
56. Roder JD, Stein HJ, Hüttl W, Siewert JR (1992) Pylorus-preserving versus standard pancreatico-duodenectomy: an analysis of 110 pancreatic and periampullary carcinomas. Br J Surg 79: 152–155

57. Roder JD, Nekarda H, Becker K, Rossmann A, Fink U, Siewert JR (1994) Ploidy and S-phase in resected ductal carcinoma of the pancreas: prognostic relevance. J Cancer Res Clin Oncol 120 [Suppl]: R73
58. Sharp KW, Ross CB, Halter SA, Morrison JG, Richards WO, Williams LF, Sawyers JL (1989) Pancreatoduodenectomy with pyloric preservation for carcinoma of the pancreas: a cautionary note. Surgery 105: 645–653
59. Tian F, Appert HE, Myles J, Howard JM (1992) Prognostic value of serum CA 19–9 levels in pancreatic adenocarcinoma. Ann Surg 215: 350–355
60. Trede M (1985) The surgical treatment of pancreatic carcinoma. Surgery 97: 28–35
61. Trede M, Schwall G, Saeger HD (1990) Survival after pancreaticoduodenectomy: 118 consecutive resections without an operative mortality. Ann Surg 211: 447–458
62. Trichopoulos D, Tzonou A, Kalapothaki V, Sparos L, Kremastinou T, Skoutari M (1990) Alpha 1-antitrypsin and survival in pancreatic cancer. Int J Cancer 45: 685–686
63. Van Heerden JA, McIlrath DC, Ilstrup DM, Weiland LH (1988) Total pancreatectomy for ductal adenocarcinoma of the pancreas: an update. World J Surg 12: 658–662
64. Warshaw AL (1991) Implications of peritoneal cytology for staging of early pancreatic cancer. Am J Surg 161: 26–30
65. Warshaw AL (1991) Implications of malignant-cell DNA content for treatment of patients with pancreatic cancer. Ann Surg 214: 645–647
66. Warshaw AL, Swanson RS (1988) What's new in general surgery? Pancreatic cancer in 1988: possibilities and probabilities. Ann Surg 208: 541–553
67. Weger AR, Falkmer VG, Schwab G, Glaser K, Kemmler G, Bodner E, Auer E, Mikuz G (1990) Nuclear DNA distribution pattern of the parenchymal cells in adenocarcinomas of the pancreas and in chronic pancreatitis. Gastroenterology 99: 237–242
68. Willet CG, Lewanbrowski K, Warshaw Al, Efird J, Compton CC (1993) Resection margins in carcinoma of the head of the pancreas. Implications for radiation therapy. Ann Surg 217: 144–148
69. Wittekind C (1993) Bedeutung von Tumorwachstum und -ausbreitung für die chirurgische Radikalität. Zentralbl Chir 118: 500–507
70. Yamaguchi K, Nishihara K, Kolodziejczyk P, Tsuneyoshi M (1992) Long survivors after pancreatoduodenectomy for pancreas head carcinoma. Aust N Z J Surg 62: 545–549
71. Yamanaka Y (1992) The immunohistochemical expression of epidermal growth factors, epidermal growth factor receptors and c-erbB-2 oncoprotein in human pancreatic cancer. J Nippon Med School 59: 51–57
72. Yamanaka Y, Friess H, Kobrin MS, Büchler M, Beger HG, Korc M (1993) Coexpression of epidermal growth factor receptors and ligands in human pancreatic cancer is associated with enhanced tumor aggressiveness. Anticancer Res 13: 565–570
73. Yasuda H, Takada T, Uchiyana K, Hasegawa H (1993) Long-term prognosis and DNA ploidy pattern after pancreatoduodenectomy for cancer of the head of the pancreas. In: Takahasi T (ed) Recent advances in management of digestive cancers. Springer, Berlin Heidelberg New York
74. Zerbi A, Fossati V, Parolini D, Carlucci M, Balzano G, Bordogna G, Staudacher C, Di Carlo V (1994) Intraoperative radiation therapy adjuvant to resection in the treatment of pancreatic cancer. Cancer 73: 2930–2935

13 Lung Carcinoma

H. Asamura and T. Naruke

Introduction

When we analyze the prognostic factors in lung carcinoma, two major issues must be taken into consideration: tumour histology and stage of the disease.

The variety of histological types of lung carcinoma complicates the analysis of prognostic factors. The current classification of lung carcinomas by the World Health Organization (WHO) recognizes four major histological types: squamous cell carcinoma, adenocarcinoma, large cell carcinoma and small cell carcinoma [51]; the first three are grouped together as non-small-cell lung carcinoma (NSCLC) and account for approximately 70%–80% of lung carcinomas. Since there are great differences in the response to systemic chemotherapy or radiation and clinical outcome between NSCLC and small cell lung carcinoma (SCLC), prognostic factors should be discussed separately for these two histological categories.

Another important issue in discussing prognostic factors in lung carcinoma is anatomic extent of disease, i.e., stage. Since the staging system itself was originally designed for the purpose of separating prognostically different groups of patients, prognostic factors should be considered vis-à-vis each stage. Although the present staging system for lung carcinoma [3, 11, 25] has been widely accepted, some previous studies used different staging systems [2] which complicate analysis. Besides the TNM classification by anatomic extent of disease, an attempt to include the clinical phenomena of patients into the staging system was also made. Feinstein and Wells [8] demonstrated that the composite "clinical severity stages" had crucial prognostic distinctions that cannot be identified with TNM staging alone. They recommended using clinical severity and TNM together for estimating prognosis, because they are independently important. Although not widely used as yet, this approach points to an important direction in this field.

Published data on prognostic factors in lung carcinoma have been based on patient populations with different tumour types and different stages. The variables selected for analysis have varied from one study to another. Published data, therefore, must be interpreted carefully.

Non-Small-Cell Lung Carcinoma

NSCLC accounts for approximately 70%–80% of all lung carcinomas. Surgical resection for patients with stage I and II NSCLC yields an acceptable clinical outcome, whereas patients with stage IV are treated mainly with systemic chemotherapy. The treatment of stage III NSCLC patients is still controversial, and new approaches of combined modality treatment such as induction systemic chemotherapy with or without radiation followed by surgical resection are under evaluation.

Stages I and II

Since surgical resection for stage I and II NSCLC patients is the treatment of choice, the analysis for this category is mainly based on resected cases. In this relatively early group, several factors have been recognized to have a significant impact on survival (Table 1) [10, 15, 23, 41].

Tumour-Related Factors

The T and N category still have great prognostic significance in these stages, although Ichinose failed to demonstrate the prognostic difference between T1 and T2 groups by multivariate analysis in resected stage I NSCLC tumours [15]. The significance of histology is controversial: Gail et al. [10] and Mountain et al. [26] showed a significantly better prognosis for squamous cell carcinoma, whereas in other analyses no difference could be identified [27, 28, 50]. Special histological types such as large cell carcinoma [23] and solid carcinoma with mucus formation [41] were significant predictors for worse survival. Although DNA ploidy has been assessed by many researchers in this category, its prognostic significance is still controversial (Table 2) [4, 5, 15, 36, 46]. Beside the factors mentioned above, grade of histological differentiation [15], giant cell component [23] and plasma cell infiltration [23] were all identified as adverse prognostic factors by multivariate analyses.

Patient-Related Factors

In stage I and II NSCLC, performance status (PS), which was significant also in advanced disease, was an important factor. Gail et al. [10] demonstrated that postoperative infection was also significant.

Summary

In this relatively early localized disease, T and N factors and PS are of major prognostic significance. DNA ploidy and special pathological features have possible significance; further investigation is required.

Table 1. Prognostic factors of independent significance for survival in stages I and II non-small-cell lung carcinoma (NSCLC)

Reference	Staging system[a]	Patients (n)	T	N	Performance status	Histological type	Postoperative infection	Miscellaneous
Gail et al. [10]	AJCC	392	+	+	+	+ (ad vs. sq)	+	–
Lipford et al. [23]	AJCC	173	+	+	+	+ (lg)	n.t.	Giant cell component, plasma cell infiltration
Sorensen [41]	UICC/AJCC	137	+	+	n.t.	+ (sc)	n.t.	–
Ichinose et al. [15]	UICC/AJCC	151	–	n.t.	n.t.	n.t.	n.t.	Differentiation, DNA ploidy

+, Statistically significant; –, not statistically significant; n.t., not tested; ad, adenocarcinoma; sq, squamous cell carcinoma; lg, large cell carcinoma; sc, solid carcinoma with mucus formation.

[a] AJCC, former American Joint Committee on Cancer (AJCC) TNM staging system [2]; UICC, present International Union Against Cancer (UICC)/AJCC TNM staging system [3,11,25].

Table 2. DNA aneuploidy as a prognostic factor in early-stage non-small-cell lung carcinoma (NSCLC)

Reference	Patients (n)	Staging system[b]	Histological type	Type of analysis	Significance
Cibas et al. [5]	93	AJCC	ad	Univariate	–
Van Bodegom et al. [46]	52	UICC/AJCC	sq	Univariate	+
Schmidt et al. [36][a]	102	UICC/AJCC	NSCLC	Multivariate	–
Asamura et al. [4][a]	46	UICC/AJCC	ad	Univariate	+
Ichinose et al. [15]	151	UICC/AJCC	NSCLC	Multivariate	–

+, Statistically significant; –, not statistically significant; ad, adenocarcinoma; sq, squamous cell carcinoma.
[a] End point is postoperative recurrence.
[b] AJCC, former American Joint Committee on Cancer (AJCC) TNM staging system [2]; UICC/AJCC, present International Union Against Cancer (UICC)/AJCC TNM staging system [3,11,25].

Stages III and IV

This group of patients is treated primarily with non-surgical modalities such as systemic chemotherapy and radiation, but without substantial success. Patients with stage IIIA disease can be cured by surgical resection alone [27, 28]. The general results of the multivariate analysis on variables for independent prediction of prognosis are presented in Table 3 [6, 7, 9, 20, 24, 29, 33, 35, 37, 41, 44].

Tumour-Related Factors

In this advanced disease, stage (limited/extensive or TNM staging system) and metastasis to various organs such as bone, liver, brain, etc. are independent prognostic factors.

Patient-Related Factors

Patient-related factors include age, gender, PS and weight loss. Laboratory data such as serum albumin, white cell count and lactate dehydrogenase (LDH) level are also included in this category. PS was uniformly mentioned in all but one study, and its importance is well recognized. Female gender is a favourable predictor for survival both in advanced NSCLC as well as SCLC.

Treatment-Related Factors

The impact of therapeutic response on survival generally has not been shown to be significant. The study by O'Connell is one of the few which demonstrated its significance [29]. On the other hand, Shinkai et al. [37] demonstrated that

Table 3. Prognostic factors of independent significance for survival in advanced non-small-cell lung carcinoma (NSCLC)

Reference	Patients (n)	PS	Gender	Stage	Age	Weight loss	Histology	Metastasis						Albumin	LDH	WBC
								Brain	Bone	Liver	Sub-cutaneous	Supra-clavicular lung	Contralateral lung			
Stanley et al. [44]	5138	+	n.t.	+	–	+	–	–	–	–	–	–	–	n.t.	n.t.	n.t.
Lanzotti et al. [20]	316	+	–	+	+	+	–	+	+	+	–	+	+	n.t.	n.t.	n.t.
Miller et al. [24]	452	+	+	+	–	n.t.	n.t.	–	–	–	n.t.	n.t.	n.t.	n.t.	n.t.	n.t.
Finkelstein et al. [9]	893	+	+	n.t.	–	+	+	n.t.	+	+	+	–	–	n.t.	n.t.	n.t.
Einhorn et al. [6]	124	+	n.t.	–	n.t.	–	–	n.t.	n.t.	n.t.	n.t.	–	n.t.	n.t.	n.t.	n.t.
Evans et al. [7]	90	–	n.t.	n.t.	n.t.	+	n.t.	n.t.	n.t.	+	n.t.	n.t.	n.t.	+	+	n.t.
O'Connell et al. [29]	378	+	+	n.t.	–	–	–	–	+	–	n.t.	n.t.	n.t.	n.t.	+	n.t.
Rapp et al. [33]	137	+	–	–	–	+	+	n.t.	n.t.	n.t.	n.t.	n.t.	n.t.	n.t.	–	n.t.
Sakurai et al. [35]	190	+	+	n.t.	–	n.t.	–	–	–	–	n.t.	n.t.	n.t.	n.t.	n.t.	n.t.
Sorensen [41]	259	+	–	–	–	–	n.t.	–	–	+	n.t.	n.t.	n.t.	n.t.	+	+

+, Statistically significant; –, not statistically significant; n.t., not tested; PS, performance status; LDH, lactate dehydrogenase; WBC, white blood cell count.

the treatment period, instead of a chemotherapeutic effect, was a significant factor.

A Prognostic Factor Index

An attempt to define special prognostic groups has been made based on the results of a multivariate analysis on 192 advanced NSCLC patients treated with cisplatin-containing chemotherapy [38]. Based on the results that the number of metastatic sites, gender, serum albumen levels, PS, and LDH were independent prognostic factors, an index was calculated to define prognostic groupings for survival. Shinkai et al. [38] have shown that this particular regression model can aid in the design and analysis of new treatment strategies and may be useful for indirect comparisons of different studies carried out in similar patient populations.

Summary

In this advanced disease, PS, stage (extent of disease) and weight loss are of definite prognostic significance, although there are a few contradictory results. Gender and LDH level might be of significance. On the other hand, age and histology probably do not have prognostic importance.

Small Cell Lung Carcinoma

SCLC is different from other types of lung carcinoma in several pathobiological and clinical features. It has a large growth fraction, grows rapidly and is usually widely disseminated at diagnosis. In contrast to NSCLC, SCLC is very responsive to radiation and single-agent or combination chemotherapy, to which over two thirds of patients, including those with advanced disease, can achieve at least a partial response. However, even with optimum treatment fewer than 10% of patients are alive after 5 years.

Several studies have been made to clarify the independent factors which are closely associated with the prognosis of SCLC patients (Table 4) (H. Bülzebruck and P. Drings, personal communication) [1, 16, 31, 37, 42, 43, 48].

Tumour-Related Factors

The extent of disease, number of metastatic sites and metastasis to brain, liver and bone are shown to be significant. Although the extent of disease (limited/ extensive disease, LD/ED, classification) is important for selection of the optimal treatment for a given patient and allocation in a randomized trial for SCLC, three of seven studies failed to demonstrate its prognostic significance. This might be partly because the LD/ED classification system lacks stringency and may not reflect the tumour burden accurately.

Table 4. Prognostic factors of independent significance for survival in small cell lung carcinoma (SCLC)

Reference	PS	Extent of disease	Gender	Age	Weight loss	Number of metastatic sites	Metastasis			Chemotherapeutic effect
							Brain	Liver	Bone	
Souhami et al. [42]	+	+	–	–	–	n.t.	n.t.	n.t.	n.t.	n.t.
Osterlind and Anderson [31]	+	+	+	+	–	–	–	–	n.t.	n.t.
Vincent et al. [48]	+	+	–	–	n.t.	n.t.	n.t.	+	–	n.t.
Johnson et al. [16]	+	–	+	–	n.t.	+	–	–	–	n.t.
Shinkai et al. [38]	+	–	–	+	n.t.	n.t.	–	–	–	+
Spiegelman et al. [43]	+	+	+	+(LD)	n.t.	+(ED)	n.t.	n.t.	n.t.	n.t.
Albain et al. [1]	+(LD)	+	+(LD)	+(LD) –(ED)	–	+(ED)	+	–	–	+
Bülzebruck and Drings, personal communication	+	–	–	+	n.t.	+	+	–	+	+

+, Statistically significant; –, not statistically significant; n.t., not tested; PS, performance status; LD, limited disease; ED, extensive disease.

Patient-Related Factors

PS of the patient was a significant factor in every study, and this is one of the most important predictors of patient survival. Therefore, PS should be carefully examined prior to treatment. The Karnofsky PS (KPS) [18] and the Eastern Cooperative Oncology Group (ECOG) scales [54] are the most widely used methods of assessing functional status in cancer patients. Most of the studies on prognostic factors in lung cancer have used one of them. Both performance scales were demonstrated to be highly correlated [30]. Therefore, in interpreting the results of analyses on the prognostic significance of PS, the scale used is not a problem. On the other hand, it is difficult to translate scores from one scale to another, especially in the lower PS range where a wide spread is observed [47]. Female gender and younger age are both favourable predictors for survival, although not all studies demonstrated their significance. A normal LDH level was also a significant independent prognostic factor both in LD and ED disease in the SWOG (Southwest Oncology Group) study data base [1].

Treatment-Related Factors

According to Shinkai and Bülzebruck, the effect of chemotherapy was a significant independent prognostic factor for survival (H. Bülzebruck and P. Drings, personal communication) [37]. Lenhard suggested that the rate of regression following initial chemotherapy predicted survival [22].

Prognostic Staging System

Sagman et al. [34] have made a prognostic classification based on 614 SCLC patients; multivariate analysis revealed the following significant prognostic factors: plasma LDH and mediastinal spread in LD, PS, number of metastatic sites, bone metastasis, brain metastasis and platelet count in ED. They introduced the RECPAM (Recursive Partition and Amalgamation Algorithm Model) to identify four distinct risk groups defined in a classification tree by the following eight attributes: disease extent, PS, serum alkaline phosphatase, serum LDH, mediastinal spread, gender, WBC count and liver metastasis. They have shown a better prognostic categorization of SCLC patients by the RECPAM classification than by conventional Cox regression techniques. The four prognostic groups had median survival times of 59, 49, 35 and 24 weeks, respectively ($p < 0.0001$).

Summary

In this unique histological category, PS and extent of disease have definite prognostic importance. Gender, age and number of metastatic sites are probably important.

Miscellaneous Factors Under Investigation

With the accumulation of recent knowledge about biological features of lung carcinoma, numerous attempts to find new prognostic factors are being made. Oncogenes and their products are of possible prognostic significance, since they are involved in cancerous proliferation or in carcinogenesis itself. However, many of these factors still require further multivariate investigation to define whether they have prognostic value. Some of the new factors are presented below.

ras Gene

A k-*ras* point mutation was demonstrated in 15%–30% of adenocarcinomas of the lung [19, 40, 45] and was determined to be an adverse prognostic factor for survival in adenocarcinoma of the lung.

p53 Gene

Tumour suppressor gene p53 is located on the short arm of chromosome 17 and is frequently mutated in lung carcinoma. The accumulation of p53 protein was shown to be an unfavourable predictor for survival in NSCLC [13, 32]. Horio et al. [14] demonstrated its prognostic significance by multivariate analysis on 71 NSCLC cancer patients. However, another study failed to demonstrate this effect [49].

Blood Group Antigens

The deletion of blood group antigens and the expression of its precursor antigen I (Ma) have been demonstrated in lung carcinoma [12]. Lee et al. [21] revealed that patients with loss of antigen A in the tumour had significantly worse prognosis than those without this loss.

Blood Coagulation Test

In LD NSCLC and ED SCLC, an activated partial thromboplastin time was a significant independent predictor of survival on multivariate analysis [52].

Nucleolar Organizer Regions

Nucleolar organizer regions (NORs) are loops of DNA which occur in the nucleoli of cells and possess ribosomal RNA genes. The numbers and/or configurations of NORs are speculated to be associated with the proliferative activity of tumour cells. Kaneko et al. [17] demonstrated that the survival rate of patients with less than 5.07 NORs was significantly better than those with 5.07 and more in NSCLC ($p < 0.001$).

Cell Proliferation-Related Factors

Some of the factors which are closely related to tumour cell proliferation have been demonstrated immunohistochemically using specific antibodies. Included in this category are bromodeoxyuridine (BrdU) [53], proliferating cell nuclear antigen (PCNA), DNA polymerase alpha and Ki-67 [39]. Although they may be of prognostic significance, further investigation is needed.

References

1. Albain KS, Crowley JJ, LeBlanc M, Livingston RB (1990) Determinants of improved outcome in small-cell lung cancer: an analysis of the 2580-patient Southwest Oncology Group data base. J Clin Oncol 8: 1563–1574
2. American Joint Committee for Cancer Staging and End-Results Reporting (1978) Manual for staging of cancer 1978. American Joint Committee, Chicago
3. American Joint Committee on Cancer (AJCC) (1992) Manual for staging of cancer. 4th edn. (Beahrs OH, Henson DE, Hutter RVP, Kennedy BJ, eds). Lippincott, Philadelphia
4. Asamura H, Nakajima T, Mukai K, Shimosato Y (1991) Nuclear DNA content by cytofluorometry of stage I adenocarcinoma of the lung in relation to postoperative recurrence. Chest 96: 312–318
5. Cibas ES, Melamed MR, Zaman MB, Kimmel M (1988) The effect of tumour size and tumour cell DNA content on the survival of patients with stage I adenocarcinoma of the lung. Cancer 63: 1552–1556
6. Einhorn LH, Lohrer PJ, Williams SD, Meyers S, Gabrys T, Nottan SR, Woodburn R, Drasga R, Songer I, Fisher W, Stephens D, Hui S (1986) Random prospective study of vindesine versus vindesine plus high-dose cisplatin versus vindesine plus cisplatin plus mitomycin C in advanced non-small-cell lung cancer. J Clin Oncol 4: 1037–1043
7. Evans WK, Nikon DW, Dally JM, Ellen SS, Gardner L, Wolfe E, Shepherd FA, Feld R, Gralla R, Fine S, Chimney N, Jeejeebhoy KH, Heymsfield S, Hoffman FA (1987) A randomized study of oral nutritional support versus ad lib nutritional intake during chemotherapy for advanced colorectal and non-small-cell lung cancer. J Clin Oncol 5: 113–124
8. Feinstein AR, Wells CK (1986) A clinical-severity staging system for patients with lung cancer. Medicine 69: 1–33
9. Finkelstein DM, Eittinger DS, Ruckedschel JC (1986) Long term survivors in metastatic non-small-cell lung cancer: an Eastern Cooperative Oncology Group study. J Clin Oncol 4: 702–709
10. Gail MH, Eagan RT, Feld R, Ginsberg R, Goodell B, Hill L, Holmes CE, Lukeman JM, Mountain CF, Olkham RK, Pearson FG, Wright PW, Lake WH (1984) Prognostic factors in patients with resected stage I non-small cell lung cancer: a report from the Lung Cancer Study Group. Cancer 54: 1802–1813
11. Hermanek P, Sobin LH (eds) (1992) UICC TNM classification on malignant tumours. 4th edn, 2nd revision 1992. Springer, Berlin Heidelberg New York
12. Hirohashi S, Ino Y, Kodama T, Shimosato Y (1984) Distribution of blood group antigens A, B, H, and I (Ma) in mucus-producing adenocarcinoma of human lung. J Natl Cancer Inst 72: 1299–1305
13. Hiyoshi H, Matsuno Y, Kato H, Shimosato Y, Hirohashi S (1992) Clinicopathological significance of nuclear accumulation of tumour suppressor gene p53 product in primary lung cancer. Jpn J Cancer Res 83: 101–106
14. Horio Y, Takahashi T, Kuroishi T, Hibi K, Suyama M, Niimi T, Shimokata K, Yamakawa K, Nakamura Y, Ueda R (1993) Prognostic significance of p53 mutations and 3p deletions in primary resected non-small cell lung cancer. Cancer Res 53: 1–4
15. Ichinose Y, Hara N, Ohta M, Yano T, Maeda K, Asoh H, Katsuda Y (1993) Is T factor of the TNM staging system a predominant prognostic factor in pathologic factor analysis of 151 patients. J Thorac Cardiovasc Surg 106: 90–94
16. Johnson BE, Steinberg SM, Phelps R, Edison M, Veach SR, Ihde DC (1988) Female patients with small cell lung cancer live longer than male patients. Am J Med 85: 194–196

17. Kaneko S, Ishida T, Sugio K, Yokoyama H, Sugimachi K (1991) Nucleolar organizer regions as a prognostic indication for stage I non-small cell lung cancer. Cancer Res 51: 4008–4011
18. Karnofsky DA, Abelmann WH, Craver LF, Burchenal JH (1948) The use of nitrogen mustards in the palliative treatment of cancer. Cancer 1: 634–656
19. Kobayashi T, Tsuda H, Noguchi M (1990) Association of point mutation in c-Ki-ras oncogene in lung adenocarcinoma with particular reference to cytologic subtypes. Cancer 66: 289–294
20. Lanzotte VJ, Thomas DR, Boyle LE, Smith TL, Gehan EA, Samuels MS (1977) Survival with inoperable lung cancer. An integration of prognostic variables based on simple clinical criteria. Cancer 39: 303–313
21. Lee JS, Ro Jy, Sahin AA, Hong WK, Brown BW, Mountain CF, Hittelman WN (1991) Expression of blood-group antigen A. A favorable prognostic factor in non-small cell lung cancer. N Engl J Med 324: 1084–1090
22. Lenhard RE, Woo KB, Abeloff MD (1983) Predictive value of regression rate following chemotherapy of small cell carcinoma of the lung. Cancer Res 43: 3013–3017
23. Lipford EH, Sears DL, Eggleston JC, Moore GW, Lillemore KD, Baker RR (1984) Prognostic factors in surgically resected limited-stage, non-small-cell carcinoma of the lung. Am J Surg Pathol 8: 357–365
24. Miller TP, Chen TT, Coltman CA, O'Bryan RM, Vance RB, Weiss GB, Fletcher WS, Stephens RI, Livingston RB (1986) Effect of alternation combination chemotherapy on survival of ambulatory patients with metastatic large-cell and adenocarcinoma of the lung. A Southwest Oncology Group Study. J Clin Oncol 4: 1037–1043
25. Mountain CF (1986) A new international staging system for lung cancer. Chest 89 [Suppl]: 225s–233s
26. Mountain CF, Lukeman JM, Hammar SP, Chamberlain DW, Coulsen SP, Page DL, Victor TA, Weiland LH, and the Lung Cancer Study Group Pathology Committee (1987) Lung cancer classification: the relationship of disease extent and cell type to survival in a clinical trial population. J Surg Oncol 35: 147–156
27. Naruke T, Goya T, Tsuchiya R, Suemasu K (1988).Prognosis and survival in resected lung carcinoma based on the new international staging system. J Thorac Cardiovasc Surg 96: 440–447
28. Naruke T, Goya T, Tsuchiya R, Suemasu K (1988) The importance of surgery to non-small cell carcinoma of lung with mediastinal lymph node metastasis. Ann Thorac Surg 46: 603–610
29. O'Connell JP, Kris MG, Gralla RJ, Groshen S, Trust A, Fiore JJ, Kelsen DP, Heelan RT, Golby RB (1986) Frequency and prognostic importance of pretreatment clinical characteristics in patients with advanced non-small-cell lung cancer treated with combination chemotherapy. J Clin Oncol 4: 1604–1614
30. Orr ST, Aisner J (1986) Performance status assessment among oncology patients: a review. Cancer Treat Rep 70: 1423–1429
31. Osterlind K, Anderson PK (1986) Prognostic factors in small cell lung cancer: multivariate model based on 788 patients treated with chemotherapy with or without irradiation. Cancer Res 46: 4189–4194
32. Quinlan DC, Davidson AG, Summers CL, Warden HE, Doshi HM (1992) Accumulation of p53 protein correlates with a poor prognosis in human lung cancer. Cancer Res 52: 4828–4831
33. Rapp E, Pater JL, Willan A, Cormier Y, Murray N, Evans WK, Hodson DI, Clark DA, Feld R, Arnold AM, Ayoub JI, Wilson KS, Latreille J, Wierzbicki FR, Hill DP (1988) Chemotherapy can prolong survival in patients with advanced non-small-cell lung cancer. Report of a Canadian multicenter randomized trial. J Clin Oncol 6: 633–641
34. Sagman U, Maki E, Evans WK, Shepherd FA, Sculier JP, Haddad R, Payne D, Pringle JF, Yeoh JL, Ciampi A, DeBoer G, McKinney S, Ginsberg R, Feld R (1991). Small-cell carcinoma of the lung: derivation of a prognostic staging system. J Clin Oncol 9: 1639–1649
35. Sakurai M, Shinkai T, Eguchi K, Sasaki Y, Tamura T, Miura K, Fujiwara Y, Otsu A, Horiuchi N, Nakano H, Nakagawa K, Hong WS, Saijo N (1987) Prognostic factors in non-small cell lung cancer: multiregression analysis in the National Cancer Center Hospital (Japan). J Cancer Res Clin Oncol 113: 563–566
36. Schmidt RA, Rusch VW, Piantadosi S (1992) A flow cytometric study of non-small cell lung cancer classified as T1N0. Cancer 69: 78–85
37. Shinkai T, Sakurai M, Eguchi K, Sasaki Y, Tamura T, Fujiwara Y, Fukuda M, Yamada K, Kojima A, Sasaki S, Soejima Y, Akiyama Y, Minato K, Nakagawa K, Ono R, Saijo N (1989) Prognostic factors in small cell lung cancer: multivariate analysis in the National Cancer Center Hospital (Japan). Jpn J Clin Oncol 19: 135–141

38. Shinkai T, Eguchi K, Sasaki Y, Tamura T, Ohe Y, Kojima A, Oshita F, Miya T, Okamoto H, Iemura K, Saijo N (1992) A prognostic-factor index in advanced non-small-cell lung cancer treated with cisplatin-containing combination chemotherapy. Cancer Chemother Pharmacol 30: 1–6

39. Simony J, Pujol JL, Radal M, Ursule E, Michel FB, Pujol H (1990) In situ evaluation of growth fraction determined by monoclonal antibody Ki-67 and ploidy in surgically resected non-small cell lung cancers. Cancer Res 50: 4382–4387

40. Slebos RJC, Kibbelaar RD (1990) K-ras oncogene activation as a prognostic marker in adenocarcinoma of the lung. N Engl J Med 323: 561–565

41. Sorensen JB (1992) Prognosis and prognostic factors in adenocarcinoma of the lung. Dan Med Bull 39: 453–463

42. Souhami RL, Bradbury I, Geddes DM, Spiro SG, Harper PG, Tobias JS (1985) Prognostic significance of laboratory parameters measured at diagnosis in small cell carcinoma of the lung. Cancer Res 45: 2878–2882

43. Spiegelman D, Maurer LH, Ware JH, Perry MC, Chahinian AP, Comis R, Eaton W, Zimmer B, Green M (1989) Prognostic factors in small-cell carcinoma of the lung: an analysis of 1,521 patients. J Clin Oncol 7: 344–354

44. Stanley K, Cox JD, Petrovich Z, Paig C (1981) Patterns of failure in patients with inoperable carcinoma of the lung. Cancer 47: 2725–2729

45. Sugio K, Ishida T, Yokoyama H, Inoue T, Sugimachi K, Sasazuki T (1992) ras gene mutation as a prognostic marker in adenocarcinoma of the human lung without lymph node metastasis. Cancer Res 52: 2903–2906

46. Van Bodegom PC, Baak JPA, Galen CSV, Schipper NW, Wisse-Brekelmans ECM, Vanderschueren RGJRA, Wagenaar SS (1989) The percentage of aneuploid cells is significantly correlated with survival in accurately staged patients with stage I resected squamous cell lung cancer and long-term follow up. Cancer 63: 143–147

47. Verger E, Salamero M, Conill C (1992) Can Karnofsky performance status be transformed to the Eastern Cooperative Oncology Group scoring scale and vice versa? Eur J Cancer 28A: 1328–1330

48. Vincent MD, Ashley SE, Smith IE (1987) Prognostic factors in small cell lung cancer: a simple prognostic index is better than conventional staging. Eur J Cancer Clin Oncol 23: 1589–1599

49. Volm M, Efferth T, Mattern J (1992) Oncoprotein (c-myc, c-erbB1, c-ercB2, c-fos) and suppressor gene product (p53) expression in squamous cell carcinomas of the lung: clinical and biological correlations. Anticancer Res 12: 11–20

50. Williams DE, Pairolero PC, Davis CS, Bernatz PE, Payne WS, Taylor WF, Uhlenhopp MA, Fontana RS (1981) Survival of patients surgically treated for stage I lung cancer. J Thorac Cardiovasc Surg 82: 70–76

51. World Health Organization (1981) Histological typing of lung tumours, 2nd edn. World Health Organization, Geneva, pp.1–41

52. Wojtukiewicz MZ, Zacharski LR, Moritz TE, Hur K, Edwards RL, Rickles FR (1992) Prognostic significance of blood coagulation tests in carcinoma of the lung and colon. Blood Coagul Fibrinolysis 3: 429–437

53. Yoshida K, Morinaga S, Shimosato Y, Hayata Y (1989) A cell kinetic study of pulmonary adenocarcinoma by an immunoperoxidase procedure after bromodeoxyuridine labeling. Cancer 64: 2284–2291

54. Zubrod CG, Schneiderman M, Frei E et al (1960) Appraisal of methods for the study of chemotherapy of cancer in man: comparative therapeutic trial of nitrogen mustard and triethylene thiophosphoramide. J Chron Dis 11: 7–33

14 Osteosarcoma

H. Fukuma

A revolutionary change in the prognosis of resectable osteosarcoma was accomplished in the 1970s with the introduction of multimodal treatment. While unresectable osteosarcoma is still not being cured, in patients treated by resective surgery and chemotherapy the 5-year disease-free survival rates have increased from 10%–20% to 60%–80%.

For patients treated using the modern multimodal concept, there are many prognostic factors considered significant in relation to survival; these factors are tumour related, patient related, and treatment related. A number of published papers have attempted to identify factors that may be significant in terms of prognosis for osteosarcoma. This review is based on published reports on osteosarcoma and on data from nationwide bone tumour registration in Japan, namely 814 patients with osteosarcoma treated with surgery and chemotherapy between 1980 and 1989.

In the search for prognostic indicators, nine variables were studied: sex, age, location of primary tumour, size of tumour, extent of tumour, regional lymph node metastasis, distant metastasis at diagnosis, serum level of alkaline phosphatase and mitotic rate. The prognostic significance of each variable was estimated by its ratio of risks as determined by multivariate analysis (Table 1). This study shows that the most important prognostic factors are distant metastasis, serum level of alkaline phosphatase, regional lymph node metastasis and tumour size.

Tumour-Related Factors

Primary Site

The primary site of the tumour has been recognized as an important prognostic factor in patients with osteosarcoma. The Memorial Hospital Group (USA) identified the location of the primary lesion as a significant predictor of survival: femoral lesions (both proximal and distal) were associated with a poorer outcome than either humeral or tibial lesions [6, 13]. Our results showed that the primary location was not significant in terms of survival and it ranked eighth in the ratio of risks (Table 1).

Table 1. Prognostic factors in osteosarcoma: unpublished results of Japanese Bone Tumour Registration ($n = 814$)

Patient characteristics (prognostic factors)	Regression coefficient (β)	Estimated standard error of β	β/STD error (t statistic)	Relative risk		Ratio of risks
				Favourable	Unfavourable	
Sex	−0.070	0.179	−0.390	Female: 0.958	Male: 1.027	1.072
Age	0.296	0.162	1.827	< 9 years: 0.705	> 20 years: 1.275	1.807
Location	−0.029	0.075	−0.388	Others: 0.913	Femur: 1.026	1.124
Tumour size	0.264	0.112	2.347	< 5cm: 0.638	> 15 cm: 1.408	2.205
Tumour extent (T)	0.125	0.389	0.322	T1: 0.890	T2: 1.008	1.133
SAP	0.287	0.090	3.179	< × 1.25: 0.683	> × 10: 2.156	3.157
Regional nodes (N)	1.097	1.160	0.945	−: 0.985	+: 2.948	2.994
Distant metastasis	2.192	0.446	4.918	−: 0.721	+: 6.461	8.958
Mitotic rate	0.363	0.109	3.325	0: 0.536	> 10: 1.593	2.972

SAP, serum alkaline phosphatase.

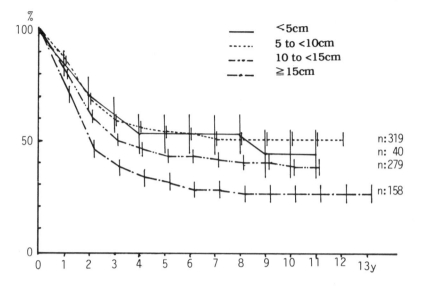

Fig. 1. Observed survival rate of osteosarcoma by tumour size. Difference between 15 cm or more and other groups significant ($p < 0.01$)

Tumour Size

Tumour size is also an important prognostic factor. Quintana et al. reported that the rate of 6-year relapse-free survival was 73.6% for those with small tumours (those measuring less than 100 cm^2) and 33.3% for those with large tumours [15]. Petrilli et al. indicated the highest survival was among women with tumours smaller than 15 cm in stage IIB osteosarcoma [14]. Our multivariate analysis of prognostic factors has shown that tumour size is an important prognostic factor: the survival rate for patients with tumours of 15 cm or more in size is significantly poorer than those with tumours of less than 15 cm (Fig. 1).

Extent of Tumour

Tumour extent has been considered an important prognostic factor in patients with osteosarcoma. Wang et al. [18] reported that osteosarcoma of long bones was classified into four stages: in stage A, the tumour is confined within the marrow cavity; in stage B, the tumour has perforated the bone cortex; in stage C, the tumour has involved the contiguous joint cartilage; and in stage D, the tumour has metastasized to the lung. Only patients in groups A and B could be expected to survive for 5 years. Our study has shown there is no significant difference in survival rate between the T1 (within cortex) (International Union Against Cancer, UICC) and the T2 group (beyond cortex) [7] (Table 1).

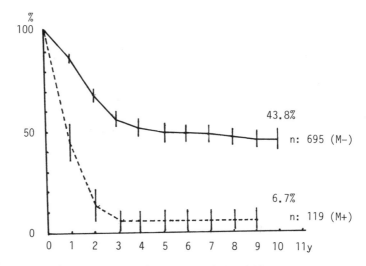

Fig. 2. Observed survival rate of osteosarcoma by distant metastasis ($p < 0.01$)

Regional Lymph Node Metastasis

Multivariate analysis in our study indicated that regional lymph node metastasis ranked third in the ratio of risks and was an important prognostic factor (Table 1). However, lymph node metastasis is very rare, occurring in only 1.4% of our cases.

Distant Metastasis

Distant metastasis at diagnosis provides the most negative prognostic factor in patients with osteosarcoma [12]. Meyers et al. reported that the 5-year survival rate of patients with osteosarcoma who presented with clinically detectable metastasis was only 11%, with a median survival of 20 months [12]. Our multivariate analysis has shown that distant metastasis ranks the highest in the ratio of risks and is associated with the poorest survival rate (Fig. 2).

Mitotic Rate

The maximal mitotic count per high power field (x200) was classified into four grades in our study: grade 1, 0; grade 2, 1–4; grade 3, 5–9; and grade 4, 10 or more. The results of this study show that mitotic rate ranks fourth in the ratio of risks and that the survival rate for patients with grade 4 was worse than that of other groups (Fig. 3).

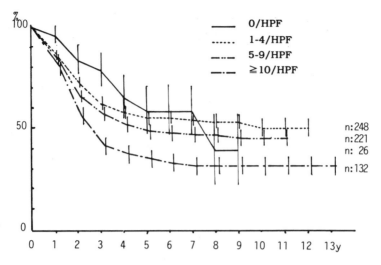

Fig. 3. Observed survival rate of osteosarcoma by mitotic rate. Difference between 10 or more/HPF and other groups statistically significant ($p < 0.05$)

Patient-Related Factors

Age

Bentzen et al. reported that patients approximately 25–30 years of age were associated with an especially good prognosis. The prognosis worsened with advancing age. Patients aged between 5 and less than 25 years had significantly poorer prognoses than those aged 25–30 years [3]. Delepine et al. showed that the worst prognostic factor was young age: 5-year disease-free survival for patients 15-years old or younger was 30%, while for those over 15 years the disease-free survival rate was 85%. These patients were treated during the period from 1978 to 1982 [5]. Our study showed that overall survival of patients under 9 years was worse than for those over 20 years; however, age ranked sixth in the ratio of risks (Table 1). It seemed that age was no longer a negative prognostic factor when patients with osteosarcoma were treated with intensive adjuvant chemotherapy [13].

Serum Alkaline Phosphatase

Some studies reported that an elevated alkaline phosphatase level was associated with a poor prognosis. Bacci et al. mentioned that the percentage of patients suffering relapse was higher in patients with high levels of the enzyme in comparison to patients with moderately elevated values (66.4% versus 47%) [1]. Meyers et al. showed that disease-free survival correlates with serum lactate dehydrogenase, alkaline phosphatase, primary tumour site, race and histological response to preoperative chemotherapy [13]. Our multivariate analysis showed that the alkaline phosphatase level ranked second in the ratio of risks. According to the value of alkaline phosphatase, patients were classified into five groups: group 1, serum alkaline phosphatase (SAP) lower than 1.25 times the upper limit of normal value; group 2, 1.25 to less than 2.5 times; group 3, 2.5 to less than five times; group 4, five to less than ten times; and group 5, ten times or more the upper limit. The survival rate of each group is shown in Fig. 4. Reverse correlation was found between survival rate and serum level of alkaline phosphatase.

Lactate Dehydrogenase

Meyers et al. and Link et al. revealed that in univariate analysis elevation of the serum lactate dehydrogenase (LDH) at diagnosis was the most adverse prognostic factor [10, 13].

Treatment-Related Factors

Local Control

The Memorial Hospital Group indicated that local control of the tumour was one of the most significant predictors of survival [6], and Bauer et al. reported that local tumour control was the most important prognostic factor [2].

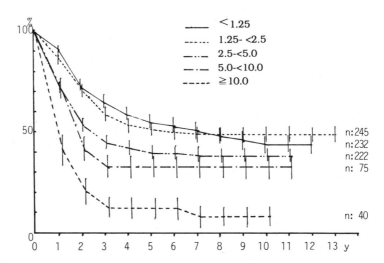

Fig. 4. Observed survival rate of osteosarcoma by value of alkaline phosphatase (multiples of upper limit of normal value). Difference between 10.0 or more and other groups statistically significant ($p < 0.01$)

Histological Tumour Response
(Treatment-Caused Tumour Regression)

Several papers have revealed that the degree of tumour regression following preoperative chemotherapy in the primary tumour was a major prognostic factor. Quintana et al. reported that the 6-year relapse-free survival rate was higher for good responders than for poor ones [15]. The Memorial Hospital Group reported that disease-free survival correlated with the histological response to preoperative chemotherapy [6, 13]. Honegger et al. showed that patients with 80%–100% tumour necrosis had a 5-year disease-free survival rate of 81% versus 44% for patients with necrosis of less than 80% [8]. Hudson et al. reported that with increasing tumour regression, the frequency of pulmonary metastasis was reduced [9]. Raymond et al. revealed that the percentage of tumour necrosis was found to be the most significant prognostic factor and that 90% or greater tumour necrosis related to high, continuous disease-free survival [16]. Davis et al. [4] reported that the most important prognostic variable for patients with osteosarcoma of the extremity was tumour necrosis following preoperative chemotherapy.

Miscellaneous

Several other prognostic factors have been reported for patients with osteosarcoma. These include DNA pattern [11], histological subtype [3], symptom duration [17] and allele loss on chromosome 17p [19]. Further investigation is required.

Summary

Distant metastasis at diagnosis is the most negative prognostic factor in osteosarcoma. Several factors, including tumour size, SAP, LDH, regional lymph node metastasis and post-chemotherapy tumour necrosis, have been found to exert significant influence on the outcome of osteosarcoma patients. The degree of histological response to preoperative chemotherapy in particular has been recognized as the most powerful predictor of disease-free survival. Chemosensitivity cannot be determined at the time of diagnosis. New techniques to identify those patients who will respond poorly to chemotherapy are needed.

References

1. Bacci G, Picci P, Ferrari S, Orlandi M, Ruggieri P, Casadei R, Ferraro A,Biagini R, Battistini A (1993) Prognostic significance of serum alkaline phosphatase measurements in patients with osteosarcoma treated with adjuvant or neoadjuvant chemotherapy. Cancer 71: 1224–1230

2. Bauer HC, Kreicbergs A, Silfversward C (1989) Prognostication including DNA analysis in osteosarcoma. Acta Orthop Scand 60: 353–360
3. Bentzen SM, Poulsen HS, Kaae S, Jensen OM, Johansen H, Mouridsen HT, Daugaard S, Arnoldi C (1988) Prognostic factors in osteosarcomas. A regression analysis. Cancer 62: 194–202
4. Davis AM, Bell RS, Goodwin PJ (1994) Prognostic factors in osteosarcoma: a critical review. J Clin Oncol 12: 423–431
5. Delepine N, Delepine G, Jasmin C, Desbois JC, Cornille H, Mathe G (1988) Importance of age and methotrexate dosage: prognosis in children and young adults with high-grade osteosarcomas. Biomed Pharmacother 42: 257–262
6. Glasser DB, Lane JM, Huvos AG, Marcove RC, Rosen G (1992) Survival, prognosis, and therapeutic response in osteogenic sarcoma. The Memorial Hospital experience. Cancer 69: 698–708
7. Hermanek P, Sobin LH (eds) (1992) UICC: TNM classification of malignant tumours, 4th edn, 2nd rev. Springer, Berlin Heidelberg New York
8. Honegger HP, Cserhati MD, Exner GU, von Hochstetter A, Groscurth P (1991) Zurich experience with preoperative, high dose methotrexate-containing chemotherapy in patients with extremity osteosarcomas (OSA). Ann Oncol 2: 489–494
9. Hudson M, Jaffe MR, Jaffe N, Ayala A, Raymond K, Carrasco H, Wallace S, Murray J, Robertson R (1990) Pediatric osteosarcoma: therapeutic strategies, results, and prognostic factors derived from a 10-year experience. J Clin Oncol 8: 1988–1997
10. Link MP, Goorin AM, Horowitz M, Meyer WH, Belasco J, Baker A, Ayala A, Shuster J (1991) Adjuvant chemotherapy of high-grade osteosarcoma of the extremity. Updated results of the Multi-Institutional Osteosarcoma Study. Clin Orthop 270: 8–14
11. Mankin HJ, Gebhardt MC, Springfield DS, Litwak GJ, Kusazaki K, Rosenberg AE (1991) Flow cytometric studies of human osteosarcoma. Clin Orthop 270: 169–180.
12. Meyers PA, Heller G, Healey JH, Huvos A, Applewhite A, Sun M, LaQuaglia M (1993) Osteogenic sarcoma with clinically detectable metastasis at initial presentation. J Clin Oncol 11: 449–453
13. Meyers PA, Heller G, Healey J, Huvos A, Lane J, Marcove R, Applewhite A, Vlamis V, Rosen G (1992) Chemotherapy for nonmetastatic osteogenetic sarcoma: the Memorial Sloan-Kettering experience. J Clin Oncol 10: 5–15
14. Petrilli S, Penna V, Lopes A, Figueiredo MT, Gentil FC (1991) IIB osteosarcoma. Current management, local control, and survival statistics – Sao Paulo, Brazil. Clin Orthop 270: 60–66
15. Quintana J, Baresi V, DelPozo H, Latorre JJ, Henriquez A, Chamas N, Diaz V, Geldres V, Sepulveda L, Macho L, Dolz G (1991) Intra-arterial cisplatin given prior to surgery in osteosarcoma: grade of necrosis and size of tumor as major prognostic factors. Am J Pediatr Hematol Oncol 13: 269–273
16. Raymond AK, Chawla SP, Carrasco CH, Ayala AG, Fanning CV, Grice B, Armen T, Plager C, Papadopoulos NE, Edeiken J et al (1987) Osteosarcoma chemotherapy effect: a prognostic factor. Semin Diagn Pathol 4: 212–236
17. Taylor WF, Ivins JC, Unni KK, Beabout JW, Golenzer HJ, Black LE (1989) Prognostic variables in osteosarcoma: a multi-institutional study. J Natl Cancer Inst 81: 21–30
18. Wang D, Wang G (1991) A staging of bone-marrow-derived osteosarcoma of long bones with a 64-cases analysis. Chin Med Sci J 6: 193–196
19. Yamaguchi Y, Toguchida J, Yamamuro T, Kotoura Y, Takada N, Kawaguchi N, Kaneko Y, Nakamura Y, Sasaki SS, Ishizaki K (1992) Allelotype analysis in osteosarcomas: frequent allele loss on 3q, 13q, 17p and 18q. Cancer Res 52: 2419–2423

15 Soft Tissue Sarcomas in Adults

S. Toma, W. Hohenberger, R. Palumbo, O. Schmidt,
G. Nicolò, G. Canavese, and F. Badellino

Soft tissue sarcomas (STS) in adults (age 16 years or more) are a heterogeneous group of malignant tumours showing great variations in histological type and grade, clinical presentation, site and biological behaviour. These tumours are relatively uncommon, and the number of patients treated at an individual institution is usually limited. Furthermore, treatment strategies vary, thus adequate experience with these tumours is restricted to relatively few centres.

As at other tumour sites, the anatomic extent of disease is generally accepted as the most powerful indicator of outcome. However, it has become clear that the histological grade strongly affects prognosis. Thus, in 1977 the AJCC (American Joint Committee on Cancer) staging system [2] added histological grade to size and anatomic extent, and this principle is adhered to by the unified TNM classification and stage grouping of the UICC (International Union Against Cancer) and AJCC now used [6, 22].

Although the UICC/AJCC stage grouping remains a valid system for STS, other prognostic factors may significantly and independently influence prognosis. It is the aim of this contribution to provide an overview of the literature on prognostic factors in STS. Unfortunately, most reports are based on univariate analyses and on limited numbers of patients. Some putative prognostic factors, evident on univariate analysis, are not significant when multivariate analysis is applied. Furthermore, the interpretation of data is difficult because study designs differ or lack exact definitions (e.g., prospective versus retrospective recruitment, treatment for first diagnosis only or recurrent tumours included, R classification, surgery alone versus multimodal treatment and definitions of surgical treatment applied). Therefore, this overview will focus on the results of relatively large studies that used multivariate analysis (Table 1).

Overall Survival

Overall 5-year survival rates of soft tissue sarcomas are at present in the range of 50%–80%. Extreme figures, e.g. 21.5% [15] or 94% [18], may be explained by selection of patients.

Table 1. Multivariate studies on prognosis of soft tissue sarcomas

Authors	Reference	Tumour sites included	Further remarks
Collin et al.	12	Extremities	
Tsujimoto et al.	55	All except mediastinum	
Lack et al.	29	Extremities	
Mandard et al.	32	All except mediastinum and retroperitoneum	
Alvegard et al.	3	Extremities, trunk	High-grade only
Berlin et al.	7	Extremities	
Chang et al.	11	Extremities	Liposarcoma only
El-Jabbour et al.	15	All except retroperitoneum	
Rööser et al.	39	All except mediastinum and retroperitoneum	G3–4 only
Stotter et al.	45	Extremities, trunk	
Jensen et al.	24	All except mediastinum and retroperitoneum	
Serpell et al.	42	Upper extremity	
Ravaud et al.	37	All except mediastinum	
Saddegh et al.	40	Extremity, trunk	
Eeles et al.	13	Head and neck	
Herbert et al.	21	Extremities	
Kraus et al.	28	Head and neck	
Tanabe et al.	51	Extremities	G1 excluded

Not included are studies with less than 50 patients (only first manifestations, not recurrences), insufficient data description, and/or exclusion of more than 30% of patients because of missing data. Tumour site is subdivided into extremities, head and neck, trunk (thoracic and abdominal wall), mediastinum and retroperitoneum.

Patient-Related Factors

Patient-related factors considered are age, gender and symptoms, especially pain in addition to a mass. Table 2 shows that no patient-related factor can be accepted as proven.

In most studies, age did not influence the prognosis of STS in adults. Only four studies showed age as an adverse prognostic factor (with different cut-off points).

Gender had, in a few studies, an independent influence on prognosis (men had a worse prognosis); most studies, however, showed no significant influence of gender on prognosis.

Pain was an independent predictor of poor outcome in the study by Collin et al. 1987 [12]; however, this was not confirmed in three other multivariate studies and was not investigated in most studies.

Table 2. Patient-related factors in the literature

Factor	Significant influence on:		No significant influence
	Overall survival	Disease-free survival only (local and/or distant recurrence)	
Age	7 (continuous) 12 (> 53 years) 24 (> 65 years)	13 (30–50/> 50 years)	3, 11, 15, 29, 37, 40, 42, 45, 55
Gender (male)	15, 29	3, 37	7, 11, 12, 24, 39, 40, 42, 45, 55
Symptoms (pain)	12		7, 11, 24

Only the results of multivariate studies listed in Table 1 are considered; adverse factors are shown in parentheses.

Tumour-Related Factors

Anatomic Extent of Sarcoma

According to general experience, prognosis is influenced by tumour size (Table 3A). This is shown by the data of Collin et al. [12] on 123 patients with STS of the extremities: the 5-year survival rates were 68% for tumours of 5 cm or less, 57% for more than 5–10 cm and 39% for more than 10 cm; the respective 10-year survival rates were 63%, 46% and 33%.

In STS the lungs are the predominant site of metastases. In some tumour types, however, metastases to the regional lymph nodes are also common. From institutions with a high frequency of therapeutic and elective lymph node dissections, regional lymph node metastases have been reported in 46%, 45% and 21% of cases of rhabdomyosarcoma, malignant fibrous histiocytoma and synovial sarcoma, respectively [23]. In epithelioid sarcoma, Enzinger and Weiss [17] observed lymph node involvement in 34%. Regional lymph node metastasis is a strong adverse prognostic factor (Table 3B); 5-year survival rates of 13% [12] are reported compared to about 50% in patients without lymph node metastasis.

Histological Grade

In STS, histological grade is one of the strongest indicators of outcome. In some STS the grade is determined by the histological type and subtype, e.g. alveolar and embryonal rhabdomyosarcoma, pleomorphic liposarcoma or extraskeletal Ewing sarcoma are always high-grade sarcomas and well-differentiated and myxoid liposarcomas are low-grade tumours. Other STS, e.g., fibrosarcoma, malignant fibrous histiocytoma or leiomyosarcoma, may be low-grade or high-grade tumours.

Table 3. Tumour-related prognostic factors in the literature

Factor	Significant influence on:		No significant influence
	Overall survival	Disease-free survival only (local and/or distant recurrence)	
A. Tumour size	11 (> 5 cm) 12 (> 10 cm) 32 (> 5 cm) 39 (> 10 cm) 40 (> 7 cm) 45 (> 10 cm) 51 (> 11 cm)	3 (> 10 cm)	7, 13, 15, 21, 24, 28, 29, 37, 42, 55
B. Regional lymph node metastases (positive)	12		
C. Histologic grade (high-grade)	7, 11, 12, 21, 24, 28, 37, 39, 40, 45, 51	3	13[a], 15[b], 29[b], 32[b], 42[a], 55[b]
D. Depth of tumour (deep)	24,32,37,55	42	7, 11, 12, 40, 45
E. Tumour site			
Extremity vs. head & neck vs. trunk	37 (head & neck, trunk)		15, 55
Extremity: upper vs. lower			7, 21
Head vs. neck	13 (neck)		
Extremity: distal vs. proximal	12 (proximal) 29 (proximal) 42 (distal, flexor side)		11, 24, 40, 45

[a] Grade not significant; however, histological subtype significant.
[b] Tumour necrosis, mitotic index or other components of grade were analyzed separately from grade and were significant.
Only results of multivariate studies listed in Table 1 are considered; adverse factors are shown in parentheses.

There is still no single system for grading STS [17, 58]. Most systems utilize cellularity, pleomorphism, mitotic rate, necrosis and the amount of intercellular substances such as collagen or mucoid material. Sometimes three and sometimes four grades are used, but there is now a trend to employ two groups, namely low grade (G1, 2) and high grade (G3, 4).

Although in the literature different grading systems have been used, the strong independent influence of histological grade on prognosis was found in nearly all multivariate studies (Table 3C). Necrosis and mitotic activity were sometimes analyzed separately and found as independent prognostic factors, but they are mostly evaluated as components of the grading system.

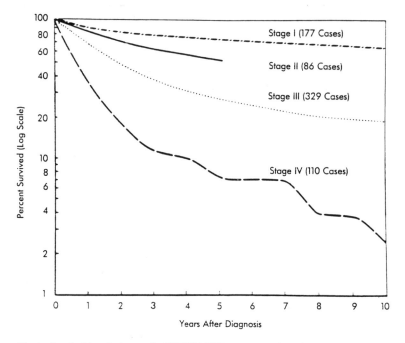

Fig. 1. Survival in relation to the UICC/AJCC stage grouping. From [17]

Stage Grouping

The UICC/AJCC stage grouping uses anatomic extent (TNM) as well as histological grade. A retrospective study of 302 STS collected from 13 different institutions in the United States diagnosed between 1954 and 1969 shows a clear correlation between stage and overall survival (Fig. 1). This can also be demonstrated in the data of the Massachusetts General Hospital regarding 5-year local control and 5-year disease-free survival (Table 4).

Table 4. Prognostic in relation to stage grouping (UICC/AJCC)

Stage	Patients (n)	Five-year local control (%)	Five-year disease-free survival (%)
IA	17	100	100
IB	30	93	88
IIA	40	88	83
IIB	66	85	52
IIIA	33	93	87
IIIB	69	79	39
IVA	3	(100)	(100)
Total	258	88	66

Data of Suit et al. [48] for patients without distant metastasis; all tumour sites except mediastinum and retroperitoneum.

Depth of Tumour

Depth of the tumour is a component of the MSKCC (Memorial Sloan-Kettering Cancer Center) Clinical Staging System for sarcomas [12, 19]. It is described as superficial or deep. Superficial STS are tumours not involving the superficial (investing) fascia; deep STS are located deep to or invading the superficial fascia. All mediastinal and retroperitoneal STS as well as those with invasion of major vessels, nerves or bone are considered deep.

Although not confirmed in all studies, depth of STS can be considered as an independent prognostic factor: deep tumours have a worse prognosis than superficial ones (Table 3D). In a recent report from Japan [20], the 5-year overall survival rate was 32% for retroperitoneal STS ($n = 181$), 43% for deep STS of the periphery (head and neck, thoracic and abdominal wall, extremities; $n = 290$) and 62% for superficial STS of the periphery ($n = 212$).

There are several reports on the adverse prognostic influence of invasion of blood vessel, nerves or bones [3, 12, 29, 32, 39]. However, such findings are associated only with deep STS and there are not sufficient data demonstrating the prognosis of deep STS worsens as a result of invasion of vessels, nerves or bones if the tumour is completely removed.

Tumour Site

Tumour site was investigated only by a limited number of multivariate studies (Table 3E). Nevertheless, general experience shows that retroperitoneal and mediastinal STS have the worst prognosis and that, on the other hand, extremity STS behave better than those of the trunk, head and neck [60]. It should be emphasized that these differences may be explained by differences in depth of tumours.

There are differences on the influence of proximal versus distal site of STS of extremities. According to Yang et al. [60], this is a generally accepted prognostic factor. However, multivariate analyses gave conflicting reports (Table 3E): sometimes no significant influence and sometimes significantly worse results were found for proximal STS, and in one study [42] worse results for distal STS of the upper extremity located on the flexor side were reported. According to one study [13], STS of the neck had a worse prognosis than those of the head.

Further Histological Factors

In a multivariate study of high-grade STS, microscopic invasion of blood or lymphatic vessels was an independent adverse factor for developing distant metastasis [3].

Mast cell infiltration – at least one mast cell per ten high fields (HF) – was demonstrated as a favourable prognostic factor by Ueda et al. [56] (in a multivariate analysis on highly selected patients) and by Katenkamp and Hünerbein [26].

Table 5. Possible biological and molecular prognostic factors

Factor	Reference
Cytometry (DNA ploidy, S-phase fraction, G1-phase fraction)	3[a,b], 41, 44, 61
Ki-67 index	44, 57[a]
Retinoblastoma gene product expression	10, 38, 59
p53 overexpression	27[a], 33, 35, 46
Amplification of c-*myc* oncogene	5
HSP-27 expression	53[a]
Mdr gene overexpression	52

[a] Correlation with prognosis observed.
[b] Further references.

Biological and Molecular Factors

Recent laboratory developments are the source of great interest in the biology and molecular pathology of STS. Some recent findings are listed in Table 5. However, the clinical significance of these findings, especially their putative independent prognostic influence, remains to be established. These biological and molecular factors may in future help in planning therapy, e.g. in the selection of patients for adjuvant treatment or choice of chemotherapy by determination of chemosensitivity in vivo [3, 44].

Treatment-Related Factors

The treatment of STS of the extremities has changed since the introduction of limb-sparing surgery (LSS) in the late 1960s. Amputation is now used for a minority of advanced, mostly complicated tumours. This explains the reported worse results following ablative surgery in comparison with LSS, e.g. 5- and 10-year survival rates of 72% and 65% for LSS ($n = 276$) and 40% and 33% for amputation ($n = 138$) [12] or 5-year survival rates of 60% for LSS ($n = 140$) compared to 13% for amputation ($n = 21$) [56].

Review of the literature with regard to quality of surgical excision is difficult because the definitions of surgical procedures are frequently unclear and terms such as adequate and inadequate or marginal, wide and radical excision (including compartmental resection) [16] are not uniformly used. The classification of resection margins is based sometimes on gross, sometimes on histological findings: frequently "close resection margins" are described without any definition.

According to several univariate studies, the width of excision and tumour-involved resection margins influence the frequency of local recurrences: about 10% after amputation, 15%–40% following wide excision, and 65%–70% after marginal or incomplete excision. Postoperative radiotherapy after tumour excision with limited margins of clearance can reduce the frequency of local recurrences [1, 25, 30, 31, 36, 43].

In some multivariate studies, the width of excision and the margin status showed an influence on local recurrence rates and disease-free survival [7, 37, 45]; in most studies overall survival was also significantly influenced [11, 12, 15, 21, 28, 29, 32, 40, 51]. For example, the data of Collin et al. [12] on 276 STS of the extremities treated by LSS show the following results: 5-year and 10-year survival rates were 76% and 71% for adequate margins, 76% and 68% for marginal margins and 52% and 25% for inadequate margins, respectively.

In optimal surgery of a STS, the surgeon does not see the tumour nor cut through the tumour. The adverse influence of intraoperative tumour violation is recognized by all surgeons; however, relevant data were published only by Tanabe et al. [51]. These authors treated 95 patients with intermediate and high-grade extremity STS by preoperative radiation therapy and LSS. Local recurrences were observed in 40% of patients (four out of ten) with tumour violation compared to 12% (ten out of 85) in patients without tumour violation. The 5-year local disease-free survival was 47% versus 87% ($p < 0.005$). In multivariate analysis intraoperative tumour violation was an adverse prognostic factor for both end points.

Adjuvant radiotherapy now has an established role in excisional surgery; it achieves a higher local control rate and a longer recurrence-free survival time [31, 45, 49, 50, 60]. In head and neck STS, local control was observed in 34% of patients treated with surgery alone versus 75% of those receiving adjuvant radiotherapy [54].

Preoperative (neoadjuvant) radiotherapy is used especially for large STS. Initially unresectable tumours might become resectable after high doses of radiotherapy, and for large tumours (more than 15 cm) the local control rate is higher [4, 8, 47, 48].

Adjuvant chemotherapy currently remains controversial in adult STS and should be considered still investigational for these tumours (for an overview see [9, 14, 34, 60]).

References

1. Abbatucci JS, Boulier N, De Ranieri J, Mandard AM, Tanguy A, Vernhes JC, Busson A (1986) Local control and survival in soft tissue sarcomas of the limbs, trunk walls and head and neck. Int J Radiat Oncol Biol Phys 12: 579–586
2. American Joint Committee for Cancer Staging and End-Results Reporting (AJC) (1977) Manual for staging of cancer. AJC, Chicago
3. Alvegard TA, Berg NO, Baldetorp B, Fernö M, Killander D, Ranstam J, Rydholm A, Akerman M (1990) Cellular DNA content and prognosis of high-grade soft tissue sarcoma: the Scandinavian Sarcoma Group experience. J Clin Oncol 8: 538–547
4. Barkley HT, Martin RG, Romsdahl MM, Lindberg HL, Zagars GK (1988) Treatment of soft tissue sarcomas by preoperative irradiation and conservative surgical resection. Int J Radiat Oncol Biol Phys 14: 693–699
5. Barrios C, Castresana JS, Ruiz J, Kreicbergs A (1994) Amplification of the c-*myc* proto-oncogene in soft tissue sarcomas. Oncology 51: 13–17

6. Beahrs OH, Henson DE, Hutter RVP, Kennedy BJ (eds) (1992) American Joint Committee on Cancer (AJCC): Manual for staging of cancer, 4th edn. Lippincott, Philadelphia
7. Berlin Ö, Stener B, Angervall L, Kindblom LG, Markhede G, Oden A (1990) Surgery for soft tissue sarcomas in the extremities. Acta Orthop Scand 61: 475–486
8. Brant TA, Parsons JT, Marcus jr RB, Spanier SS, Heare TV, van der Griend RA, Enneking WK, Million RR (1992) Preoperative irradiation for soft tissue sarcomas of the trunk and extremities in adults. Int J Radiat Oncol Biol Phys 19: 899–906
9. Brennan MF, Casper ES, Harrison LB, Shiu MH, Gaynor J, Hajdu SI (1991) The role of multimodality therapy in soft tissue sarcoma. Ann Surg 214: 328–338
10. Cance WG, Brennan MF, Dudas ME, Huang CM, Cordon-Cardo C (1990) Altered expression of the retinoblastoma gene product in human sarcomas. N Engl J Med 323: 1457–1462
11. Chang HR, Gaynor J, Tan C, Hajdu SI, Brennan MF (1990) Multifactorial analysis of survival in primary extremity liposarcoma. World J Surg 14: 610–618
12. Collin C, Godbold J, Hajdu S, Brennan M (1987) Localized extremity soft tissue sarcoma: an analysis of factors affecting survival. J Clin Oncol 5: 601–612
13. Eeles RA, Fisher C, A'Hern RP, Robinson M, Rhys-Evans P, Henk JN, Archer D, Harmer CL (1993) Head and neck sarcomas: prognostic factors and implications for treatment. Br J Cancer 68: 201–207
14. Elias AD (1993) Chemotherapy for soft-tissue sarcomas. Clin Orthop 289: 94–105
15. El-Jabbour JN, Akhtar SS, Kerr GR, McLaren KM, Smyth JF, Rodger A, Leonard RCF (1990) Prognostic factors for survival in soft tissue sarcoma. Br J Cancer 62: 857–861
16. Enneking WF, Spanier SS, Malawer MM (1981) The effect of anatomic setting on the results of surgical procedures for soft part sarcomas of the thigh. Cancer 47: 1005–1022
17. Enzinger FM, Weiss SW (1988) Soft tissue sarcomas, 2nd edn. Mosby, St Louis
18. Geer RJ, Woodruff J, Casper ES, Brennan MF (1992) Management of small soft-tissue sarcoma of the extremity in adults. Arch Surg 127: 1285–1289
19. Hajdu SI (1985) Differential diagnosis of soft tissue and bone tumors. Lea and Febiger, Philadelphia
20. Hashimoto H, Daimaru Y, Takeshita A, Tsuneyoshi M, Enjoji M (1992) Prognostic significance of histologic parameters of soft tissue sarcomas. Cancer 70: 2816–2822
21. Herbert SH, Corn BW, Soling LJ, Lanciano MM, Schultz DJ, Gillies McKenna W, Coia LR (1993) Limb-preserving treatment for soft tissue sarcomas of the extremities. Cancer 72: 1230–1238
22. Hermanek P, Sobin LH (eds) (1992) UICC: TNM classification of malignant tumours, 4th edn, 2nd rev. Springer, Berlin Heidelberg New York
23. Hohenberger W, Göhl J, Kessler C, Hermanek P (1990) Behandlung von Weichteilsarkomen. Ein Erfahrungsbericht anhand des Erlanger Krankengutes. In: Gall FP, Göhl J, Hohenberger W (eds) Weichteilsarkome. Zuckschwerdt, Munich
24. Jensen OM, Hogh J, Ostgaard SE, Nordentoft AM, Sneppen O (1991) Histopathological grading of soft tissue tumors. Prognostic significance in a prospective study of 278 consecutive cases. J Pathol 163: 19–24
25. Karakousis CP, Emrich LJ, Rao U, Krishnamsetty RM (1986) Feasibility of limb salvage and survival in soft tissue sarcomas. Cancer 56: 484–491
26. Katenkamp D, Hünerbein R (1992) Untersuchungen zur prognostischen Bedeutung von Entzündungszellen in malignen Weichgewebstumoren des Menschen. Zentralbl Pathol 138: 21–25
27. Kawai A, Noguchi M, Beppu J, Yokoyama R, Mukai K, Hiroshashi S, Inoue H, Fukuma H (1994) Nuclear immunoreaction of p53 protein in soft tissue sarcomas. Cancer 73: 2499–2505
28. Kraus DH, Dubner S, Harrison LB, Strong EW, Hajdu SI, Kher U, Begg C, Brennan MF (1994) Prognostic factors of recurrence and survival in head and neck soft tissue sarcomas. Cancer 74: 697–702
29. Lack EE, Steinberg SM, White DE, Kinsella T, Glatstein E, Chang AE, Rosenberg SA (1989) Extremity soft tissue sarcomas: analysis of prognostic variables in 300 cases and evaluation of tumor necrosis as a factor in stratifying higher-grade sarcomas. J Surg Oncol 41: 263–273
30. Leibel SA, Tranbaugh RF, Wara WM, Beckstead JH, Bovill EG, Phillips TL (1982) Soft tissue sarcomas of the extremities. Cancer 50: 1076–1083
31. Lindberg RD, Martin RG, Romsdahl MM, Barkley HT (1981) Conservative surgery and postoperative radiotherapy in 300 adults with soft tissue sarcomas. Cancer 47: 2391–2397

32. Mandard AM, Petiot JF, Marnay J, Mandard JC, Chasle J, De Ranieri E, Dupin P, Herlin P, De Ranieri J, Tanguy A, Boulier N, Abbatucci JS (1989) Prognostic factors in soft tissue sarcomas. Cancer 63: 1437–1451

33. Menon AG, Anderson KM, Riccardi VM, Chang RV, Whaley JM, Yandell DW (1990) Chromosome 17p deletions and p53 gene mutations associated with the formation of malignant neurofibrosarcomas in von Recklinghausen neurofibromatosis. Proc Natl Acad Sci USA 87: 5435–5439

34. Mertens WC, Bramwell VH (1993) Adjuvant chemotherapy in the treatment of soft tissue sarcomas. Clin Orthop 289: 81–93

35. Porter PL, Gown AM, Kramp SG, Coltera MD (1992) Widespread p53 overexpression in human malignant tumors. Am J Pathol 140: 145–153

36. Potter DA, Kinsella T, Glatstein E, Wesley R, White DE, Seipp CA, Chang AE, Lack EE, Costa J, Rosenberg SA (1986) High-grade soft tissue sarcomas of the extremities. Cancer 58: 190–205

37. Ravaud A, Bui NB, Coindre JM, Lagarde P, Tramond P, Bonichon F, Stöckle E, Kantor G, Trojani M, Chauvergne J, Maree D (1992) Prognostic variables for the selection of patients with operable soft tissue sarcomas to be considered in adjuvant chemotherapy trials. Br J Cancer 66: 961–969

38. Reissmann PT, Simon MA, Lee WH, Slamon D (1989) Studies of the retinoblastoma gene in human sarcomas. Oncogene 4: 839–843

39. Rööser BO, Berg NO, Ranstam J, Rydholm A, Willen H (1990) Prediction of survival in patients with high-grade soft tissue sarcoma. Int Orthop 14: 199–204

40. Saddegh MK, Lindholm J, Lundberg A, Nilsome U, Kreicbergs A (1992) Staging of soft-tissue sarcomas. Prognostic analysis of clinical and pathological features. J Bone Joint Surg 74B: 495–500

41. Schmidt RA, Conrad EU, Collins C, Rabinovitch P, Finney A (1993) Measurement and prediction of the short-term response of soft tissue sarcomas to chemotherapy. Cancer 72: 2593–2601

42. Serpell JW, Ball BS, Robinson MH, Fryatt I, Fischer C, Thomas JM (1991) Factors influencing local recurrence and survival in patients with soft tissue sarcoma of the upper limb. Br J Surg 78: 1368–1372

43. Shiu MH, Castro EB, Hajdu SI, Fortner JG (1975) Surgical treatment of 297 soft tissue sarcomas of the lower extremity. Ann Surg 182: 172–179

44. Stenfert Kroese MC, Rutgers DH, Wils IS, van Unnik JAM, Rokoll PJM (1990) The relevance of the DNA index and proliferation rate in the grading of benign and malignant soft tissue tumors. Cancer 65: 1782–1788

45. Stotter AT, A'Hern RP, Fisher C, Mott AF, Fallowfield M, Westbury G (1990) The influence of local recurrence of extremity soft tissue sarcoma on metastasis and survival. Cancer 65: 1119–1129

46. Stratton MR, Moss S, Warren W, Patterson H, Clark H, Fisher C, Fletcher CDM, Ball A, Thomas M, Gusterson BA, Cooper CS (1990) Mutation of the p53 gene in human soft tissue sarcomas: association with abnormalities of the RB1 gene. Oncogene 5: 1297–1301

47. Suit HD, Mankin HJ, Wood WC, Proppe KH (1985) Preoperative, intraoperative and postoperative radiation in the treatment of primary soft tissue sarcoma. Cancer 55: 2659–2667

48. Suit HD, Mankin HJ, Willert CG, Gebhardt MC, Wood WC, Skates S (1988) Limited surgery and external irradiation in soft tissue sarcomas. In: Ryan JR, Baker LH (eds) Recent concepts in sarcoma treatment. Kluwer Academic, Dorddrecht

49. Suit HD, Mankin HJ, Wood WC, Gebhardt MC, Harmon DC, Rosenberg A, Tepper JE, Rosenthal D (1988) Treatment of the patient with stage M0 soft tissue sarcoma. J Clin Oncol 6: 854–862

50. Suit HD, Proppe KH, Mankin HG, Wood WC (1981) Preoperative radiation therapy for sarcoma of soft tissue. Cancer 47: 2269–2274

51. Tanabe KK, Pollock RE, Ellis LM, Murphy A, Sherman N, Romsdahl NM (1994) Influence of surgical margins on outcome in patients with preoperatively irradiated extremity soft tissue sarcomas. Cancer 73: 1652–1659

52. Tawa A, Inoue M, Ishihara S, Hara J, Yumura-Yagi K, Okada A, Nihei A, Taguchi J, Kanai N, Tsuruo T, Kawa-Ha K (1990) Increased expression of the multidrug-resistance gene in undifferentiated sarcoma. Cancer 66: 1980–1983

53. Tetu B, Lacasse B, Bouchard HL, Lagace R, Hout J, Landry J (1992) Prognostic influence of HSP-27 expression in malignant fibrous histiocytoma: a clinicopathological and immunohistochemical study. Cancer Res 52: 2325–2328

54. Tran LM, Mark R, Meier R, Calcaterra T, Parker RG (1992) Sarcomas of the head and neck. Prognostic factors and treatment strategies. Cancer 70: 169–177
55. Tsujimoto M, Aozasa K, Ueda T, Morimura Y, Komatsubara Y, Doi T (1988) Multivariate analysis for histologic prognostic factors in soft tissue sarcomas. Cancer 62: 994–998
56. Ueda T, Aozasa K, Tsujimoto M, Hamada H, Hayashi H, Ono K, Matsumoto K (1988) Multivariate analysis for clinical prognostic factors in 163 patients with soft tissue sarcoma. Cancer 62: 1444–1450
57. Ueda T, Aozasa K, Tsujimoto M, Ohsawa M, Uchida A, Aoki J, Ono K, Matsumoto K (1989) Prognostic significance of Ki-67 reactivity in soft tissue sarcomas. Cancer 63: 1607–1611
58. Weiss SW in collaboration with LH Sobin and pathologists in 9 countries (1994) Histological typing of soft tissue tumors, 2nd edn. Springer, Berlin Heidelberg New York
59. Wunder JS, Czitrom AA, Kandel R, Andrulis IL (1991) Analysis of alterations in the retinoblastoma gene and tumor grade in bone and soft-tissue sarcomas. J Natl Cancer Inst 83: 194–200
60. Yang JC, Glatstein EJ, Rosenberg SA, Antman KH (1993) Sarcomas of soft tissues. In: de Vita VT Jr, Hellmann S, Rosenberg SA (eds) Cancer. Principles and practice of oncology, 4th edn. Lippincott, Philadelphia
61. Zalupski MM, Macioroaski Z, Ryan JR, Ansley JF, Hussein ME, Sundareson AS, Baker LH (1993) DNA content parameters of paraffin-embedded soft tissue sarcomas: optimization of retrieval technique and comparison to fresh tissue. Cytometry 14: 327–333

16 Skin Carcinoma

P. Hermanek and H. Breuninger

The favourable overall prognosis of skin carcinoma can be illustrated by a comparison of incidence and mortality. In the United States, more than 60 000 newly diagnosed skin carcinomas and about 2100 deaths from this tumour were reported in 1990 [1].

The biological behaviour varies according to the histological type. In basal cell carcinoma, the most common type in Caucasians (three quarters of all skin carcinomas), metastasis is extremely uncommon and was observed in Australia and New Zealand in only 0.0028% [16]. In contrast, in squamous cell carcinoma, the second most common type, metastasis develops in about 2%–6% of patients [2, 4, 14, 15]. In the uncommon histological types, such as apocrine, eccrine, sebaceous and Merkel cell carcinomas, a higher risk of metastasis exists.

Basal Cell Carcinoma

Prognosis is influenced by tumour size (T) and also by the clinical and histological subtype. The superficial basal cell carcinoma and the fibroepithelial tumour of Pinkus are the most favourable subtypes; the nodulo-ulcerative and pigmented subtypes correspond to the common behaviour; the morphea-like or fibrosing subtype and the uncommon infiltrative subtype [17] show a worse prognosis. Related to the histological subtypes [11], the adenoid seems worse than the solid, keratotic and cystic subtypes. Dense fibrous stroma and loss of peripheral palisading indicate tumours which are locally more aggressive than the common basal cell carcinoma with its loose stroma [9].

The metatypical carcinoma (metatypical basal cell carcinoma, basosquamous carcinoma) is a basal cell carcinoma with foci of atypical squamous cells. It shows a biological behaviour between that of basal cell and squamous cell carcinoma [5, 12].

Squamous Cell Carcinoma

Squamous cell carcinomas of the mucocutaneous junctions (lip, vulva, penis) have a more unfavourable prognosis than those of skin and are therefore not included in the TNM classification of skin carcinoma.

According to univariate analyses, in patients with non-metastasized squamous cell carcinoma of the skin, the prognosis is influenced by

- Size
- Level of invasion
- Tumour thickness
- Histological grade of differentiation
- Development in pre-existent skin lesion.

The T classification considers primarily the tumour size and in addition the invasion of deeper structures. However, there are good data demonstrating that tumour thickness and level of invasion influence prognosis also within the individual size-determined T categories, i.e. T1–3 [2, 6]. Therefore, an extension of the T classification by ramification has been proposed [7].

The verrucous carcinoma, an extremely well-differentiated squamous cell carcinoma, is characterized by a good prognosis despite occasional advanced local invasion [10, 13]. In contrast, the very uncommon true adenosquamous carcinoma of the skin is more aggressive than the usual squamous cell carcinoma [18].

An influence of the histological grade of differentiation on prognosis was reported by several authors [2, 6, 8]. However, its independence has yet to be confirmed by multivariate studies. The same is true for the reported worse prognosis of so-called secondary squamous cell carcinoma developing in burn scars (Marjolin ulcer), draining sinuses from chronic osteomyelitis, irradiated skin, etc. [14]. A possible prognostic influence of tumour localization (except for mucocutaneous carcinomas, see above) is still controversial.

Other Skin Carcinomas

Skin carcinomas other than basal and squamous cell carcinomas are very uncommon. In general, prognosis is less favourable than in squamous cell carcinoma of the skin. In extramammary Paget disease, an associated visceral cancer occurs in 10%–15% of cases [3].

References

1. Boring CC, Squires TS, Tong T (1992) Cancer statistics. CA 42: 19–38
2. Breuninger H, Black B, Rassner G (1990) Microstaging of squamous cell carcinoma. Am J Clin Pathol 94: 624–627
3. Chanda JJ (1985) Extramammary Paget's disease. Prognosis and relationship to internal malignancy. J Am Acad Dermatol 13: 1009–1013
4. Epstein E, Epstein NE, Bragg K et al (1968) Metastases from squamous cell carcinoma of the skin. Arch Dermatol 97: 245–251
5. Farmer ER, Helwig EB (1980) Metastatic basal cell carcinoma. A clinicopathologic study of 17 cases. Cancer 46: 748–757

6. Friedman HI, Cooper PH, Wanebo HJ (1985) Prognostic and therapeutic use of microstaging of cutaneous squamous cell carcinoma of the trunk and extremities. Cancer 56: 1099–1105
7. Hermanek P, Henson DE, Hutter RVP, Sobin LH (eds) (1993) UICC: TNM supplement 1993. A commentary on uniform use. Springer, Berlin Heidelberg New York
8. Immerman SC, Scanlon EF, Christ M, Knox KL (1983) Recurrent squamous cell carcinoma of the skin. Cancer 51: 1537–1540
9. Jacobs GH, Rippey JJ, Altini M (1982) Prediction of aggressive behaviour in basal cell carcinoma. Cancer 49: 533–537
10. Kao GF, Graham JH, Helwig EB (1982) Carcinoma cuniculatum (verrucous carcinoma of the skin). A clinicopathologic study of 46 cases with ultrastructural observations. Cancer 49: 2395–2403
11. Lever WF, Schaumburg-Lever G (1983) Histopathology of the skin, 6th edn. Lippincott, Philadelphia
12. Lopes de Faria J (1985) Basal cell carcinoma of the skin with areas of squamous cell carcinoma. A basosquamous cell carcinoma? J Clin Pathol 38: 1273–1277
13. McKee PH, Wilkinson JD, Black MM, Whimster IW (1980) Carcinoma (epithelioma) cuniculatum. Histopathology 5: 425–436
14. Moller R, Reymann F, Hou-Jensen K (1979) Metastases in dermatological patients with squamous-cell carcinoma. Arch Dermatol 115: 703–705
15. Murphy GF, Elder DE (1991) Non-melanocytic tumours of the skin. Atlas of tumour pathology, 3rd series, fasc 1. Armed Forces Institute of Pathology, Washington DC
16. Paver K, Poyzer K, Burry N (1973) The incidence of basal cell carcinoma and their metastases in Australia and New Zealand. Aust J Dermatol 14: 53
17. Siegle RJ, MacMillan J, Pollack S (1986) Infiltrative basal cell carcinoma: a nonsclerosing subtype. J Dermatol Surg Oncol 12: 830–836
18. Weidner N, Foucar E (1985) Adenosquamous carcinoma of the skin. An aggressive mucin- and gland-forming squamous carcinoma. Arch Dermatol 121: 775–779

17 Malignant Melanoma of Skin

P. Hermanek and N.N. Blinov

This compilation of prognostic factors in malignant melanoma of the skin is predominantly based on the updated comprehensive overview on prognosis published in 1992 by Balch et al. [3, 4]. The authors' data from the University of Erlangen, Germany (more than 850 patients) [26, 48, 49], and from the N.N. Petrov Research Institute of Oncology, St.Petersburg, Russia (614 patients) [53], are widely comparable with the data from the University of Alabama, Birmingham, USA, and the Sydney Melanoma Unit, Australia (over 8500 patients) [3], and are therefore not presented separately. In 1989, an analysis of 54 multivariate studies of melanoma was published by Vollmer [52]. The methodological differences and deficiencies of various studies and the importance of patient selection were discussed, especially with regard to different results. In Vollmer's analysis of the literature, patients of different stages have been combined. However, it should always be taken into account that anatomic extent is the main prognostic factor and that analysis of further prognostic factors has to be performed separately for the following subgroups defined by anatomic extent:

– Localised melanoma (any pT N0 M0)
– Melanoma with regional lymph node metastasis (any pT N1, 2a M0)
– Melanoma with in transit metastasis (any pT N2b, c M0)
– Melanoma with distant metastasis (any pT any N M1)

There are also differences according to the method of staging (clinical only versus pathological). With regard to these differences the patients with melanoma in the following are subdivided into four groups. The definition and the corresponding TNM stage grouping [25] together with the 10-year survival rates are shown in Table 1.

Prognostic Factors in Clinically Localised Melanoma (Without Consideration of Pathological Findings in Elective Lymphadenectomy Specimens)

For analysis of patients with localised melanoma it is essential to consider survival data with a minimum of 7–10 years of follow-up. This applies especially for less aggressive melanomas which have been diagnosed with increasing

Table 1. Subgroups of patients with malignant melanoma for whom prognostic factors are different

Subgroups	Definition by TNM/pTNM [25]	TNM/pTNM stage groups [25]	Ten-year survival rates		
			Balch et al. [3, 4]	ECC[a]	Häffner et al. [24]
Localised melanoma	pT1, 2 N0 M0	I	— $\Big\}$ 79%	84% $\Big\}$ 71%	92% $\Big\}$ 31%
	pT3 N0 M0	II	— (65%—85%)	68%	68%
	pT4 N0 M0		—	41%	—
Melanoma with in transit metastasis	Any pT N2b, c/pN2b, c M0		20%	—	—
Melanoma with regional lymph node metastasis	Clinical: any pT N1, 2a M0 Pathological: any pT any N pN1, 2 aM0	III	12% 27%—48%	28% $\Big\}$ 36% 35%	—
Melanoma with distant metastasis	Any pT any N/pN M1	IV	0% (median survival time, 6 months)		

[a] Erlangen Cancer Center (unpublished data, 1992).

frequency in recent years. In these patients recurrences frequently occur more than 5 years after initial treatment.

The overall 10-year survival rates for clinically localised melanomas were 71% for 6515 patients treated at the University of Alabama, USA, and the Sydney Melanoma Unit, Australia, between 1955 and 1986 [3] and 75.5% for 5093 patients treated at four German University Hospitals between 1968 and 1988 [22].

Table 2 shows the results of 14 large studies using multivariate analysis. There is general consensus that tumour thickness is the most important single prognostic factor; it is demonstrable in all studies listed in Table 2. It remains effective in all subgroup analyses [3] and is considered in the pT classification.

The classes used to describe tumour thickness have been the subject of discussion [19, 24]; however, the subsets proposed by the UICC (International Union Against Cancer) and AJCC (American Joint Committee on Cancer) in 1987 [25] are well proven and should be retained until decisive new findings make it necessary to reassess them.

Tumour thickness is a more relevant prognostic factor than the level of invasion [4, 19, 37]. However, the level is also included in the pT classification not only because of its additional prognostic information [34], but also for two further reasons:

1. In cases in which, for technical reasons, there are difficulties in measuring the thickness the level may be helpful.
2. In cases in which there is ulceration, tumour thickness underestimates the aggressive potential of the tumour; this can be corrected by consideration of the level.

The prognostic significance of the pT classification is shown in Fig. 1 and Table 3 for patients with clinically localised melanoma.

Prognostic factors other than those considered in pT are shown in Table 2; they include ulceration, site, sex and melanoma type (growth pattern).

Of these factors ulceration is the one which shows influence in all the subgroups, while the other factors are independently effective only in some subgroups [3].

The influence of tumour site on prognosis was demonstrated in ten of 13 multivariate studies. However, the question of how site should be classified with regard to prognosis is still being discussed. According to summarised data from Balch et al. [4], the extremities have a better prognosis than an axial tumour site (trunk, head and neck), the face and neck a better prognosis than the scalp, and extremities other than the hands and feet a better prognosis than the hands and feet.

Melanoma type (growth pattern) was demonstrated as an independent factor in only four of 11 multivariate studies (Table 2). The melanoma type is strongly correlated with tumour thickness: nodular melanomas are generally thicker than superficial spreading and lentigo maligna melanoma. Lentigo maligna melanoma is probably associated with a more favourable prognosis even after accounting

Table 2. Prognostic factors in clinically localised melanoma (excluding pathological stage and elective lymphadenectomy)

Reference/institution	Patients (n)	Tumour thickness	Ulceration	Site	Gender	Melanoma type	Level of invasion
Balch et al. [3] Sydney, Australia, and Alabama, USA	Over 8500	1	2	3	5	n.s.	4
Garbe et al. [22] Germany (four institutions)	5093	1	6	3	2	5	4
Morton et al. [34] Santa Monica, USA	3323	1	n.a.	3	2	n.a.	4
McCarthy et al. [30] Sydney, Australia	3025	3	1	2	n.s.	n.s.	4
Cox et al. [10] Duke University, USA	2470	3	4	2	n.s.	1	n.s.
Sondergaard and Schou [43] Copenhagen, Denmark	1469	+	+	+	+	n.a.	+
Balch et al. [2] Alabama, USA	783	1	2	3	n.s.	n.s.	n.s.
Ronan et al. [37] Chicago, USA	740	1	3	n.s.	n.a.	n.s.	2
Drzewiecki et al. [18] Odense, Denmark	632	+	1	n.s.	+	n.a.	+
Sober et al. [42] Harvard and New York University, USA	598	1	+	2	n.s.	n.s.	n.s.
Eldh et al. [21] Göteborg, Sweden	573	2	1	n.s.	n.s.	+	+
Tonak et al. [48] Erlangen, Germany	455	1	n.s.	2.5	2.5	n.s.	n.s.

Table 2 (*Contd.*)

Reference/institution	Patients (n)	Tumour thickness	Ulceration	Site	Gender	Melanoma type	Level of invasion
Meyskene et al. [32] Arizona, USA	377	1	2	n.s.	n.s.	n.s.	n.s.
Cascinelli et al. [7] Milan, Italy	234	1	n.s.	3	n.s.	2	n.s.
Centres with significant influence of the respective factor (n)		14	11	10	6	4	8
Centres in which this factor was analysed (n)		14	13	13	13	11	14

Numbers 1–6 indicate relative strength of the factor, with 1 being the highest. Age is not considered because it influences observed survival but not relative survival.

n.s., not significant; n.a., not analysed; +, significant, but rank order not stated.

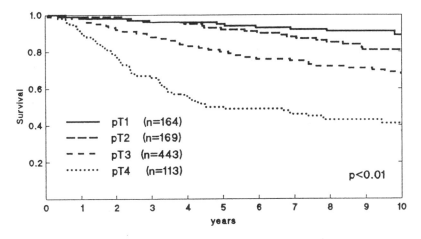

Fig. 1. Prognosis of patients with clinically localised malignant melanoma – observed survival curves. Dependence on pT classification [25]. Data of the Erlangen Cancer Center 1970–1986 (Dec. 31, 1991). Calculation according to Kaplan-Meier. See also Table 3

Table 3. Prognosis of patients with clinically localised malignant melanoma (see Fig.1 and legend)

Curve	TNM/ pTNM	Patients (n)	Five-year survival rates with standard deviations		Ten-year survival rates with standard deviations		Median survival (months)
			Observed	Relative	Observed	Relative	
1	pT1N0M0	164	95 ± 2%	100 ± 2%	89 + 5%	100 ± 7%	n.d.
2	pT2N0M0	169	92 ± 2%	98 ± 2%	81 + 6%	94 ± 7%	n.d.
3	pt3N0M0	443	80 ± 4%	87 ± 7%	58 + 8%	83 ± 10%	n.d.
4	pT4N0M0	113	50 ± 5%	56 ± 5%	41 + 7%	53 ± 10%	56.9

n.d., not determined.

for other prognostic factors [50]. In contrast, the prognosis for patients with acral lentiginous melanoma seems to be worse than for those with other melanoma types comparable in tumour thickness [3].

Another probably independent prognostic factor evaluated only in some studies (not listed in Table 2) is the mitotic rate [8, 11, 12, 20, 23, 35, 37, 44, 51]. It is considered together with tumour thickness in the so-called prognostic index by Schmoeckel et al. [38, 39] and seems to be a further useful predictor of prognosis [28]. Elder and Murphy [19] emphasised that only mitoses in the vertical growth phase are relevant to prognosis (not those in the radial growth phase). The failure of some studies to separate this may account for the discrepancies in reported results.

In four multivariate studies an independent prognostic influence of host response (inflammatory lymphocytic reaction) has been reported [8, 18, 37, 44]. The host response to the radial growth phase should be distinguished from that of the vertical phase, the latter being further characterised as infiltrative (tumour-infiltrating lymphocytes) and non-infiltrating and – according to the extent – as "brisk" and "non-brisk" [8, 19]. A brisk tumour-infiltrating lymphocytic reaction correlates with improved prognosis.

Other possible independent prognostic factors for which further investigation and confirmation are needed include:

– Horizontal tumour diameter [20, 38, 39]
– Cell type [1, 14, 17, 37, 44, 51]
– Microsatellites [13, 43]
– Regression [9, 19, 36]
– Timing of biopsy (prior to definitive treatment) [18]
– Width of local excision [47]
– Aneuploidy [27] and proliferative indices [31]

Prognostic Influence of Elective Lymphadenectomy and Pathological Staging in Clinically Localised Melanoma

Patients with clinically localised melanoma may show occult regional lymph node metastases after pathological examination of an elective lymphadenectomy specimen. The incidence of such clinically undetectable regional lymph nodes depends predominantly on pT: it is not significant in pT1 and pT2 (under 5%) and increases in pT3 and pT4 (16% and 19%, respectively) according to unpublished data from the University of Erlangen from 1970 to 1986.

The relatively high frequency of occult lymph node metastasis in pT3 and 4 explains why the pathological N classification, i.e. absence or presence of regional lymph node metastasis, is an important independent prognostic factor for patients with clinically localised melanoma treated with elective lymphadenectomy: the 10-year survival rate for patients with occult regional lymph node metastasis was 48% compared with 65% for those without lymph node metastasis [3].

For certain subgroups of patients the type of initial surgical management – local excision only or local excision with elective lymphadenectomy – also independently influences prognosis [3, 5, 16].

Prognostic Factors in Melanoma with Regional Lymph Node Metastasis

According to the diagnostic methods used there are two groups of melanoma patients with regional lymph node metastasis:

1. Manifest regional lymph node metastasis
   a) Clinically detected and microscopically confirmed node metastasis
   b) Clinically detected but not histologically confirmed metastasis (only very few patients: group may be disregarded)

2. Occult regional lymph node metastasis: clinically not detected but histologically diagnosed metastasis, i.e. node metastasis detected by pathological examination of elective lymphadenectomy specimens

At the University of Alabama, USA, and the Sydney Melanoma Unit, Australia, patients with occult lymph node metastasis had a 48% 10-year survival rate compared with only 12% for those patients with clinically evident nodal metastasis [3]. Similar figures have been reported from Germany: 49% versus 28% [26].

An overview of the predominant independent prognostic factors in patients with regional lymph node metastasis as revealed by multivariate analyses is shown in Table 4. These data relate to N1 or pN1 only, because for the most part regional lymph nodes 3 cm or less (greatest dimension) are observed (N1) (according to Drepper et al. [15] in 98%). There are at present no reliable data for N2 or pN2.

Table 4 demonstrates that the number of involved nodes is the most important prognostic factor identified in all studies that included this variable in their analysis.

The number of involved nodes can be most usefully divided into one, two to four and more than four [3, 26]. Cochran et al. [9] showed that prognosis is also influenced by the extent of involvement of the individual nodes, i.e. tumour burden.

The prognostic influence of the other factors listed in Table 4 could be proven only in a smaller proportion of studies. Differences may be explained by the different number of patients, the different clinicopathological stages and different limits of classes in the individual factors [15].

According to summarised data from Alabama and Sydney [3], the site of the primary tumour is an independent prognostic factor (extremity more favourable than axial). In the Sydney series, the type of melanoma (growth pattern) turned out to be a prognostic factor.

Prognostic Factors in Melanoma with In Transit Metastasis

According to the TNM classification [25], in transit metastasis is classified as N2b or c. Today, in transit metastasis is nearly always observed as regional recurrence after previous treatment of the primary tumour. The current frequency is approximately 2%–3%. Factors influencing occurrence are the site of primary tumour (especially in melanoma of the lower extremity), thickness and ulceration of the primary tumour and recurrent nodal metastases [6].

Prognosis after occurrence of in transit metastasis is poor: the overall survival rate is about 30% after 5 years and 20% after 10 years, and the median survival time 30–40 months [41].

The single multivariate study on prognosis from the M.D. Anderson Hospital [40] revealed three independent prognostic factors:

Table 4. Predominant prognostic factors in melanoma with regional lymph node metastasis

Reference/institution	Patients (n)	Nodes involved[a] (n)	Ulceration	Tumour thickness[b]	Peri-nodular growth	Patient selection[c]
Cascinelli et al. [7] Milan, Italy	530	+	n.a.	n.a.	+	Pathological
Cox et al. [10] Duke University, USA	418	+	+	n.s.	n.s.	Pathological
McCarthy et al. [30] Sydney, Australia	366	n.a.	+	+	n.s.	Clinical
Morton et al. [33] Los Angeles, USA	150	+	n.s.	n.s.	+	Pathological
Balch et al. [2] Alabama, USA	119	+	+	n.s.	n.s.	Pathological
Sober et al. [43] Harvard and New York University, USA	46	+	n.s.	+	n.s.	Clinical N0, pathological lymph node metastasis
Centres with significant influence of the respective factor (n)		5	3	2	2	
Centres in which the factor was analysed (n)		5	5	5	6	

n.s., not significant; n.a., not analysed; +, significant.
[a] One, two to four or five or more nodes.
[b] 4 mm or less versus more than 4 mm.
[c] Pathological, pathologically detected nodal metastasis irrespective of clinical staging; clinical, clinically detected nodal metastasis irrespective of microscopic confirmation.

1. Location of in transit metastasis (subcutaneous only was worse than intradermal or intradermal and subcutaneous)
2. Presence or absence of concomitant recurrence within the regional basin
3. Gender (prognosis in men was worse than in women)

Prognostic Factors in Melanoma with Distant Metastasis

The overall prognosis for patients with distant metastasis is very poor: their median survival time is only about 6 months [3].

Data from Alabama, USA [2, 3], and from Milan, Italy [7], show that the number of metastatic sites (one, two or three or more) and the site of metastasis (non-visceral versus visceral) are the predominant prognostic factors. According to these factors, the median survival time varies from 2 to 8 months, and the 1-year survival rate from 0 (three or more sites) to 46% (non-visceral) [3].

Other factors which are significant according to multivariate analysis by a single institution include remission duration (less than 12 versus 12 or more months) [3], high performance status and gender (male worse than female) [35].

In a recently published comprehensive multivariate study [42] on 248 patients with advanced metastatic malignant melanoma, 54 factors were analysed (e.g. age, performance status, remission duration, site of the primary, 11 pretreatment laboratory values, prior treatment, number and site of metastases). The following five features were found to be significant independent factors indicating a poor prognosis:

1. Elevated serum value of lactate dehydrogenase (LDH)
2. Low serum albumin
3. High platelet count
4. Visceral organ involvement
5. Male gender

Prognostic Index

Malignant melanoma is the tumour type for which the development of a prognostic index has made the greatest progress.

The computerised mathematical model and scoring system for patients with localised melanoma published in 1985 by Soong [45] was the first example of a prognostic index with the primary aim to predict patient outcome *and* to be applied for the design and analysis of clinical trials. The updated and extended model of Soong [46] makes the following possible:

– Disease management decisions
– Expanded staging in the sense of prognostic grouping
– Analysis of clinical studies including subgroup analysis

Another model for prognostic index was developed by Clark et al. 1989 [8]. It is also applicable for patients with localised melanoma, but it was developed only on cases with tumour vertical growth phase because survival is 100% in radial growth phase melanoma.

For patients with advanced metastatic melanoma, two prognostic models have recently been proposed by Sirott et al. [42].

Further research is needed on the development of reproducible prognostic indices and their prospective evaluation. We agree with the statement made by Elder and Murphy [19] that to date none of the models that have been presented can be considered to be definitive.

References

1. Baak JP, Tan GJ (1986) The adjuvant prognostic value of nuclear morphometry in stage I malignant melanoma of the skin: a multivariate analysis. Anal Quant Cytol Histol 8: 241–244
2. Balch CM, Urist MM, Maddox WA, Soong S-J (1985) Melanoma in the Southern United States: experience at the University of Alabama in Birmingham. In: Balch CM, Milton GW (eds) Cutaneous melanoma. Lippincott, Philadelphia
3. Balch CM, Soong S-J, Shaw HM, Urist MM, McCarthy WH (1992) An analysis of prognostic factors in 8500 patients with cutaneous melanoma. In: Balch CM, Houghton AN, Milton GW, Sober AJ, Soong S-J (eds) Cutaneous melanoma, 2nd edn. Lippincott, Philadelphia
4. Balch CM, Cascinelli N, Drzewiecki KT, Eldh J, MacKie RM, McCarthy WH, McLeod GR, Morton DL, Seigler HF, Shaw HM, Sim FH, Sober AJ, Soong S-J, Takematsu H, Tonak J, Wong J (1992) A comparison of prognostic factors worldwide. In: Balch CM, Houghton AN, Milton GW, Sober AJ, Soong S-J (eds) Cutaneous melanoma, 2nd edn. Lippincott, Philadelphia
5. Balch CM, Milton GW, Cascinelli N, Sim FH (1992) Elective lymph node dissection. Pros and cons. In: Balch CM, Houghton AN, Milton GW, Sober AJ, Soong S-J (eds) Cutaneous melanoma, 2nd edn. Lippincott, Philadelphia
6. Calabro A, Singletary SE, Balch CM (1989) Patterns of relapse in 1001 consecutive patients with melanoma nodal metastases. Arch Surg 124: 1051–1055
7. Cascinelli N, Nava M, Vaglini M, Marolda R, Santinami M, Rovini D, Clemente C (1985) Melanoma in Italy: experience at the National Cancer Institute of Milan. In: Balch CM, Milton GW (eds) Cutaneous melanoma. Lippincott, Philadelphia
8. Clark WH, Elder DE, Guerry D, Braitman LE, Trock BJ, Schultz D, Synnestvedt M, Halpern AC (1989) A model predicting survival in stage I melanoma based upon tumor progression. J Natl Cancer Inst 81: 1893–1904
9. Cochran AJ, Lana AMA, Wen D-R (1989) Histomorphometry in the assessment of prognosis in stage II malignant melanoma. Am J Surg Pathol 13: 600–604
10. Cox EB, Vollmer RT, Seigler HF (1985) Melanoma in the Southeastern United States: experience at the Duke Medical Center. In: Balch CM, Milton GW (eds) Cutaneous melanoma. Lippincott, Philadelphia
11. Day CL Jr, Sober AJ, Kopf AW, Lew RA, Mihm MC Jr, Golomb FM, Postel A, Hennessey P, Harris MN, Gumport SL, Raker JW, Malt RA, Cosimi AB, Wood WC, Roses DF, Gorstein F, Fitzpatrick TB, Postel A (1981) A prognostic model for clinical stage I melanoma of the lower extremity. Surgery 89: 599–603
12. Day CL Jr, Sober AJ, Kopf AW, Lew RA, Mihm MC Jr, Golomb FM, Postel A, Hennessey P, Harris MN, Gumport SL, Raker JW, Malt RA, Cosimi AB, Wood WC, Roses DF, Gorstein F, Fitzpatrick TB, Postel A (1981) A prognostic model for clinical stage I melanoma of the trunk: location near the midline is not an independent risk factor for recurrent disease. Am J Surg 142: 247–251
13. Day CL Jr, Harrist TJ, Gorstein F, Sober AJ, Lew RA, Friedman RJ, Pasternack BS, Kopf AW, Fitzpatrick TB, Mihm MC Jr (1981) Malignant melanoma: prognostic significance of microscopic satellites in the reticular dermis and subcutaneous fat. Ann Surg 194: 108–112

14. Day CL Jr, Harrist TJ, Lew RA, Mihm MC Jr (1982) Classification of malignant melanomas according to the histologic morphology of melanoma nodules. J Dermatol Surg Oncol 8: 874–890
15. Drepper H, Biess B, Hofherr B, Hundeiker M, Lippold A, Otto F, Padberg G, Peters A, Wiebelt H (1992) The prognosis of patients with stage III melanoma. Prospective long-term study on 286 patients of the Fachklinik Hornheide. Cancer 71: 1239–1246
16. Drepper H, Köhler CO, Bastian B, Breuninger H, Bröcker E-B, Göhl J, Groth W, Hermanek P, Hohenberger W, Lippold A, Kölmel K, Landthaler M, Peters A, Tilgen W (1993) Benefit of elective lymph node dissection in subgroups of melanoma patients. Cancer 72: 741–749
17. Drzewiecki KT, Andersen PK (1982) Survival with malignant melanoma. A regression analysis of prognostic factors. Cancer 49: 2414–2419
18. Drzewiecki KT, Poulsen H, Vibe P, Ladefoged C, Andersen PK (1985) Melanoma in Denmark: experience at the University Hospital, Odense. In: Balch CM, Milton GW (eds) Cutaneous melanoma. Lippincott, Philadelphia
19. Elder DE, Murphy GF (1991) Melanocytic tumors of the skin. Atlas of tumor pathology, 3rd series, fascicle 2. AfiP, Washington DC
20. Eldh J, Boeryd B, Peterson LE (1978) Prognostic factors in cutaneous malignant melanoma in stage I. A clinical, morphological and multivariate analysis. Scand J Plast Reconstr Surg 12: 243–255
21. Eldh J, Boeryd B, Suurküla M, Peterson LE, Holmström H (1985) Melanoma in Sweden: experience at the University of Göteborg. In: Balch CM, Milton GE (eds) Cutaneous melanoma. Lippincott, Philadelphia
22. Garbe C, Büttner P, Bertz J, Burg G, d'Hoedt B, Drepper H, Guggenmoos-Holzmann I, Lechner W, Lippold A, Orfanos CE, Peters A, Rassner G, Schwermann M, Stadler R, Stroebel W (1990) Die Prognose des primären malignen Melanoms. Eine multizentrische Studie an 5093 Patienten. In: Orfanos CE, Garbe C (eds) Das maligne Melanom der Haut. Zuckschwerdt, Munich
23. Hacene K, Le Doussal V, Brunet M, Lemoine F, Guerin P, Hebert H (1983) Prognostic index for clinical stage I cutaneous malignant melanoma. Cancer Res 43: 2991–2996
24. Häffner AC, Garbe C, Burg G, Büttner P, Orfano CE, Rassner G (1992) The prognosis of primary and metastasising melanoma. An evaluation of the TNM classification in 2,495 patients. Br J Cancer 66: 856–861
25. Hermanek P, Sobin LH (eds) (1992) UICC TNM classification of malignant tumours, 4th edn, 2nd rev. Springer, Berlin Heidelberg New York
26. Hohenberger W, Göhl J, Kessler C (1993) Prophylaktische und therapeutische Lymphknoten-dissektion bei malignem Melanom. Chirurg 32: 7–9
27. Kheir SA, Bines SD, Vonroenn JH, Soong S-J, Urist MM, Coon JS (1988) Prognostic significance of DNA aneuploidy in stage I cutaneous melanoma. Ann Surg 207: 455–461
28. Kopf AW, Gross DF, Rogers DS, Rigel DS, Hellman LJ, Levenstein M, Welkovich B, Friedman RJ, Roses DF, Bart RS, Mintzis MM, Gumport SL (1987) Prognostic index for malignant melanoma. Cancer 59: 1236–1241
29. Kopf AW, Welkovich B, Frankel RE, Stoppelmann EJ, Bart RS, Rogers GS, Rigel DS, Friedman RJ, Levenstein MJ, Gumport SL, Hennessey P (1987) Thickness of malignant melanoma: global analysis of related factors. J Dermatol Surg Oncol 13: 345–420
30. McCarthy WH, Shaw HM, Milton GW, McGovern VJ (1985) Melanoma in New South Wales, Australia: experience at the Sydney Melanoma Unit. In: Balch CM, Milton GW (eds) Cutaneous melanoma. Lippincott, Philadelphia
31. Merkel DE, McGuire WL (1990) Ploidy, proliferative activity and prognosis. DNA flow cytometry of solid tumors. Cancer 65: 1194–1205
32. Meyskens FL Jr, Berdeaux DH, Parks B, Tong T, Loescher LS, Moon TE (1988) Cutaneous malignant melanoma (Arizona Cancer Center experience). Cancer 62: 1207–1214
33. Morton DL, Roe DJ, Cochran AJ (1985) Melanoma in the Western United States: experience with stage II melanoma at the UCLA Medical Center. In: Balch CM, Milton GW (eds) Cutaneous melanoma. Lippincott, Philadelphia
34. Morton DL, Davtyan DG, Wanek LA, Foshag LJ, Cochran AJ (1993) Multivariate analysis of the relationship between survival and the microstage of primary melanoma by Clark level and Breslow thickness. Cancer 71: 3737–3743
35. Presant CA, Bartolucci AA, Southeastern Cancer Study Group (1982) Prognostic factors in metastatic malignant melanoma. Cancer 49: 2192–2196

36. Ronan SG, Eng AM, Briele HA, Shioura NN, Gupta TK (1987) Thin malignant melanomas with regression and metastases. Arch Dermatol 123: 1326–1330
37. Ronan SG, Han MC, Das Gupta TK (1988) Histologic prognostic indicators in cutaneous malignant melanoma. Semin Oncol 15: 558–565
38. Schmoeckel C, Bockelbrink A, Bockelbrink H, Koutsis J, Braun-Falco O (1983) Low- and high-risk malignant melanoma. I. Evaluation of clinical and histological prognostic factors in 585 cases. Eur J Cancer Clin Oncol 19: 227–236
39. Schmoeckel C, Bockelbrink A, Bockelbrink H, Braun-Falco O (1983) Low- and high-risk malignant melanoma. II. Multivariate analyses for a prognostic classification. Eur J Cancer Clin Oncol 19: 237–243
40. Singletary SE, Tucker SL, Boddie AW (1988) Multivariate analysis of prognostic factors in regional cutaneous metastases of extremity melanoma. Cancer 61: 1437–1440
41. Singletary SE, Balch CM (1992) Recurrent regional metastases and their management. In: Balch CM, Houghton AN, Milton GW, Sober AJ, Soong S-J (eds) Cutaneous melanoma, 2nd edn. Lippincott, Philadelphia
42. Sirott MN, Bajorin DF, Wong GYC, Tao Y, Chapman PB, Templeton MA, Houghton A (1993) Prognostic factors in patients with metastatic malignant melanoma. Cancer 72: 3091–3098
43. Sober AJ, Day CL Jr, Koh HK, Lew RA, Mihm MC Jr, Kopf AW, Fitzpatrick TP (1985) Melanoma in the Northeastern United States: experience of the Melanoma Clinical Cooperative Group. In: Balch CM, Milton GW (eds) Cutaneous melanoma. Lippincott,Philadelphia
44. Sondergaard K, Schou G (1985) Therapeutic and clinico-pathological factors in the survival of 1,469 patients with primary cutaneous malignant melanoma in clinical stage I. Virchows Arch [A] 408: 249–258
45. Soong S-J (1985) A computerized mathematical model and scoring system for predicting outcome in melanoma patients. In: Balch CM, Milton GW (eds) Cutaneous melanoma. Lippincott, Philadelphia
46. Soong S-J (1992) A computerized mathematical model and scoring system for predicting outcome in patients with localized melanoma. In: Balch CM, Houghton AN, Milton GW, Sober AJ, Soong S-J (eds) Cutaneous melanoma, 2nd edn. Lippincott, Philadelphia
47. Timmons MJ, Thomas JM (1993) The width of excision of cutaneous melanoma. Eur J Surg Oncol 19: 313–315
48. Tonak J, Hermanek P, Weidner F, Guggenmoos-Holzmann I, Altendorf A (1985) Melanoma in Germany: experience at the University of Erlangen-Nürnberg. In: Balch CM, Milton GW (eds) Cutaneous melanoma. Lippincott, Philadelphia
49. Tonak J (1986) Malignes Melanom der Haut. In: Gall FP, Hermanek P, Tonak J (eds) Chirurgische Onkologie. Springer, Berlin Heidelberg New York
50. Urist MM, Balch CM, Soong S-J, Milton GW, Shaw HM, McGovern VJ, Murad TM, McCarthy WH, Maddox WA (1984) Head and neck melanoma in 536 clinical stage I patients. Ann Surg 200: 769–775
51. Van der Esch EP, Cascinelli N, Preda F, Morabito A, Bufalino R (1981) Stage I melanoma of the skin: evaluation of prognosis according to histologic characteristics. Cancer 48: 1668–1673
52. Vollmer RT (1989) Malignant melanoma. A multivariate analysis of prognostic factors. Pathol Annu 24: 383–407
53. Wagner RI, Blinov NN, Anisimov VV (1987) Clinical diagnostic and prognosis of primary malignant skin melanoma. In: Actual problems of diagnostic and treatment of malignant skin melanoma. Research Works of the Petrov Research Institute of Oncology, Leningrad

18 Breast Carcinoma

H.B. Burke, R.V.P. Hutter, and D.E. Henson

There has been a proliferation of prognostic factors in breast cancer. Currently there are at least 76 putative breast cancer prognostic factors reported in humans. In this chapter the literature for 37 factors is reviewed. The factors that are supported in the literature are not necessarily the final prognostic factors for breast cancer. They deserve further study in an integrative model. The prognostic factors are presented in three tables, each representing a level of analysis, i.e., epidemiologic, anatomic–cellular, and molecular–genetic.

Before proceeding it is necessary to mention factors that are not reviewed. Treatment (physician, therapeutic modality, compliance, etc.) is a large domain that cannot be adequately addressed in a chapter that is primarily a compilation of prognostic factors. Psychological prognostic factors, e.g., adverse life events [2], have not been well supported in the literature, probably because of the poor sensitivity of the assessment instruments. Performance status has not been shown to be a powerful prognostic factor [70]. Quality of life during chemotherapy may be a predictor of overall survival [14].

The following serum biochemical markers are not discussed because they have been recently reviewed elsewhere [60,68]: the adenocarcinoma marker carcinoembryonic antigen (CEA), the breast mucin markers CA 15–3, CA 549, CA M26, CA M29, mucin-like carcinoma-associated antigen (MCA), mammary serum antigen (MSA), cancer-associated serum antigen (CASA), the reaction products hydroxyproline, ferritin, and isoferritin (p43), tumor-associated trypsin inhibitor (TATI), C-reactive protein (CRP), orosomucoid, erythrocyte sedimentation rate (ESR), and the proliferation marker tissue polypeptide antigen (TPA). Many of these markers are a nonspecific host response to the tissue damage caused by the cancer. Their utility has not been well studied, but the available research suggests that most lack adequate sensitivity and specificity for outcome prediction. With sequential testing, some may be useful for the quantification of tumor burden, the monitoring of disease, and the determination of therapeutic effect.

Other prognostic factors are not discussed because each has only a few reports in the literature or are from one research group. These include vitamin D, urokinase-type plasminogen activator, tetranectin, TRPM-2, multicentricity, tumor necrosis factor alpha (not the same as histologic tumor necrosis), tubule formation, laminin, type 2 carbohydrate, haptoglobin-related protein, natural killer cells, chromosome 11q13, alterations in chromosome 1, nuclear volume,

Table 1. Epidemiologic prognostic factors

Name	Literature support	Properties	References
Age	+	Age is usually a significant predictor because of its small measurement variability. A recent study suggests worse prognosis in premenopausal women	47, 49
Co-morbidity	+	Worse outcome regardless of early diagnosis	52
Dietary fat	0	Relationship between dietary fat and outcome is unclear, research is in progress to clarify relationship	29
Obesity	+	Poor prognosis in women receiving adjuvant chemotherapy	3
Race	+	African-Americans have lower survival rates, possibly due to economic status	1, 59

+, Well supported; 0, equivocal support.

tumor-infiltrating lymphocytes, glutathione level, Glut-1 glucose transporter, cyclic adenosine monophosphate (cAMP)-binding proteins, Bcl-2 protein, and matrix metalloproteinase-2. Epidemiologic prognostic factors are listed in Table 1, anatomic and cellular factors in Table 2, while molecular-genetic prognostic factors are shown in Table 3.

Discussion

Many researchers are actively engaged in the search for new prognostic factors for breast cancer patients. Their research efforts have the potential to dramatically increase predictive accuracy; however, the proliferation of putative prognostic factors has given rise to two problems, the poor reproducibility of results (interstudy variability) and the inability of prognostic factors to be integrated into a predictive system.

There are a number of reasons for the interstudy variability. They include: sampling error, the use of different laboratory assays for a prognostic factor, varying levels of laboratory skill and quality control, different cut-off points for the definition of a positive finding, the enrollment of small populations and special patient subgroups, capturing too few outcome events, providing limited follow-up, employing different end points, using different statistical models, and testing for independence with ad hoc groups of prognostic factors.

A review of the significance, independence, and clinical usefulness [8] of a putative prognostic factor requires, for a specific end point, a description of the sampling method, a description of the assay, assessment of intraobserver, interobserver, and interlaboratory variability, a description of the cut-off point criteria and whether the cut-off point was selected before the data were analyzed, a listing of the subject enrollment criteria, subject characteristics, the number of subjects and outcome events, the therapeutic intervention(s), the duration of

Table 2. Anatomic and cellular prognostic factors

Name	Literature support	Properties	References
Tumor size, extent (T)	+	Pathologic more reliable than clinical	47
Regional lymph node involvement (N)	+	Pathologic more reliable than clinical	9
Metastasis (M)	+	Radiographic tests acceptable	31
Histology: Type	+	Most breast cancer is ductal	19
Grade	+	Problems with uniformity of criteria	7, 21, 27
Chromatin	+	Nuclear morphology	33
Tumor necrosis	+	Cell degeneration and death	20
Mitotic counts	+	Cell activity, fixative problems, only M-phase cells	13, 30
DNA ploidy	0	Conflicting results	36
Thymidine labeling index	+	Cell proliferation, thymidine a DNA precursor, thymidine analogue 5-bromodeoxyuridine also used, predicts recurrence	39, 41, 56
S-phase; flow cytometry	+	Cell proliferation, no standardized cut-off point	36
Ki-67 antibody	+	Recognizes nuclear antigen expressed only in proliferating cells	64, 67
Proliferating cell nuclear antigen (PCNA)	0	Cell cycle-dependent protein that accumulates in the nucleus of replicating cells during S-phase, conflicting results	6
Angiogenesis[a]	+	Related to tumor angiogenesis factors	66
Peritumoral lymphatic vessel invasion	+	Significant for relapse-free survival but not overall survival	19

+, Well supported; 0, equivocal support.

[a] Factor VIII-related antigen and CD 31 are vascular detection techniques for quantifying tumor angiogenesis. Basic fibroblast growth factor is an angiogenic peptide and can be measured in the urine [40]. The degree of correlation between vascular antigens and angiogenic peptide in tumor angiogenesis is not known.

follow-up, justification for the type of multivariate model used, a description of the factors placed in the model, and of those factors retained in the final model with their significance values. Such a detailed review is beyond the scope of this chapter.

The capability to measure a prognostic factor reliably and accurately is a prerequisite for its clinical use. The clinical applicability of a prognostic factor is based on a cost–effectiveness analysis, i.e., determining the relationship between the improvement in prognostic accuracy provided by the factor and the cost of determining the factor. In addition, if a prognostic factor is to be useful its analysis must be timely, and it cannot be so complex that it is restricted to research laboratories.

For over 40 years the International Union Against Cancer [28]/American Joint Committee on Cancer [4] have developed the TNM staging system. This system combines the variables tumor size and local extension (T), regional lymph node involvement (N), and metastatic spread (M). The TNM staging system has been very useful, but although it is the best system available, it is not extremely accurate.

Table 3. Molecular–genetic prognostic factors

Gene name[a]	Chromosome	Gene product	Literature support	Function	Expression	Properties	Detection method	References
nm23-H1 (current name NME-1)	17q1.1–2.1	nm23 protein[b]	+	Metastasis suppressor	Increased expression associated with good prognosis	Related to histologic grade and stage	Immunohistochemical	26,50
p53 (current name TP53) Proto-oncogene	17q13.1	p53 protein[b]; nuclear phosphoprotein	+	Suppressor gene; expressed in all cells late in late G1 phase	Accumulation of p53 protein associated with metastasis and reduced survival	Inversely associated with number of hormone receptors	Immunohistochemical; detect p53 antibodies	15, 55
c-myc[b] (current name CMYC) Proto-oncogene	8q24	DNA-binding protein	+	Implicated in control of cell growth, differentiation and apoptosis	Amplification associated with poor prognosis; amplification occurs in 6%–10% of patients studied	Regulated by estrogen in hormone-dependent cells, also associated with hormone-independent cells	Quantitative polymerase chain reaction-based assay	44, 65
	6p21.3	Heat shock protein[b], hsp70, aka hspa1, 70 kDa	+	Involved in protein–protein interactions	High levels associated with shorter disease-free survival in node-negative patients, not overall survival	Associated with c-myc and p53; hormone related	Western blot, immunohistochemical	10
	3, 9, X Three related human genes, not fully sequenced yet	Heat shock protein[b] hsp27, 27 kDa, aka p29, stress response protein srp-27	0		Does not have independent prognostic significance at 8-year follow-up	Hormone related	Northern and western blot, immunohistochemical	11, 12, 61

RAS (Ha-, Ki-, N-) Proto-oncogene	Ha- 11p15 Ki – 12p12.1 N- 1p13	p21 RAS protein, 21 kDa	0	Related to cell division	Expressed in non-neoplastic breast; highest levels found in carcinomas	Intra-cytoplasmic vs. plasma membrane localization; equivocal relationship with ER	Semi-quantitative immuno-histochemical; different methods produce different results	23, 58
	11p15 (near Ha-RAS)	Cathepsin D[b] (three active forms), 34 kDa	0	Lysosomal protease	Increased expression associated with poor prognosis	Estrogen-regulated, can be induced by growth factors	Cytosolic preparations support; western blot, immuno-histochemical methods do not support	32, 46
	17q21-22	DNA Topo-isomerase II enzyme[b]	0	Marker of cellular proliferation; required for DNA replication, present in S-phase	Low levels suggest chemotherapeutic drug resistance	Prediction not well supported yet; inversely associated with ER, PR	Immuno-histochemical	53, 63
PS2	21q	PS2 protein[b], 84 amino acids aka pNR2, BCE1	+	Growth factor	Expression is associated with longer DFS and OS; may be a better predictor than estrogen	Gene expression controlled by estrogen; structurally similar to IGF	Northern blot; Immuno-histochemical	17, 48

Table 3 (*Contd.*)

Gene name[a]	Chromosome	Gene product	Literature support	Function	Expression	Properties	Detection method	References
	6q24-27	ER[b]	+	Growth factor	Predicts response to hormonal therapy; expression associated with improved DFS and OS	Hormone related	Immuno-histochemical	16, 25, 37
	11q23	PR[b]	+	Growth factor	In association with ER, improved DFS and OS in premenopausal women	Hormone related	Immuno-histochemical	5, 16, 62
C-*erb*B-2 (HER-2/neu) Proto-oncogene	17q21	p185[erbB2] 185-kDa transmembrane protein, 50% homology to EGF-R	+	Tyrosine kinase activity; possibly a growth factor receptor	Amplification or overexpression associated with decreased survival	Expressed in a minority of patients; most studies retrospective	Immuno-histochemical	43, 57
	7p13-p12	EGF-R[b]	+	Hormonally regulated positive growth factor (autoregulatory autocrine secretion)	Presence is associated with early recurrence and death	EGF secreted by macrophages; EGF-R is negatively correlated with ER and PR status	Immuno-histochemical	24, 42, 51
	IGF1–12q23 IGF2–11p15.5	IGF I, II, aka Somatomedin C[b]	0	Stimulates cell proliferation in vitro (mitogenic)	Increased expression associated with poor prognosis	Associated with estrogen and progesterone	Western blot; radio-immunoassay	38, 45

Gene[a]	Location		Function	DFS/OS association	Hormone related	Detection method	Ref.
Aromatase[b]		0	Mediates conversion of precursors to estrone and estradiol	Not associated with DFS or OS		Quantification of tritiated water released from 1b-tritiated-androstene-dione	34
Tissue polypeptide antigen[b]		+	Measures tumor activity	Expression associated with longer DFS and OS; also used to detect treatment response	Not hormone regulated	Immuno-histochemical	22,35
CSF-1	5q33	+	Stimulates the survival, proliferation, and differentiation of mononuclear phagocytes	Presence association with poor survival	CSF-1R expressed in monocytes and tumor cells	Immuno-histochemical	54

DFS, disease-free survival; OS, overall survival; ER, estrogen receptor; PR, progesterone receptor; IGF, insulin-like growth factor; CSF, colony-stimulating factor; EGF, epidermal growth factor; EGF-R, epidermal growth factor receptor; aka, also known as; +, well supported; 0, equivocal support.

[a] The gene name in the literature on prognostic factors is not always the current name for the gene.

[b] The aspect that is prognostic in the literature.

The integration of additional factors in the TNM stage model cannot easily occur for several reasons [8]. The TNM stage model is a look-up table based on a "bin" model. In a bin model, continuous variables are divided into discrete ranges (e.g., tumor size of 0–2 cm, 2.1–5 cm, more than 5 cm) and binary variables remain binary. One range of each variable (class) is placed in a bin, resulting in a mutually exclusive and exhaustive partitioning of the data space. Thus, in breast cancer, the TNM staging system is composed of 40 bins (five tumor classes × regional four lymph node classes × two metastasis classes). The bins are then grouped into stages by decreasing survival. In a bin model the number of bins increases exponentially with the number of variables. For example, if we added the variable histologic grade, with its four types, to the TNM staging system, the result is 160 bins (5 × 4 × 2 × 4). Thus, for any set of new variables, the number of bins that would have to be organized into stages would be enormous, the number of stages would increase, and the look-up table would become too complex to be useful. Further, because the accuracy of a bin/stage model depends on the number of patients in each bin, as the number of variables increase the number of bins increase, and the number of patients must increase exponentially to retain enough patients per bin to maintain accuracy.

This is not meant to suggest that the TNM variables should be eliminated. They are of major prognostic importance and will probably remain part of any prognostic system. What this does suggest is that, other than for anatomic extent, new prognostic factors should not be added to the TNM staging system to increase its predictive accuracy. However, prognostic factors may be integrated with the TNM variables in a new prognostic system for greater accuracy in predicting outcome.

As noted in the introduction, at least 76 putative prognostic factors for human breast cancer patients have been reported, and 37 are noted in Tables 1, 2, and 3. The American Joint Committee on Cancer has adopted criteria for the definition of a prognostic factor [8]. A prognostic factor is (1) statistically significant, i.e., its prognostic value only rarely occurs by chance, (2) independent, i.e., retains its prognostic value when combined with other factors, and (3) clinically relevant, i.e., has a major impact on prognostic accuracy.

With these criteria in mind, the College of American Pathologists (CAP) convened a multidisciplinary conference of invited participants, entitled the "*CAP Conference XXVI: Clinical Relevance of Prognostic Markers in Solid Tumors*", in Snowbird, Utah in June 1994. Prognostic markers for cancer of the breast, colorectum, and prostate were considered. The proceedings of this conference are being prepared for publication.

A large number of prognostic factors for breast cancer were reviewed, although epidemiologic factors were not considered. The participants identified two subsets of relevant prognostic factors that have been used clinically, as deemed appropriate by the managing physician.

Group I includes those prognostic factors that are well supported biologically and clinically in the scientific literature. These include the TNM variables. Also included are histologic type, grade (histologic/nuclear), and steroid receptors (estrogen, progesterone). Group II includes prognostic factors extensively studied both biologically and clinically, and this group is divided into two subsets. The first of these, group IIA, includes prognostic factors that have been used in clinical trials, e.g., proliferation markers such as S-Phase fraction and Ki-67 (M1B1), and mitotic index (thymidine labeling index has been validated, but the complexity of the procedure does not lend itself to general clinical use at this time). The second subset, group IIB, includes prognostic factors in which biologic and clinical correlative studies have been carried out, but where there are few outcome studies, e.g., p53, c-*erbB*-2 (HER-2/neu), vascular invasion (lymphatic or venous), and angiogenesis. Group III includes others that do not currently meet the criteria for group I or group II. A large number of factors were discussed at the conference, including many of those in Tables 2 and 3 that are not in groups I or II. The conference participants concluded that these would not be listed since such a listing would be no more than a status report for June 24, 1994. With additional research, some may eventually meet the criteria for groups I or II, and others will doubtless be added to group III.

The CAP Snowbird Conference has effectively given perspective to the galaxy of putative prognostic factors for physicians responsible for the management of breast cancer patients. However, we must be cognizant that other prognostic factors that satisfy the criteria described may be assimilated into clinical practice when their value is proven.

References

1. Ansell D, Whitman S, Lipton R, Cooper R (1993) Race, income, and survival from breast cancer at two public hospitals. Cancer 72: 2974–2978
2. Barraclough J, Pinder P, Cruddas M, Osmond C, Taylor I, Perry M (1992) Life events and breast cancer prognosis. BMJ 304: 1078–1081
3. Bastarrachea J, Hortobagyi GN, Smith TL, Kau SC, Buzdar AU (1993) Obesity as an adverse prognostic factor for patients receiving adjuvant chemotherapy for breast cancer. Ann Intern Med 119: 18–25
4. Beahrs OH, Henson DE, Hutter RVP, Kennedy BJ (eds) (1992) Manual for staging of cancer, 4th edn. Lippincott, Philadelphia
5. Berger U, McClelland RA, Wilson P, Greene GL, Haussler MR, Oike JW et al (1991) Immunocytochemical determination of estrogen receptor, progesterone receptor, and 1,25-dihydroxyvitamin D3 receptor in breast cancer and the relationship to prognosis. Cancer Res 51: 239–244
6. Bianchi S, Paglierani M, Zampi G, Cardona G, Cataliotti L, Bonardi R et al (1993) Prognostic value of proliferating cell nuclear antigen in lymph node-negative breast cancer patients. Cancer 72: 120–125
7. Bloom H, Richardson W (1957) Histological grading and prognosis in breast cancer. Br J Cancer 9: 359–377
8. Burke HB, Henson DE (1993) Criteria for prognostic factors and for an enhanced prognostic system. Cancer 72: 3131–3135
9. Carter CL, Allen C, Henson DE (1988) Relation of tumor size, lymph node status, and survival in 24,740 breast cancer cases. Cancer 63: 181–187
10. Ciocca DR, Clark GM, Tandon AK, Fuqua SAW, Welch WJ, McGuire WL (1993) Heat shock protein hsp70 in patients with axillary lymph node-negative breast cancer: prognostic implications. J Natl Cancer Inst 85: 570–574

11. Ciocca DR, Luque EH (1991) Immunological evidence for the identity between the hsp27 estrogen-regulated heat shock protein and the p29 estrogen receptor-associated protein in breast and endometrial cancer. Breast Cancer Res 20: 33–42
12. Ciocca DR, Oesterreich S, Chamness GC, McGuire WL, Fuqua SAW (1993) Biological and clinical implications of heat shock protein 27 000 (Hsp27): a review. J Natl Cancer Inst 85: 1558–1570
13. Clayton F, Hopkins CL (1993) Pathologic correlates of prognosis in lymph node-positive breast carcinomas. Cancer 67: 11780–11790
14. Coates A, Gebski V, Signorini D, Murray P, McNeil D, Byrne M et al (1992) Prognostic value of quality-of-life scores during chemotherapy for advanced breast cancer. J Clin Oncol 10: 1833–1838
15. Davidoff AM, Herndon JE, Glover NS, Kerns BM, Pence JC, Inglehart JD, Marks JR (1991) Relation between p53 overexpression and established prognostic factors in breast cancer. Surgery 110: 259–264
16. Fisher B, Redmond C, Fisher ER, Caplan R (1988) Relative worth of estrogen and progesterone receptors and pathologic characteristics of differentiation as indicators of prognosis in node negative breast cancer patients. J Clin Oncol 6: 1076–1087
17. Foekens JA, van Putten WJ, Portengen H, de Koning H, Thirion B, Alexieva-Figusch J, Klijn JM (1993) Prediction of relapse and survival in breast cancer patients by pS2 protein status. J Clin Oncol 11: 899–908
18. Garne JP, Aspegren K, Linell F, Rank F, Ranstam J (1994) Primary prognostic factors in invasive breast carcinoma with special reference to ductal carcinoma and histologic malignancy grade. Cancer 73: 1438–1448
19. Gaspirini G, Weidner N, Bevilacqua P, Maluta S, Palma PD, Caffo O et al (1994) Tumor microvessel density, p53 expression, tumor size, and peritumoral lymphatic invasion are relevant prognostic markers in node-negative breast carcinoma. J Clin Oncl 12: 454–466
20. Gilchrist KW, Gray R, Fowble B, Tormey DC, Taylor SG (1993) Tumor necrosis is a prognostic predictor for early recurrence and death in lymph node-positive breast cancer: a 10-year follow-up study of 728 eastern cooperative oncology group patients. J Clin Oncol 11: 1929–1935
21. Gilchrist KW, Kalish L, Gould VE, Hirschl S, Imbriglia JE, Levy WM et al (1985) Interobserver reproducibility of histopathology features in stage II breast cancer: an ECOG study. Breast Cancer Res Treat 5: 3–10
22. Gion M, Mione R, Pappagallo GL, Gatti C, Nascimben O, Brandes A et al (1992) Tissue polypeptide antigen in breast cancer cytosol: a new effective prognostic factor. Eur J Cancer 29A: 66–69
23. Going JJ, Anderson TJ, Wyllie AH (1992) Ras p21 in breast tissue: association with pathology and cellular localization. Br J Cancer 65: 45–50
24. Gullick WJ (1991) Prevalence of aberrant expression of the epidermal growth factor receptor in human cancers. Br Med Bull 47: 87–98
25. Hahnel R (1983) Oestrogen receptors and breast carcinoma. Med J Aust 1: 350–351
26. Hennessy C, Henry JA, May FEB, Westley BR, Angus B, Lennard TW (1991) Expression of the antimetastatic gene nm23 in human breast cancer: association with good prognosis. J Natl Cancer Inst 83: 281–285
27. Henson DE, Ries L, Freedman LS, Carriaga M (1991) Relationship among outcome, stage of disease, and histologic grade for 22,616 cases of breast cancer. Cancer 68: 2142–2149
28 Hermanek P, Sobin LH (eds) (1992) UICC TNM classification of malignant tumours, 4th edn, 2nd revision. Springer, Berlin Heidelberg New York Tokyo
29. Ip C (1993) Controversial issues of dietary fat and experimental mammary carcinogenesis. Prev Med 22: 728–737
30. Joensuu H, Toikkanen S (1992) Identification of subgroups with favorable prognosis in breast cancer. Acta Oncol 31: 293–301
31. Kamby C (1990) The pattern of metastases in human breast cancer: methodologic aspects and influence of prognostic factors. Cancer Res Treat 17: 37–61
32. Kandalaft PL, Chang KL, Ahn CW, Traweek ST, Mehta P, Battifora H (1993) Prognostic significance of immunohistochemical analysis of Cathepsin D in low-stage breast cancer. Cancer 71: 2756–2763
33. Komitowski D, Janson C (1990) Quantitative features of chromatin structure in the prognosis of breast cancer. Cancer 65: 2725–2730
34. Lipton A, Santen RJ, Santner SJ, Harvey HA, Sanders SI, Matthews MA (1992) Prognostic value of breast cancer aromatase. Cancer 70: 1951–1955

35. Mansour O, Motawi T, Khaled H, el-Ahmady O (1993) Clinical value of thymidine kinase and tissue polypeptide specific antigen in breast cancer. Dis Markers 11: 171–177
36. McGuire WL, Clark GM (1992) Prognostic factors and treatment decisions in axillary-node-negative breast cancer. N Engl J Med 326: 1756–1761
37. McGuire WL, Clark GM, Dressler LG, Owens MA (1986) Role of steroid hormone receptors as prognostic factors in primary breast cancer. NCI Monogr 1: 19–23
38. McGuire WL, Jackson JG, Figueroa JA, Shimasaki S, Powell DR, Yee D (1992) Regulation of insulin-like growth factor-binding protein (IGFBP) expression by breast cancer cells: use of IGFBP-1 as an inhibitor of insulin-like growth factor action. J Natl Cancer Inst 84: 1336–1341
39. Meyer JS, Koehm SL, Hughes JM, Higa E, Wittliff JL, Lagos JA, Manes JL (1993) Bromo-deoxyuridine labeling for S-phase measurement in breast carcinoma. Cancer 71: 3531–3540
40. Nguyen M, Watanabe H, Budson AE, Richie JP, Hayes DF, Folkman J (1994) Elevated levels of an angiogenic peptide, basic fibroblast growth factor, in urine of patients with a wide spectrum of cancers. J Natl Cancer Inst 86: 356–361
41. O'Neill KL, Hoper M, Odling-Smee GW (1992) Can thymidine kinase levels in breast tumors predict disease recurrence? J Natl Cancer Inst 84: 1825–1828
42. O'Sullivan C, Lewis CE, Harris AL, McGee JO (1993) Secretion of epidermal growth factor by macrophages associated with breast carcinoma. Lancet 342:148–149
43. Perren TJ (1991) c-erbB-2 oncogene as a prognostic marker in breast cancer. Br J Cancer 63: 328–332
44. Pertschuk LP, Feldman JG, Kim DS, Nayeri K, Eisenberg KB, Carter AC et al (1993) Steroid hormone receptor immunochemistry and amplification of c-myc protooncogene. Cancer 71: 162–171
45. Pollak M, Costantino J, Polychronakos C, Blauer S, Guyda H, Redmond C et al (1990) Effects of tamoxifen on serum insulin-like growth factor I levels in stage I breast cancer patients. J Natl Cancer Inst 82: 1693–1697
46. Ravdin PM, Tandon AK, Allred DC, Clark GM, Fuqua AW, Hilsenbeck SH et al (1994) Cathepsin D by western blotting and immunohistochemistry: failure to confirm correlations with prognosis in node-negative breast cancer. J Clin Oncol 12: 467–474
47. Ries LA, Henson DE, Harras A (1994) Survival from breast cancer according to tumor size and nodal status. Semin Surg Oncol 3: 35–53
48. Rio MC, Chambon P (1990) The pS2 gene, mRNA and protein: a potential marker for human breast cancer. Cancer Cells 2:269–274
49. Rochefordiere AD, Asselain B, Campana F, Scholl SM, Fenton J, Vilcoq JR et al (1993) Age as prognostic factor in premenopausal breast carcinoma. Lancet 341: 1039–1043
50. Royds JA, Stephenson TJ, Rees RC, Shorthouse AJ, Silcocks PB (1993) Nm23 protein expression in ductal in situ and invasive human breast carcinoma. J Natl Cancer Inst 85: 727–731
51. Sainsbury JR, Farndon JR, Needham GK, Malcolm AJ, Harris AL (1987) Epidermal-growth-factor receptor status as predictor of early recurrence of and death from breast cancer. Lancet 1 (8547): 1398–1402
52. Satariano WA, Ragland DR (1994) The effect of comorbidity on 3-year survival of women with primary breast cancer. Ann Intern Med 120: 104–110
53. Schneider E, Horton JK, Yang CH, Nakagawa M, Cowen KH (1994) Multidrug resistance-associated protein gene overexpression and reduced drug sensitivity to topoisomerase II in a human breast carcinoma MCF7 cell line selected for etoposide resistance. Cancer Res 54: 152–158
54. Scholl SM, Pallud C, Beuvon F, Hacene K, Stanley ER, Rohtschneider L et al (1994) Anti-colony-stimulating-factor-1 antibody staining in primary breast adenocarcinomas correlates with marked inflammatory cell infiltrates and prognosis. J Natl Cancer Inst 86: 120–126
55. Silvestrini R, Benini E, Daidone MG, Veneroni S, Boracchi P, Cappelletti V et al (1993) p53 as an independent prognostic marker in lymph node-negative breast cancer patients. J Natl Cancer Inst 85: 965–970
56. Silvestrini R, Daidone MG, Gasparini G (1985) Cell kinetics as a prognostic marker in node-negative breast cancer. Cancer 56:1982–1987
57. Slamon DJ, Clark GM, Wong SG, Levin WJ, Ullrich A, McGuire WL (1987) Human breast cancer: correlation of relapse and survival with amplification of the HER-2/neu oncogene. Science 235: 177–182
58. Spandidos DA, Agnantis NJ (1984) Human malignant tumours of the breast, as compared to their respective normal tissue, have elevated expression of the Hervey ras oncogene. Anticancer Res 4: 269–272

59. Steele GD, Winchester DP, Menck HR, Murphy GP (eds) (1993) National Cancer Data Base annual review of patient care, 1993. American Cancer Society, Atlanta
60. Stenman U, Heikkinen R (1991) Serum markers for breast cancer. Scand J Clin Lab Invest 206: 52–59
61. Thor A, Benz C, Moore D, Goldman E, Edgerton S, Landry J et al (1991) Stress response protein (srp-27) determination in primary human breast carcinomas: clinical, histologic, and prognostic correlations. J Natl Cancer Inst 83: 170–178
62. Thorpe SM, Rose C (1986) Oestrogen and progesterone receptor determinations in breast cancer: technology and biology. Cancer Serv 5: 505–525
63. Tuccari G, Rizzo A, Giuffre G, Barresi G (1993) Immunohistochemical detection of DNA topoisomerase type II in primary breast carcinomas: correlation with clinico-pathological features. Virchows Arch [A] 423: 51–55
64. Veronese SM, Gambacorta M, Gottardi O, Scanzi F, Ferrari M, Lampertico P et al (1993) Proliferation index as a prognostic marker in breast cancer. Cancer 71: 3926–3931
65. Watson PH, Safneck JR, Le K, Dubik D, Shiu RPC (1993) Relationship of c-myc amplification to progression of breast cancer from in situ to invasive tumor and lymph node metastasis. J Natl Cancer Inst 85: 902–907
66. Weidner N, Folkman J, Pozza F, Bevilacqua P, Allred EN, Moore DH et al (1992) Tumor angiogenesis: a new significant and independent prognostic indicator in early-stage breast cancer. J Natl Cancer Inst 84: 1875–1887
67. Weikel W, Beck T, Mitze M, Knapstein PG (1991) Immunohistochemical evaluation of growth fractions in human breast cancers using monoclonal antibody Ki-67. Breast Cancer Res Treat 18: 149–154
68. Werner M, Faser C, Silverberg M (1993) Clinical utility and validation of emerging biochemical markers for mammary adenocarcinoma. Clin Chem 39: 2386–2396
69. Yahan SR, Neuberg DS, Dieffenbach A, Yacoub L (1993) Prediction of early relapse and shortened survival in patients with breast cancer by proliferating cell nuclear antigen score. Cancer 71: 3552–3559
70. Yates JW, Chalmer B, McKegney FP (1980) Evaluation of patients with advanced cancer using the Karnofsky performance status. Cancer 45: 2220–2224

19 Vulvar Carcinoma

J.L. Benedet, D.M. Miller, E. Kovacs, and H. Ludwig

Vulvar cancer is an uncommon malignancy accounting for approximately 4%–5% of all female genital tract cancers. It is predominantly a disease of the elderly, although reports of young, reproductive age group women with this disease appear in the literature. The external location of the vulva should prompt early presentation, but traditionally significant delays in diagnosis have been associated with this cancer.

The past decade has seen a better understanding of the prognostic factors for vulvar carcinoma which, in turn, has led to a more individualised approach to therapy. This has led to less aggressive surgery in the earlier stage of the disease with better cosmetic and functional results. It might be expected that, with the increasing life-expectancy in many countries and the concomitant ageing of the population, an increase in the number of cases diagnosed will occur in the future. Table 1 summarizes the factors that are predictors for survival in vulvar carcinoma.

Tumour-Related Factors

Anatomic Extent of Disease

In 1988, FIGO (International Federation of Gynaecology and Obstetrics) revised the staging classification to a surgical system [7, 12]. Shanbour et al. [29] compared the distribution and survival of 109 patients using the clinical staging system with the newer surgical staging system and found that 21% of clinical stage I and 48% of clinical stage II patients were upstaged because of clinically unrecognised nodal involvement. Conversely, 45% of clinical stage III and 60% of clinical stage IV patients were down-staged. Frankmann et al. [9] found that survival was related to stage of disease. Despite the inherent limitations of clinical staging for vulvar cancers, particularly as they relate to the ability to accurately assess the presence or absence of disease in the regional lymph nodes, virtually all studies to date have consistently shown the extent of the disease as measured by the size of the tumour and the presence or absence of involvement of adjacent structures, e.g. urethra and/or rectum, as well as nodal disease to be the major predictors for survival and recurrence. In a study of the current staging system for vulvar carcinoma relative to prognostic factors for survival, Homesley [15] found

Table 1. Vulvar carcinoma factors as predictors for survival

Stage	Lymph node involvement
	Tumour size
Histological grade	
Lymphatic/vascular involvement	
Pattern of invasion	
Age	

that the status of the groin nodes (number positive and laterality) and the lesion diameter were the only two important independent prognostic factors. Overall, the current staging system did properly assign patients into appropriate risk categories; however, Homesley did note that further refinements of the stage III grouping might be possible, as this group contains some individuals who are low risk, i.e. only one positive node, as well as patients with three or more positive nodes who have an extremely poor prognosis.

The involvement of lymph nodes has been shown to be the single most significant prognostic factor for vulvar carcinoma. The presence of metastatic disease in the inguinal lymph nodes has consistently been identified as the most important prognostic factor for survival. Homesley [15, 16] reported that independent risk factors for inguinal node involvement were the clinical status of the nodes, capillary–lymphatic space involvement, tumour differentiation, age and tumour thickness. He also found that, with increasing age, the patient's risk for nodal involvement increased. Podratz [25] noted that bilateral nodal involvement was associated with a 29% 5-year survival rate, as compared to 51% in patients with unilateral involvement. Similarly, Rutledge [27] noted that patients with bilaterally positive inguinal nodes were 20.3 times less likely to survive and 7.4 times more likely to have a recurrence than those with bilaterally negative nodes. As well as bilaterality, the number of positive nodes is a powerful predictor of outcome as individuals with one to two unilateral nodes involved have a significantly different relative survival rate than individuals with three or more nodes involved. Although involvement of contralateral inguinal nodes with negative ipsilateral nodes is uncommon, this has also been reported as a factor associated with a dramatically decreased relative survival rate. Origoni et al. [24] reported that the size and location of metastatic foci within positive nodes appeared to be a significant prognostic predictor in patients with stages III and IV disease. Extracapsular spread has generally been regarded as an indicator of increased risk for recurrence. The presence of metastatic disease to involved pelvic lymph nodes has also been associated with both decreased survival and increased recurrence.

The size of the primary tumour has been shown to be a significant predictor for both survival and recurrence and for nodal metastasis [1, 8, 10, 16, 25, 27]. Rutledge et al. [27] found that patients with lesions over 6 cm were 2.4 times less likely to survive and 2.1 times more likely to have a recurrence than those with tumours 2 cm or less in size. Podratz et al. [25] and Andreasson et al. [1], using a multivariate analysis, found that tumour size was an excellent predictor for survival when this was set at 3 or 4 cm in diameter. Fioretti et al. [8] also found the 3-cm size to be statistically significant. Homesley et al. [15] found that lesions up to 8 cm in diameter were at low risk as long as the groin nodes were negative. However, the risk of recurrence was increased in patients with negative groin nodes who had lesions greater than 8 cm in diameter. Tumour size correlates with survival and as such can be used as a prognostic factor. However, tumour size was not an independent predictor of inguinal node status in the Gynecologic Oncology Group (GOG) studies, as 19% of patients with lesions of 2 cm or more had positive nodes.

Depth of invasion has been studied extensively as a predictor for lymph node metastasis and also for survival and recurrence [3, 9]. Frankmann et al. [9] found that the 5-year disease-free survival rate was 98% for those lesions with invasion of 5 mm or less and only 58% for those in which the depth of invasion exceeded this value. Sedlis [28] studied a series of patients with superficial vulvar carcinoma with tumours 5 mm or less thick. He found a definite correlation between tumour thickness and nodal disease, with the proportion of patients with positive nodes increasing steadily with each millimeter of thickness, from 3.1% in tumours 1 mm or less thick to 8.9% in 2-mm-thick tumours, reaching 33.3% in a cancer 5 mm thick. Hopkins [17] found no deaths in 29 stage I patients with disease invasive 2 mm or less, although one patient with 1 mm of invasion developed a recurrence 2 years later. Berman [2] noted that 11% of patients with depth of invasion of 1 mm or less developed recurrence, as compared to 17% of those with invasion of more than 1 mm.

Histological Type

Squamous cell carcinoma is the most common histological type of vulvar carcinoma, accounting for approximately 85% of lesions. Most of the knowledge and experience obtained regarding prognostic factors with vulvar carcinoma has come from studying squamous cell carcinomas, but it would appear that the main prognostic factors identified with squamous cell carcinomas, namely tumour size and presence or absence of lymph node involvement, are also operative for the other more uncommon forms of vulvar malignancy. Verrucous carcinoma is a rare malignancy of the genital tract with metastasis being uncommon in these patients. Basal cell carcinoma is a relatively rare vulvar tumour with a tendency to local recurrence and infrequent nodal metastasis. Adenocarcinoma is another extremely uncommon form of vulvar carcinoma which may arise in Bartholin gland, vestibular gland and rarely sweat gland structures. This lesion appears to have similar prognostic factors to the squamous cell variants.

Histological Grade

Studies by both Rutledge [27] and Podratz [25] have reported that histological grade did not significantly influence survival and recurrence. Hopkins [17] found that patients with poorly differentiated tumours had a significantly worse survival than those with well-differentiated or moderately differentiated tumour in stages I and II disease; however, grade did not appear to be a factor for patients with stages III or IV disease. Homesley [15], in studying prognostic factors as they relate to the current staging system for vulvar carcinoma, found that histological differentiation was not significant for survival when adjusted for extent of groin node metastasis and lesion diameter. He showed, however, that tumour differentiation was a highly significant predictor for groin node involvement. It should be noted that the GOG grading system, which is based on the proportion of the tumour that is undifferentiated, was used in this study. Husseinzadeh et al. [18] found cytological grading to be more significant than histological grading with regards to nodal metastasis.

Other Histological Features

Several authors [15, 16, 23, 25, 28] have reported that capillary-like space involvement is an adverse prognostic factor and that it is a significant predictor for survival and recurrence. Onnis [23] reported that lymphatic vascular space invasion correlates with lymph node involvement, and similar findings were also reported by Sedlis and Binder [3, 28], who noted that in patients with superficially invasive tumours, in spite of only 21 of 272 patients (7.7%) having capillary-like space involvement, positive groin nodes occurred five times as frequently as in patients with negative capillary-like space findings. Although the results of the multivariate analysis have shown capillary space involvement to be a significant prognostic factor for superficially invasive tumours, this is only of limited practical use because it appeared to be present in a small proportion of patients. Homesley [16], reporting on a larger series of 588 patients, found that 15% had positive capillary-like space involvement. Also, with this study, the frequency of positive groin nodes amongst patients with positive capillary-like space involvement was almost three times greater than that for patients with negative capillary-like space disease.

Hacker et al. [11], in a review of stage I vulvar carcinomas, noted that the pattern of invasion largely reflected depth of invasion. He also noted that, of those with non-confluent patterns, with spray patterns of infiltration, 28.6% had nodal metastasis. Similarly, Magrina [21] found that with stage I tumours microscopic confluence did correlate with patient survival. Kürzl and Messerer [20] found that predictive survival was affected by a dissociated tumour growth.

Biological and Molecular Factors

Van Der Sijde [31] studied a series of 94 women with squamous cell carcinoma to see the significance of serum squamous cell carcinoma antigen (SCC) and found that the levels varied from 10% in patients with stage I disease to 40% in those with stage IV disease. No correlation was noted between elevated pretreatment squamous cell carcinoma values and the presence of lymph node metastasis. Forty-two per cent of patients with recurrent or progressive disease had elevated levels, but 25% of patients without demonstrable tumour activity were also noted to have elevated serum SCC levels. Rose et al. [26] reported that 29% of patients with advanced vulvar carcinoma had an elevated SCC level. Similar to the study by Van Der Sijde, the levels appeared to be mainly elevated in individuals with stage III and IV disease, where 41% and 44%, respectively, had elevated levels. Also in this study, there appeared to be no association with nodal metastasis.

Dolan et al. [5] reported that DNA ploidy and S-phase fraction analyses did not appear to be useful prognostic factors for vulvar squamous carcinomas. Similar results were noted by Siracky et al. [30], who found that 80% had diploid content and yet many had regional lymph node disease.

Patient-Related Factors

The prognostic significance of age in the literature has been contradictory. Several authors have found that age was a significant predictor for survival and recurrence [1, 9, 20, 22]. Frankmann et al. [9] found a 5-year disease-free survival rate of 87% in patients up to 79 years of age and 48% in patients older than 80 years. However, Rutledge et al. [27], using a univariate Cox proportional hazards model, found that age is a non-significant predictor for survival and recurrence. Hopkins [17] also reported that age was not prognostic for survival, either with early- or late-stage diseases. Homesley [15], in a GOG study, found that the odds ratio of increased risk for nodal involvement was related to age with the risk increasing fivefold between the ages 55 and 65. He also noted that a 75-year-old woman was 13 times more likely to have positive groin nodes than a 55-year-old woman and that although age was predictive for nodal disease, it had no independent impact on relative survival. Podratz [25] found that increasing age was directly related to increasing stage and recurrence.

One of the problems in assessing the impact of age as a prognostic variable for vulvar carcinoma has been that the more elderly patients with the disease are often treated less aggressively because of poor general medical conditions and thus treatment and subsequent pathological assessment is incomplete.

Treatment-Related Factors

Data from the 1950s and 1960s clearly indicate that radical vulvectomy with inguinal–femoral lymphadenectomy provided the best cure rates and the lowest evidence of recurrence in contrast to patients treated in a less aggressive fashion. Several studies have shown that, in patients with negative groin nodes, a 5-year disease-free survival of 85%–90% could be expected. Conversely, in individuals found to have inguinal node metastasis, the overall 5-year survival rate has been reported as approximately 55%. In the past, a routine pelvic lymphadenectomy was recommended as an attempt to improve results. As pelvic node metastasis is extremely rare in the absence of inguinal node involvement, most individuals have abandoned the routine use of pelvic lymphadenectomy. Currently, postoperative radiotherapy is recommended for patients with positive inguinal lymph nodes.

With a better understanding of the various prognostic factors in this disease has come a more individualised approach to the management of early vulvar carcinoma. This is particularly true for patients with early-stage disease in which, after careful histological assessment, the tumour has been shown to be not only small but also superficially invasive. Also, a lateral location of the lesion in these situations has led to more conservative tissue-sparing surgery at the primary site. Several authors [2, 11, 13, 27] have shown that this approach has not compromised survival in carefully selected patients. Iversen et al. [19] showed that the omission of contralateral groin dissection was possible in the presence of a lateral lesion that did not involve midline structures, providing that the ipsilateral nodes themselves were negative for metastasis.

Radiation therapy plays an important role in the treatment and management of vulvar carcinoma. Most centres [4, 6, 11, 14, 28] have used radiation therapy either as an adjunct to primary surgical management in patients with positive resection margins or metastatic disease to groin lymph nodes. In certain situations, radiotherapy has also been used in a preoperative fashion as an adjunct to surgery for individuals with large lesions or lesions involving central structures such as rectum and/or bladder. In the GOG study, Sedlis et al. [28] studied patients with positive inguinal lymph nodes, randomised to pelvic node resection or radiation therapy; those treated with radiation therapy had an estimated 2-year survival rate of 68% as compared to 54% for those who underwent pelvic lymphadenectomy. Malmström et al. [22] reported on a series of patients treated with vulvectomy followed by radiotherapy to the vulvar area and groins and noted survival rates similar to those reported for more aggressive surgery.

Conclusion

A clearer understanding of the prognostic factors in vulvar carcinoma has been achieved in the past decade with the presence of disease in regional lymph nodes being identified as the single most important predictor for survival and recurrence. This understanding has led to a more individualised and less radical treatment for patients with early-stage, superficially invasive tumours. In turn, this has resulted in less morbidity and better cosmetic and functional results, without compromising cure. Identification of new prognostic factors in the future should result in further refinement in treatment policies with improved cure rates and decreased morbidity.

References

1. Andreasson JA, Nyboe J (1985) Value of prognostic parameters in squamous cell carcinoma of the vulva. Gynecol Oncol 22: 341–351
2. Berman ML, Super JT, Creasman WT et al (1989) Conservative surgical management of superficially invasive stage I vulvar carcinoma. Gynecol Oncol 35: 352–357
3. Binder SW, Huang I, Fu YS (1990) Risk factors for the development of lymph-node metastases in vulvar squamous-cell carcinoma. Gynecol Oncol 37: 9–16
4. Boronow RC, Hickman BT, Reagan MT et al (1987) Combined therapy as an alternative to exenteration for locally advanced vulvovaginal cancer. II. Results, complications, and dosimetric and surgical considerations. Am J Clin Oncol 10: 171–181
5. Dolan JR, McCall AR, Gooneratne S et al (1993) DNA ploidy, proliferation index, grade, and stage as prognostic factors for vulvar squamous cell carcinomas. Gynecol Oncol 48: 232–235
6. Fairey RN, MacKay P, Benedet JL et al (1985) Radiation treatment of carcinoma of the vulva, 1950–1980. Am J Obstet Gynecol 151: 591–595
7. FIGO (1990) Changes in gynecologic cancer staging by the International Federation of Gynecology and Obstetrics. Am J Obstet Gynecol 162: 610–611
8. Fioretti P, Gadducci A, Prato B et al (1992) The influence of some prognostic factors on the clinical outcome of patients with squamous cell carcinoma of the vulva. Eur J Gynaecol Oncol 13: 97–104
9. Frankmann O, Kabulski Z, Nilsson B et al (1991) Prognostic factors in invasive squamous cell carcinoma of the vulva. Int J Gynaecol Obstet 36: 219–228
10. Grimshaw RN, Murdoch JB, Monaghan JM (1993) Radical vulvectomy and bilateral inguinal-femoral lymphadenectomy through separate incisions – experience with 100 cases. Int J Gynecol Cancer 3: 18–23
11. Hacker NF, Berek JS, Juillard GJF et al (1984) Preoperative radiation therapy for locally advanced vulvar cancer. Cancer 54: 2056–2061
12. Hermanek P, Sobin LH (eds) (1992) UICC International Union Against Cancer: TNM classification of malignant tumors, 4th edn, 2nd rev. Springer, Berlin Heidelberg New York
13. Hoffman MS, Roberts WS, Lapolla JP et al (1989) Recent modifications in the treatment of invasive squamous cell carcinoma of the vulva. Obstet Gynecol Surv 44: 227–233
14. Homesley HD, Bundy BN, Sedlis A et al (1986) Radiation therapy versus pelvic node resection for carcinoma of the vulva with positive groin nodes. Obstet Gynecol 68: 733–740
15. Homesley HD, Bundy BN, Sedlis A et al (1991) Assessment of current International Federation of Gynecology and Obstetrics staging of vulvar carcinoma relative to prognostic factors for survival (a Gynecologic Oncology Group Study). Am J Obstet Gynecol 164: 997–1004
16. Homesley HD, Bundy BN, Sedlis A et al (1993) Prognostic factors for groin node metastasis in squamous cell carcinoma of the vulva (a Gynecologic Oncology Group study). Gynecol Oncol 49: 279–283
17. Hopkins MP, Reid GC, Vettrano I et al (1991) Squamous cell carcinoma of the vulva: prognostic factors influencing survival. Gynecol Oncol 43: 113–117
18. Husseinzadeh N, Wesseler T, Schneider D et al (1990) Prognostic factors and the significance of cytologic grading in invasive squamous cell carcinoma of the vulva: a clinicopathologic study. Gynecol Oncol 36: 192–199
19. Iversen T, Abeler V, Aalders J (1981) Individualized treatment of stage I carcinoma of the vulva. Obstet Gynecol 57: 85–89
20. Kurzl R, Messerer D (1989) Prognostic factors in squamous cell carcinoma of the vulva: a multivariate analysis. Gynecol Oncol 32: 143–150
21. Magrina JF, Webb MJ, Gaffey TA et al (1979) Stage I squamous cell cancer of the vulva. Am J Obstet Gynecol 134: 453–459

22. Malmstrom H, Janson H, Simonsen E et al (1990) Prognostic factors in invasive squamous cell carcinoma of the vulva treated with surgery and irradiation. Acta Oncol 29: 915–919
23. Onnis A, Marchetti M, Maggino T (1992) Carcinoma of the vulva: critical analysis of survival and treatment of recurrences. Eur J Gynaecol Oncol 13: 480–485
24. Origoni M, Sideri M, Garsia S et al (1992) Prognostic value of pathological patterns of lymph node positivity in squamous cell carcinoma of the vulva stage III and IVA FIGO. Gynecol Oncol 45: 313–316
25. Podratz KC, Symmonds RE, Taylor WF et al (1983) Carcinoma of the vulva: analysis of treatment and survival. Obstet Gynecol 61: 63–74
26. Rose PG, Nelson BE, Fourner L et al (1992) Serum squamous cell carcinoma antigen levels in invasive squamous vulvar cancer. J Surg Oncol 50: 183–186
27. Rutledge FN, Mitchell MF, Munsell MF et al (1991) Prognostic indicators for invasive carcinoma of the vulva. Gynecol Oncol 42: 239–244
28. Sedlis A, Homesley H, Bundy BN et al (1987) Positive groin lymph nodes in superficial squamous cell vulvar cancer: a Gynecologic Oncology Group study. Am J Obstet Gynecol 156: 1159–1164
29. Shanbour KA, Manne RS, Morris PC et al (1992) Comparison of clinical versus surgical staging systems in vulvar cancer. Obstet Gynecol 80: 927–930
30. Siracky J, Kysela B, Siracka E (1989) Flow cytometric analysis of primary cervical and vulvar carcinomas and their metastases. Neoplasma 36: 437–445
31. Van Der Sijde R, De Bruijn HWA, Krans M et al (1989) Significance of serum SCC antigen as a tumor marker in patients with squamous cell carcinoma of the vulva. Gynecol Oncol 35: 227–232

20 Cervix Uteri Carcinoma

A. Fyles and P. Kirkbride

Carcinoma of the cervix accounts for approximately one fifth of all gynecologic cancers and 2% of all malignancies in women. Numerous prognostic factors have been studied in patients with cervical carcinoma, using both univariate and multivariate analyses. Differences in end points of analysis, whether survival (disease-free or overall), relapse-free rate or local control rate, make comparisons of such studies difficult. Stage, histologic type and histologic grade are the commonly considered factors and have recently been joined by biologic factors including DNA ploidy, S-phase fraction and oncogene expression. Not all factors are relevant to all patients; for example, depth of tumor invasion and presence of vascular space invasion may only be reliably determined in patients treated with surgery, whereas hemoglobin level is important in patients treated with radiation. This review will concentrate largely on those factors identified using multivariate techniques, such as log rank or Cox regression analysis, in order to account for interactions between various factors and will present estimates such as hazard ratios, where available, in order to indicate the strengths of individual variables.

Patient-Related Factors

The influence of the age of the patient on relapse and survival is somewhat controversial. Young age (typically less than 40 years) has been associated with an increased risk of relapse in FIGO (International Federation of Gynecology and Obstetrics) stages I and II disease [26] and in all stages [8, 23] and with a decrease in the overall survival in FIGO stage III disease [3] and in all stages [9]. These data were largely derived from patients referred to tertiary care institutions and may reflect some degree of referral bias. A population-based analysis using data from a regional cancer registry comprising over 10 000 patients with invasive cervical carcinoma found a contrary result, with young age significantly associated with a small improvement in survival [27].

A number of retrospective series have demonstrated an adverse effect of low hemoglobin, or hematocrit level, in patients treated primarily with radiotherapy, possibly due to increased tumor hypoxia. Although the level of anemia required to demonstrate an adverse effect has ranged between less than 10 g/dl and as high as 12 g/dl, a multivariate analysis found levels less than 10 g/dl occurring during radiation therapy to be associated with an increased risk of local and distant failure [10]. Another study of a large group of patients of all stages treated primarily with radiation has found an independent effect of hematocrit on locoregional control and survival and demonstrated that the best results were obtained in patients with levels of 40% or more [23]. In addition, in a study of 113 patients treated with radiation therapy, thrombocytosis (platelet count greater than 400 000/μl) was found to be an independent indicator of poor overall survival [16].

Other patient-related factors studied in multivariate analyses and found to be significant adverse prognostic influences include low Karnofsky performance status [26] and lack of compliance with screening recommendations [38].

Tumor-Related Factors

Anatomic Extent of Disease

Stage has long been recognized as the most important determinant of outcome in patients with cervical carcinoma [9, 20, 21, 23, 26, 27, 32, 36, 38]. Although the TNM categories now correspond to FIGO stages [15], the majority of the reports in the literature have used the FIGO system only. Relative risk (RR) of relapse by FIGO stage for two representative studies are shown in Table 1. Furthermore, several studies have shown a prognostic effect of substages, particularly within FIGO stages II and III, differentiating between unilateral or bilateral parametrial involvement and unilateral or bilateral extension to pelvic wall [3, 9, 26]. Patients with bilateral parametrial infiltration in FIGO stage II and bilateral extension to pelvic wall in FIGO stage III have poorer rates of survival and pelvic control compared to those with unilateral parametrial disease or extension to pelvic wall.

The size of the primary tumor has most frequently been studied in FIGO stage I disease, but as the exact dimensions of the tumor may be difficult to estimate in more advanced cases, substage may be a more accurate estimate of tumor volume and probably acts as a surrogate for size in the studies noted above. Several analyses have demonstrated an independent effect of tumor size in early

Table 1. Effect of FIGO stage on relapse and survival

Covariate	Relative risk	
	Relapse[a]	DFS[b]
Stage I	1.00	1.00[c]
Stage II	2.66	2.00
Stage III	7.08	3.03
Stage IV	18.80	7.41

DFS, disease-free survival.
[a] From [3].
[b] From [2].
[c] Includes stage IIA.

Table 2. Tumor size and risk of recurrence in FIGO stage I

Tumor size (cm)	Relative risk
Preclinical	1.0
1	1.6
2	1.9
3	2.4
4	2.9
6	4.4
8	6.6

stage alone [1, 6, 22, 35, 37] and in patients of all stages [23, 27, 29, 31, 36]. The inferior survival reported in patients with barrel-shaped tumors is also probably due to larger tumor volume [30]. The RR of recurrence as a function of tumor size in FIGO stage IB as estimated from a Cox regression model is shown in Table 2 [6].

Disease-free interval (DFI) was independently correlated with depth of tumor invasion into the cervical stroma in a large prospective study from the Gynecologic Oncology Group (GOG) of FIGO stage IB carcinoma of the cervix treated by radical hysterectomy [6, 43]. When the thickness of the cervical wall was divided into thirds, the RR of relapse was 4.74 for deep third involvement and 1.71 for middle third involvement compared to an RR of 1.0 for inner third involvement only.

Lymph node metastasis is of course included in the TNM staging classification system, but not in the FIGO scheme. In the TNM system regional lymph node involvement is categorized as N1 and staged as IIIB. Para-aortic lymph node involvement is categorized as M1 disease. In patients staged according to FIGO guidelines, involvement of pelvic lymph nodes assessed either by surgical dissection or by lymphangiogram is associated with poorer survival and increased risk of relapse [22, 24, 27, 36]. The number of nodal metastases was found to correlate with survival in one study [1], but not in another [6]. Para-aortic nodal metastases detected by lymphangiography are associated with an increased RR of relapse of 2.62 [21] and an RR for disease-free survival of 1.6 [9].

Other Histologic Features

Squamous cell and adenocarcinomas are the most commonly occurring histologic types of cervical carcinoma and account for approximately 80% and 15% of all cases, respectively. Controversy exists as to the prognostic significance of these two tumor types, although two studies have shown an independent and adverse effect of adenocarcinoma histology in patients with stage I and II tumors treated by surgery with or without radiation [12, 22]. A population-based study did not demonstrate an adverse effect of adenocarcinoma or adenosquamous carcinomas

[38], nor did an analysis from Stanford University which included patients with all stages [21]. Whether these discrepancies are due to differences in the populations studied, referral bias, or an effect of treatment is unclear at present. Small cell carcinomas are known for their aggressive behavior, although their rarity limits further analysis using multivariate techniques [41].

The GOG study did not identify histologic grade to be of independent prognostic significance [6, 43] in patients with FIGO stage IB tumors. An alternative grading system based on eight pathologic elements including tumor structure, differentiation, nuclear polymorphism, frequency of mitotic figures, and measures of the tumor–host relationship such as vascular invasion was found to be the most important factor in a study of FIGO stages IB and IIA patients [42], but was not confirmed in another study of FIGO stage IB–III patients [20].

The GOG study [6] found capillary–lymphatic space invasion to be predictive of failure with a 3-year DFS of 88.9% in patients without capillary–lymphatic space involvement versus 77% for patients with this feature (RR, 1.7). Vascular space invasion was also an adverse independent factor for survival in patients with FIGO stage IB and IIA tumors and positive lymph nodes at lymphadenectomy [12].

DNA Ploidy

The significance of DNA ploidy as a prognostic indicator is currently controversial. Although it was of significance in two multivariate analyses, one in FIGO stages IB–III [20] and another in all stages [39], it had no independent effect in another study of IB and IIA tumors [24]. A study of 53 patients with FIGO stage IB cervical carcinoma found no independent significance of ploidy on recurrence or survival [4].

Biologic and Molecular Factors

A large study of 307 patients found S-phase fraction (SPF) to be a significant covariate for survival in cervical carcinoma in a Cox regression analysis, when considered either as a continuous variable – relative hazard (RH), 2.59; 95% confidence limits (CL), 1.30–4.92 – or as a categorical variable when the SPF was greater than 20% (RH, 4.26; CL, 1.36–13.32) [39]. A smaller study quoted above found no correlation between SPF and outcome [4]. A study of mitotic index failed to demonstrate a relationship with survival in a univariate analysis [19].

Positive staining for PC10 (a monoclonal antibody to proliferating cell nuclear antigen, PCNA) was the strongest predictive indicator of survival in a Cox regression analysis of 194 patients with FIGO stage III squamous carcinoma of the cervix treated by radiation therapy [28].

As yet there are few published studies evaluating oncogenes as prognostic factors in cervical carcinoma, but in 55 patients with FIGO stage III and IV tumors no relationship was found between expression of c-*myc*, *ras*, or c-*jun* oncogenes and survival or time to distant or local recurrence [40]. However, another study found c-*myc* overexpression to be an independent predictor of distant metastases (RR 11.7) [35]. The univariate analyses of epithelial growth factor receptor (EGFR) and HER-2/neu oncogenes have suggested an increased death rate with overexpression in two studies [13, 14].

Although many studies have suggested an adverse effect of human papilloma virus (HPV) in cervical tumors (particularly HPV 18), three published multivariate analyses have convincingly shown that HPV negativity is associated with increased risk of recurrence (RR, 2.6) [34] and death (RR, 1.9) [5, 17], and a further Cox regression analysis demonstrated that HPV negativity was independently associated with a greater risk of distant metastases (RR, 13.8) than of pelvic recurrence (RR, 2.0) [35].

Other features that have been studied as prognostic factors include tumor estrogen and progesterone receptor levels, which have been reported as being correlated with an improved overall survival rate [32], and decreased intratumoral oxygen tension, which adversely predicts for survival in advanced cases treated with radiation therapy [18]. Other markers studied include elevated serum levels of squamous cell antigen (SCC) and CA 125 levels, both of which were found to be independently associated with poor survival in a study of 60 patients [2].

Treatment-Related Factors

In patients with FIGO stage IB cervical carcinoma treated by radical hysterectomy and postoperative radiation, the presence of positive surgical margins and tumor size were the only independent prognostic factors in predicting survival [37], a positive surgical margin being associated with a hazard ratio of 14.02.

A Patterns of Care study established that the use of intracavitary radiation therapy in addition to external beam treatment was a significant independent prognostic factor for survival and pelvic control [26]. The same analysis determined that total doses of more than 8500 cGy were associated with improved pelvic control in FIGO stage III cervical carcinoma. To some extent these two features may be surrogates for one another, as patients who are not treated with intracavitary brachytherapy generally receive lower total doses due to the limitations of normal tissue toxicity with external beam radiation. This may explain why the radiation dose was significant only in FIGO stage III and not in all stages.

The overall treatment time in radiation therapy is inversely correlated with pelvic control and survival in two recent studies [8, 25] and is consistent with data from other squamous cell carcinoma such as head and neck tumors.

Table 3. Summary of major prognostic factors

Stage	Factor
Overall	Anatomic extent
	Size
	HPV negativity
	Radiation treatment duration
Stage I	Size
	Depth of stromal invasion
	Capillary–lymphatic space invasion
Stage II/III	Extent of parametrial involvement or
	extension to pelvic wall
	PCNA
	Radiation treatment duration

HPV, human papilloma virus; PCNA, proliferating cell nuclear antigen.

Conclusions

Numerous prognostic factors have been studied in cervical carcinoma, and it is possible that many of the factors identified as significant may be surrogates for other variables. Therefore, the use of data from multivariate analyses may allow a clearer determination of the root causes of treatment failure and death by exposing interactions between covariates. Nevertheless, caution must be used in interpreting some of these results as analyses of similar patient groups may not examine the same covariates, thereby resulting in discrepancies. Prognostic factors identified in at least two multivariate analyses are shown in Table 3. Clearly anatomic extent of disease represented by stage is the most important feature and further stratification of prognostic groups within stages can be achieved by assessing tumor size in early stages and extent of parametrial involvement or extension to pelvic wall in FIGO stages II and III, respectively. In stage I, the depth of tumor invasion and the presence of capillary–lymphatic space invasion appear to be independent factors. Nodal involvement is important, but histologic grade and ploidy do not appear to be independently significant. Histologic type, apart from small cell carcinoma, does not have a major impact, although there is some suggestion that adenocarcinomas have a worse outcome than squamous cell carcinoma when treated by radical hysterectomy.

Conflicting results exist as to whether age is a determinant of outcome; this may reflect patterns of referral or possibly geographic differences in tumor biology. Hemoglobin level, positive surgical margins, radiation treatment duration, and the use of intracavitary radiation appear to be independent factors, although data is more limited.

Biologic markers have the potential to determine the outcome in patients with a good prognosis, although this potential has not yet been fully realized. In addition, assays such as PCNA may identify patients with rapidly proliferating tumors who may benefit from novel therapeutic strategies such as accelerated fractionation in radiation therapy. At present it appears that the absence of HPV

DNA in cervical tumors is associated with a poor outcome, compared with HPV positivity. Whether this seemingly counterintuitive result is due to more aggressive behavior in tumors arising from carcinogens other than HPV, as yet unknown HPV subtypes, or simply that more aggressive lesions are more apt to lose the viral genome [7] can only be speculated. More information on the role of biologic markers as independent prognostic factors will emerge as more studies are published. Interesting factors not yet assessed in a multivariate fashion include vascular density [33] and radiosensitivity [11].

References

1. Alvarez RD, Soong SJ, Kinney WK et al (1989) Identification of prognostic factors and risk groups in patients found to have nodal metastasis at the time of radical hysterectomy for early-stage squamous carcinoma of the cervix. Gynecol Oncol 35: 130–135
2. Avall-Lundqvist EH, Sjovall K, Nilsson BR et al (1992) Prognostic significance of pretreatment serum levels of squamous cell carcinoma antigen and CA 125 in cervical carcinoma. Eur J Cancer 28A: 1695–1702
3. Benstead K, Cowie VJ, Blair V et al (1986) Stage III carcinoma of cervix. The importance of increasing age and extent of parametrial infiltration. Radiother Oncol 5: 271–276
4. Connor JP, Miller DS, Bauer KD et al (1993) Flow cytometric evaluation of early invasive cervical cancer. Obstet Gynecol 81: 367–371
5. DeBritton RC, Hildesheim A, De LS et al (1993) Human papillomaviruses and other influences on survival from cervical cancer in Panama. Obstet Gynecol 81: 19–24
6. Delgado G, Bundy B, Zaino R et al (1990) Prospective surgical-pathologic study of disease-free interval in patients with stage IB squamous cell carcinoma of the cervix: a Gynecologic Oncology Group study. Gynecol Oncol 38: 352–357
7. Franco EL (1992) Prognostic value of human papillomavirus in the survival of cervical cancer patients: an overview of the evidence. Cancer Epidemiol Biomarkers Prev 1: 499–504
8. Fyles A, Keane TJ, Barton M et al (1992) The effect of treatment duration in the local control of cervix cancer. Radiother Oncol 25: 273–279
9. Fyles A, Kirkbride P, Levin W et al (1995) Prognostic factors for survival in patients with cervix cancer treated by radiation therapy: results of a multiple regression analysis. Radiother Oncol (in press)
10. Girinski T, Pejovic-Lenfant MH, Bourhis J et al (1989) Prognostic value of hemoglobin concentrations and blood transfusions in advanced carcinoma of the cervix treated by radiation therapy: results of a retrospective study of 386 patients. Int J Radiat Oncol Biol Phys 16: 37–42
11. Girinsky T, Lubin R, Pignon JP et al (1992) Predictive value of in vitro radiosensitivity parameters in head and neck cancers and cervical carcinomas: preliminary correlations with local control and overall survival. Int J Radiat Oncol Biol Phys 25: 3–7
12. Gonzalez D, Ketting BW, van Bunningen B et al (1989) Carcinoma of the uterine cervix stage IB and IIA: results of postoperative irradiation in patients with microscopic infiltration in the parametrium and/or lymph node metastasis. Int J Radiat Oncol Biol Phys 16: 389–395
13. Hale RJ, Buckley CH, Fox H et al (1992) Prognostic value of c-erbB-2 expression in uterine cervical carcinoma. J Clin Pathol 45: 594–596
14. Hale RJ, Buckley CH, Gullick WJ et al (1993) Prognostic value of epidermal growth factor receptor expression in cervical carcinoma. J Clin Pathol 46: 149–153
15. Hermanek P, Sobin LH (eds) (1992) UICC TNM classification of malignant tumours 4th edn, 2nd revision 1992. Springer, Berlin Heidelberg New York
16. Hernandez E, Lavine M, Dunton CJ et al (1992) Poor prognosis associated with thrombocytosis in patients with cervical cancer. Cancer 69: 2975–2977
17. Higgins GD, Davy M, Roder D et al (1991) Increased age and mortality associated with cervical carcinomas negative for human papillomavirus RNA. Lancet 338: 910–913
18. Höckel M, Knoop C, Schlenger K et al (1993) Intratumoral pO2 predicts survival in advanced cancer of the uterine cervix. Radiother Oncol 26: 45–50

19. Ireland D, Monaghan JM (1985) A critical evaluation of three methods of studying cell proliferation in human cervical epithelium. Obstet Gynecol 65: 227–234
20. Jakobsen A, Bichel P, Vaeth M (1985) New prognostic factors in squamous cell carcinoma of cervix uteri. Am J Clin Oncol 8: 39–43
21. Johnson DW, Cox RS, Billingham G et al (1983) Survival, prognostic factors, and relapse patterns in uterine cervical carcinoma. Am J Clin Oncol 6: 407–415
22. Kamura T, Tsukamoto N, Tsuruchi N et al (1992) Multivariate analysis of the histopathologic prognostic factors of cervical cancer in patients undergoing radical hysterectomy. Cancer 69: 181–186
23. Kapp DS, Fischer D, Gutierrez E et al (1983) Pretreatment prognostic factors in carcinoma of the uterine cervix: a multivariable analysis of the effect of age, stage, histology and blood counts on survival. Int J Radiat Oncol Biol Phys 9: 445–455
24. Kenter GG, Cornelisse CJ, Aartsen EJ et al (1990) DNA ploidy level as prognostic factor in low stage carcinoma of the uterine cervix. Gynecol Oncol 39: 181–185
25. Lanciano RM, Pajak TF, Martz M et al (1993) The influence of treatment time on outcome for squamous cell cancer of the uterine cervix treated with radiation: a Patterns of Care study. Int J Radiat Oncol Biol Phys 25: 391–397
26. Lanciano RM, Won M, Coia LR et al (1991) Pretreatment and treatment factors associated with improved outcome in squamous cell carcinoma of the uterine cervix: a final report of the 1973 and 1978 Patterns of Care studies. Int J Radiat Oncol Biol Phys 20: 667–676
27. Meanwell CA, Kelly KA, Wilson S et al (1988) Young age as a prognostic factor in cervical cancer: analysis of population based data from 10,022 cases. Br Med J (Clin Res Ed) 296: 386–391
28. Oka K, Hoshi T, Arai T (1992) Prognostic significance of the PC10 index as a prospective assay for cervical cancer treated with radiation therapy alone. Cancer 70: 1545–1550
29. Perez CA, Grigsby PW, Nene SM et al (1992) Effect of tumor size on the prognosis of carcinoma of the uterine cervix treated with irradiation alone. Cancer 69: 2796–2806
30. Perez CA, Kao MS (1985) Radiation therapy alone or combined with surgery in the treatment of barrel-shaped carcinoma of the uterine cervix. Int J Radiat Oncol Biol Phys 11: 1903–1909
31. Podczaski ES, Palombo C, Manetta A et al (1989) Assessment of pretreatment laparotomy in patients with cervical carcinoma prior to radiotherapy. Gynecol Oncol 33: 71–75
32. Potish RA, Twiggs LB, Adcock LL et al (1986) Prognostic importance of progesterone and estrogen receptors in cancer of the uterine cervix. Cancer 58: 1709–1713
33. Révész L (1991) Vascular density in relation to the outcome of radiation therapy: a review. Int J Radiat Oncol Biol Phys 60: 179–182
34. Riou G, Favre M, Jeannel D et al (1990) Association between poor prognosis in early-stage invasive cervical carcinomas and non-detection of HPV DNA. Lancet 335: 1171–1174
35. Riou G, Le MG, Favre M et al (1992) Human papillomavirus-negative status and c-myc gene overexpression: independent prognostic indicators of distant metastasis for early-stage invasive cervical cancers. J Natl Cancer Inst 84: 1525–1526
36. Rutledge FN, Mitchell MF, Munsell M et al (1992) Youth as a prognostic factor in carcinoma of the cervix: a matched analysis. Gynecol Oncol 44: 123–130
37. Seong J, Loh JJ, Kim G et al (1990) Postoperative radiotherapy for stage IB carcinoma of the uterine cervix. Yonsei Med J 31: 367–374
38. Sigurdsson K, Hrafnkelsson J, Geirsson G et al (1991) Screening as a prognostic factor in cervical cancer: analysis of survival and prognostic factors based on Icelandic population data, 1964–1988. Gynecol Oncol 43: 64–70
39. Strang P, Stendahl U, Bergstrom R et al (1991) Prognostic flow cytometric information in cervical squamous cell carcinoma; a multivariate analysis of 307 patients. Gynecol Oncol 43: 3–8
40. Symonds RP, Habeshaw T, Paul J et al (1992) No correlation between ras, c-myc and c-jun proto-oncogene expression and prognosis in advanced carcinoma of cervix. Eur J Cancer 28: 1615–1617
41. Van Nagell JR, Donaldson ES, Wood EG et al (1977) Small cell cancer of the uterine cervix. Cancer 40: 2243–2249
42. Willen H, Eklund G, Johnsson JE et al (1985) Invasive squamous cell carcinoma of the uterine cervix. VIII. Survival and malignancy grading in patients treated by irradiation in Lund 1969–1970. Acta Radiol (Oncol) 24: 41–50
43. Zaino R, Ward S, Delgado G et al (1992) Histopathologic predictors of the behavior of surgically treated stage IB squamous cell carcinoma of the cervix. Cancer 69: 1750–1758

21 Corpus Uteri Carcinoma

J.L. Benedet, T.G. Ehlen, E. Kovacs, and H. Ludwig

In many countries, carcinoma of the corpus uteri (endometrial carcinoma) has now surpassed cervical carcinoma as the most common form of malignancy affecting the female genital tract. This has occurred as the result of two factors. Firstly, the effective population-based cervical carcinoma screening programs have effectively identified the preclinical phases of this disease with a subsequent reduction in its incidence and mortality rates. Second, the increased life-expectancy in many countries today has, in turn, led to an increased number of patients being diagnosed with endometrial carcinoma, which is predominantly a disease of post-menopausal women. Endometrial carcinoma most often presents as post-menopausal bleeding, which results in women presenting promptly for investigation of this complaint. The majority of endometrial carcinomas are diagnosed as stage I lesions [37]. Nonetheless, this condition has the potential to behave in an aggressive fashion, resulting in recurrence and ultimately death. The identification of prognostic factors has been the primary focus of the research on this condition in the past 20 years. Prognostic factors in stage I and II and in stage III and IV disease are shown in Tables 1 and 2, respectively.

Tumour-Related Factors

Anatomic Extent of Disease

In 1988, the International Federation of Gynaecology and Obstetrics (FIGO) changed the staging for endometrial carcinoma from a clinical to a surgical pathological system [15]. The new system was changed to emphasise both intra- and extra-uterine factors which were felt to be important in the prognosis of this condition. Clinical staging was most important when patients were treated primarily with either preoperative irradiation or exclusively with radiotherapy. Uterine size, cervical involvement by tumour and histological grade of the tumour were all important prognostic factors emphasised by the previous staging system. The clinical staging system for endometrial carcinoma recognised uterine size as a predictor for survival and incorporated this into the subgrouping of stage I patients with IA and IB disease, with 8 cm selected as the reference point. Creasman et al. [12] showed a progressive increase in lymph node metastasis to pelvic and para-aortic nodes with an increase in uterine size. DeMuelenaere [13]

Table 1. Prognostic factors in stage I and II disease

Factor	Unfavourable variant
Anatomic extent of disease	Stage II
	Depth of myometrial invasion
Histological type	Clear cell, papillary serous
Histological grade	3
Lympho-vascular invasion	Present
Age	Advanced
Ploidy	Aneuploid tumour
Oncogene amplification	HER-2/neu

Table 2. Prognostic factors in stage III and IV disease

Factor	Unfavorable variant
Anatomic extent of disease	Stage III C, IV
	Depth of myometrial invasion
	Number of sites involved
Histological type	Clear cell, papillary serous
Histological grade	3
Age	Advanced
Hormone receptor	Absence of progesterone receptors
Ploidy	Aneuploid tumour

reported that 10 cm is a better discriminator for assessing survival as opposed to the 8-cm size in the FIGO clinical classification. It should be noted that the histological grade of tumour and the degree of myometrial invasion within these subgroups are factors which may have more significance for prognosis. The degree of myometrial penetration has been noted to be a consistent indicator of survival and recurrence for endometrial carcinoma [3, 6, 7, 10, 12, 14, 20, 26, 30, 32]. Lutz et al. [31] noted that the depth of myometrial penetration appeared to be less important than the proximity of the tumour extension to the uterine serosa. Patients whose tumours invaded to within 5 mm of serosa had a 65% 5-year survival as compared to 97% for those whose tumours were greater than 10 mm from the serosal surface. Lurain et al. [30] found the depth of myometrial invasion to be associated with disease recurrence in a univariate analysis, but not in a multivariate analysis. This probably reflects the fact that the histology and grade are more important predictors of both lymph node metastasis and recurrence and that the myometrial invasion is closely linked to tumour grade. Genest et al. [20] were able to show that tumours invading the outer third of the myometrium in stage I cases had a significantly poorer prognosis than lesions involving the inner one third (95% 5-year survival versus 70%). Similarly, DiSaia et al. [14] noted that 8% of patients with endometrial involvement only experienced a recurrence and 5% died of disease, as compared to 36% of deaths in patients with deep muscle involvement.

When the disease does involve the cervix (stage II), prognosis is poorer, and survival drops from approximately 80% to the 50% range when this occurs. One reason for this appears to be related to a 12% frequency of para-aortic node metastasis in this group of patients [29]. Several studies [12, 14, 19, 30, 38] have shown that the presence of extra-uterine disease affecting adnexal or other intra-pelvic or abdominal structures carries with it a poor prognosis for survival and a high likelihood of recurrence. These patients have also been noted to account for a significant proportion of those patients with positive peritoneal washings and, if the latter prognostic indicator is corrected for this finding, then its significance is greatly diminished [25].

Cytological sampling of peritoneal fluid or washing has become routine as an adjunct to staging for patients with endometrial carcinoma. Creasman [12] noted that 12% of their patients had positive washings, and Morrow [32] noted that, in 32 patients with positive washings as the only positive risk factor, recurrence was observed in 18.8%. Similar findings have also been reported by others [30, 36], but Kadar [26] found it was only important when there was extra-uterine disease.

In the past, it was thought that early-stage endometrial carcinoma infre-quently spread to lymph nodes and, when it did, the para-aortic lymph nodes were the primary site of metastasis. In 1970, Lewis, Stallworthy and Cowdell [29] reported a series of 129 patients with adenocarcinoma of the corpus uteri treated by radical hysterectomy and lymphadenectomy. In this study, 13.2% of patients had lymph node involvement, or 11.2% when the cervix was free of disease. They also noted that the frequency of node involvement was related to the degree of differentiation of the tumour and the depth of myometrial invasion. They noted that the survival rate in patients with positive nodes was significantly less than in patients where no evidence of metastasis could be demonstrated. In an excellent review of the role of radical hysterectomy in adenocarcinoma of the endometrium [33], Rutledge retrospectively surveyed the literature for the preceding 20 years and noted that approximately 10% of patients with stage I disease had metastasis to the pelvic lymph nodes. He also noted that the frequency of nodal metastasis increased as the degree of myometrial invasion increased, as well as the tumours being more undifferentiated. In a more recent study, Creasman [12] reported on the Gynecologic Oncology Group (GOG) results and noted an 11% frequency of pelvic node metastasis in stage I carcinomas and 6% with para-aortic metastasis. He also found that the grade of tumour and the depth of myometrial invasion correlated well with nodal disease. In analysing the site of tumour location with regards to lymph node metastasis, he noted that, if only the fundus was involved, 8% of the patients had pelvic node metastasis. This doubled if the lower uterine segment was also involved and 4% of fundal lesions metastasised to para-aortic nodes, while lower segment lesions had over three times the frequency of para-aortic metastasis. Morrow [32] noted that patients with positive para-aortic node metastasis accounted for nearly 25% of all recurrences. He also found that para-aortic and pelvic node positivity correlated well with clinical findings. In pathological stage III, the depth of myometrial invasion and the number of sites involved were predictors of distant failure [21].

Histological Type

The histological type of endometrial carcinoma is a prognostic factor for survival. The vast majority, however, are adenocarcinoma with an endometrioid pattern with or without benign squamous metaplasia (adenoacanthoma). When compared on a stage-for-stage basis, patients with these lesions have a much better prognosis than patients with clear cell carcinoma or papillary serous carcinoma of the endometrium [2, 9, 21, 35, 38]. Lurain et al. [30] noted that, in a study of 227 patients with adenocarcinoma or adenoacanthoma, 8.8% suffered a recurrence, compared to 35.7% of patients with adenosquamous, 25% of 16 papillary adenocarcinomas and four of seven patients with the clear cell variety. Symonds [35] also noted that these types of tumours were more likely to metastasise and have an adverse outcome. In a detailed review of 1224 cases, Christopherson [9] noted that 5.5% were clear cell adenocarcinomas and this histological type was found to have a particularly poor outcome. Similarly, Wilson et al. [38], in a review of patients treated at the Mayo Clinic, noted that 13% of patients in their series had these uncommon histological subtypes and the overall survival in these patients was only 33%, in contrast to that of patients with endometrioid lesions, in which the survival rate was 92%.

Hendrickson et al. [22] called attention to papillary serous endometrial carcinoma and indicated its highly aggressive behaviour. Since then, several reports [2, 19, 34, 38] have confirmed the aggressive nature of this particular subtype of endometrial carcinoma. Abeler and Kjorstad [2] reviewed all endometrial carcinomas treated at the Norwegian Radium Hospital between 1970 and 1977 and found the frequency of papillary serous carcinoma of the endometrium to be 1.1% of all patients. They concluded that this tumour occurred more frequently in older women and was extremely aggressive. They were unable, however, to relate this to a higher proportion having lymphatic invasion or deep myometrial infiltration as reported by others. Gallion and co-workers [19], in reporting their experience with papillary serous endometrial carcinoma, noted that 38% had more extensive disease than had been appreciated clinically. They also noted a 50% frequency of lymphatic involvement as compared to 14% for non-papillary serous tumours. Furthermore, 75% of these patients developed a recurrence and all eventually died of disease. They also noted that 70% of patients with any degree of myometrial invasion developed recurrence.

Histological Grade

The grade of tumour has been universally accepted as one of the more sensitive indicators for prognosis in endometrial carcinomas. The histological differentiation has also been correlated with depth of myometrial invasion [3, 7, 12] and lymph node metastasis [29]. Creasman et al. [12] noted a higher percentage of pelvic and para-aortic lymph node involvement with both increasing stage and grade, but the largest percentage increase was noted when grade 3 lesions were compared to grade 2 ones. Several studies [10, 12, 26, 29, 30, 32] have shown that, within the stage I group [10, 20], tumour differentiation as expressed by grade 3 versus grades 1 and 2 is a most significant independent variable for survival and recurrence. Lurain and co-workers [30], in studying prognostic factors in patients with stage I tumours that recurred, found that those with grade 3 tumours were five times as likely to develop recurrence than patients with grade 1 or 2 tumours.

Other Histological Features

Several studies [1, 3, 12, 18, 26] have identified lymphatic or blood vessel (lympho-vascular space, LVS) invasion as an important prognostic factor for endometrial carcinoma. Gal et al. [18] noted that LVS invasion correlated well with other prognostic indicators such as tumour grade, depth of myometrial invasion, peritoneal spread and lymph node involvement. It also proved to be an independent indicator for decreased survival in patients with clinical stage I endometrial carcinoma. In this study, it proved to be the only prognostic indicator that was positive in all patients who died from endometrial adenocarcinoma. Similarly, the study by Creasman et al. [12] also identified LVS invasion as an important prognostic factor and found that this was present in 15% of their patients. Pelvic lymph nodes were positive approximately four times more often when this finding was present. This relative risk of nodal disease increased sixfold for para-aortic nodes when present. In a recent review of the GOG data, Morrow [32] reported that, in those patients where lymphatic space invasion was the single positive risk factor, the recurrence rate was 26.5%.

Biological and Molecular Factors

Hormone Receptors

It would appear that the presence of steroid receptors, particularly progesterone receptors, may be associated with lesser virulence of these tumours. Endometrial carcinoma has been known to be a hormone-sensitive and -dependent tumour and, when steroid receptors are present, this would tend to indicate that the tumour has retained some of the biological properties of the host tissue, which in turn might lead to a better outcome [11]. Kadar et al. [27] studied 137 surgically staged women with clinical stage I and II endometrial carcinomas and noted that increasing steroid receptor concentrations were associated with an increase in survival. They felt that, in studying their data with a multivariate analysis, only the progesterone receptor concentration affected survival independently, but that effect was apparent only in patients with extra-uterine involvement. They concluded that the receptor status of the primary tumour was of limited prognostic significance unless advanced disease was present. Kleine et al. [28] noted that receptor status correlated with clinical stage and grade of tumour, but not with myometrial invasion. When they subjected their data to a multivariate analysis, progesterone receptor emerged as a significant prognostic factor next to clinical stage, whereas oestrogen receptor had no significant prognostic relevance. Friberg and Norén, [16] in studying the prognostic value of steroid receptors in stage II patients, concluded that patients who died did not have significantly different oestrogen and progesterone receptor concentrations from those that survived. One of the main values of receptor study and assays at this time is to help determine which patients might or might not be suitable for hormone therapy.

Flow Cytometry

The use of flow cytometry and estimation of tumour ploidy has been consistent in indicating the prognostic value of these factors with regards to survival and recurrence [4, 8, 24, 35]. Symonds [35] noted that DNA analysis appeared to be most useful when histological studies were inconclusive in terms of risk assignment and noted a definite correlation between DNA index and the risk of metastasis. Iversen et al. [24] studied both the DNA ploidy and steroid receptors as predictors for the disease course in patients with endometrial carcinoma. Both the death and recurrence rates were significantly lower among patients with diploid and receptor-rich tumours. Single-factor analysis in the first data set of this study showed significant prognostic value for ploidy, surgical stage, grade and depth of myometrial invasion. In a stepwise analysis, tumour grade lost significance and myometrial invasion became of borderline significance. When the receptor data were included, both oestrogen and progesterone receptor values were of significance in the univariate analysis; however, in the stepwise analysis, only ploidy and surgical stage were significant. This would suggest that the prognostic information of receptor status on survival seemed to be dependent on and included in the information already obtained by ploidy.

Amplification of certain oncogenes and increases in their oncoproteins have been shown to be prognostic in a variety of carcinomas. Berchuck et al. [5] noted that, although only 9% of endometrial carcinomas had overexpression of HER-2/neu, when present it was associated with an increased frequency of death from persistent or recurrent cancer. Similarly, Hetzel et al. [23] showed that HER-2/neu overexpression was a major prognostic factor in endometrial carcinoma when subjected to multivariate analysis. Fujimoto et al. [17] studied *ras* oncogene activation in endometrial carcinoma and found that there did not appear to be any relationship between point mutation and clinical prognostic factors such as clinical stage, depth of myometrial invasion, grade, histological type and ascitic cytology.

Patient-Related Factors

The significance of age as a prognostic factor for endometrial carcinoma has been recognised for many years. Several authors [3, 10, 20, 25, 30] have shown that younger patients have improved survival as compared to older patients. In a multivariate analysis, Abeler and Kjorstad [3] showed that age at the time of diagnosis was the most important single prognostic factor. These observations may be related to the fact that the younger women, in general, tend to have earlier, better differentiated lesions with less myometrial invasion. In addition, a relative lack of immunocompetence may be more prevalent in older patients. Approximately 5%–10% of endometrial carcinomas will occur in premenopausal women, often in association with altered gonadal steroid function. These patients may have some delay in diagnosis because the symptom of bleeding or spotting from these lesions often is not fully appreciated at the outset, permitting the tumours to theoretically invade deeper into the myometrium. Nonetheless, there is no evidence to suggest that these patients have a worse prognosis than the postmenopausal woman.

Endometrial carcinoma has not only been regarded as a disease of postmenopausal women, but also as a disorder that is more common in women who are obese, hypertensive and diabetic. Bokhman [6] postulated that there were two main types of endometrial carcinoma. The first and most common type was associated with these factors, as well as other manifestations of abnormal function of the hypothalamic hypophyseal complex. The second type occurred in women in whom these factors were either not prominent or absent. He noted that the latter type accounted for 35% of patients and that they were more likely to be higher grade with a tendency to deep myometrial invasion and a much poorer prognosis than patients in the former type (58.8% 5-year survival rate versus 85.6%).

Treatment-Related Factors

Total abdominal hysterectomy and bilateral salpingo-oophorectomy (TAH/BSO) has generally been accepted as the mainstay of therapy for early-stage endometrial carcinoma. Combinations of this surgery with and without irradiation treatment have also been used extensively in an attempt to improve survival and lower recurrences. Irradiation, either pre- or postoperatively or on occasion both, has also been used to treat endometrial carcinoma. Radiotherapy has often been an adjuvant therapy, but it has also been used as primary treatment for this disease. What has emerged from the literature on endometrial carcinoma is that no one treatment method is superior with respect to survival. Rutledge [33] noted that the recurrence and survival rates were no different for patients treated by radical hysterectomy or TAH/BSO, but the site of recurrence was different. This review indicated that there are subsets and groups of patients in whom disease spreads early beyond the local site and is not detected by the usual clinical means, and that the treatment methods employed can affect local recurrence but not survival in such patients.

Aalders et al. [1] carried out a study randomising patients to TAH/BSO with postoperative intracavitary radium alone or with external beam radiation therapy. This study concluded that only patients with poorly differentiated tumours (grade 3) which infiltrated more than half the myometrial thickness might benefit from additional external therapy. There was no difference in survival or recurrence rates, but patients who received external beam therapy had a 1.9% vaginal or pelvic wall recurrence, as compared to 6.9% for those who did not receive external beam therapy. This study also emphasised the significance of tumour cells in endothelial lined spaces. These patients had a death and recurrence rate of 26.7% and no difference was found between the two treatment groups in regards to the death rate.

Conclusions

Most patients with endometrial carcinoma present with stage I disease and it is this group of patients in which the prognostic factors have been studied so that therapy can be tailored to the risks for recurrence and/or death from disease. The papillary serous endometrial carcinoma and clear cell carcinoma have a poor prognosis, but these comprise only a small proportion of endometrial carcinoma patients. The current surgical staging system for endometrial carcinoma is based on previously identified intra- and extra-uterine factors that influence the prognosis. However, much of the information regarding prognosis, such as uterine size, histological type and grade and radiological evidence of disease beyond the uterus can be gleaned from careful preoperative assessment of these patients. Information regarding ploidy and receptor status is available from curettage specimens and, with increasing use of hysteroscopy, a more precise assessment of the extent of disease in the uterine cavity and involvement of the cervix may be possible.

A major concern regarding surgical staging has been the fact that many patients are elderly and obese with significant medical problems and the risk that the pelvic and para-aortic node sampling may increase morbidity. Most studies have shown that this has not been a factor. Similarly, concerns have been expressed regarding those patients who may require postoperative radiation which may be compromised by postoperative adhesions. It is yet to be demonstrated that in disease extending outside the pelvis the currently available treatments affect survival. Undoubtedly, recurrence patterns will be affected but clear demonstration of survival advantage is not available. Intraoperative immediate histological assessment of the uterine specimen with careful clinical assessment of nodal areas and the abdominal cavity may provide sufficient information regarding the risk of nodal metastasis without resorting to routine lymphadenectomy in all patients with this disease.

References

1. Aalders J, Abeler V, Kolstad P et al (1980) Postoperative external irradiation and prognostic parameters in stage I endometrial carcinoma: clinical and histopathologic study of 540 patients. Obstet Gynecol 56: 419–427
2. Abeler VM, Kjorstad KE (1990) Serous papillary carcinoma of the endometrium: a histopathological study of 22 cases. Gynecol Oncol 39: 266–271
3. Abeler VM, Kjorstad KE (1991) Endometrial adenocarcinoma in Norway. Cancer 67: 3093–3103
4. Ambros RA, Kurman RJ (1992) Identification of patients with stage I uterine endometrioid adenocarcinoma at high risk of recurrence by DNA ploidy, myometrial invasion, and vascular invasion. Gynecol Oncol 45: 235–239
5. Berchuck A, Rodriguez G, Kinney RB et al (1991) Overexpression of HER-2/neu in endometrial cancer is associated with advanced stage disease. Am J Obstet Gynecol 164: 15–21
6. Bokhman JV (1983) Two pathogenetic types of endometrial carcinoma. Gynecol Oncol 15: 10–17
7. Boronow RC, Morrow CP, Creasman WT et al (1984) Surgical staging in endometrial cancer: clinical-pathological findings of a prospective study. Obstet Gynecol 63: 825–832
8. Britton LC, Wilson TO, Gaffey TA et al (1989) Flow cytometric DNA analysis of stage I endometrial carcinoma. Gynecol Oncol 34: 317–322
9. Christopherson W, Alberhasky RC, Connelly PJ (1982) Carcinoma of the endometrium. I. A clinicopathologic study of clear-cell carcinoma and secretory carcinoma. Cancer 49: 1511–1523
10. Connelly PJ, Alberhasky RC, Christopherson WM (1982) Carcinoma of the endometrium. III. Analysis of 865 cases of adenocarcinoma and adenoacanthoma. Obstet Gynecol 59: 569–575
11. Creasman WT (1993) Prognostic significance of hormone receptors in endometrial cancer. Cancer 71: 1467–1470
12. Creasman WT, Morrow CP, Bundy BN et al (1987) Surgical pathologic spread patterns of endometrial cancer: a Gynecologic Oncology Group study. Cancer 60: 2035–2041
13. DeMuelenaere GF (1975) Prognostic factors in endometrial carcinoma. S Afr Med J 49: 1695
14. DiSaia PJ, Creasman WT, Boronow RC et al (1985) Risk factors and recurrent patterns in stage I endometrial cancer. Am J Obstet Gynecol 151: 1009–1015
15. FIGO (1990) Changes in gynecologic cancer staging by the International Federation of Gynecology and Obstetrics. Am J Obstet Gynecol 162: 610–611
16. Friberg L, Noren H (1993) Prognostic value of steroid hormone receptors for 5-year survival in stage II endometrial cancer. Cancer 71: 3570–3574
17. Fujimoto I, Shimizu Y, Hirai Y et al (1993) Studies on ras oncogene activation in endometrial carcinoma. Gynecol Oncol 48: 196–202
18. Gal D, Recio FO, Zamurovic D et al (1991) Lymphvascular space involvement – a prognostic indicator in endometrial adenocarcinoma. Gynecol Oncol 42: 142–145
19. Gallion HH, Van Nagell JR, Powell DF et al (1989) Stage I serous papillary carcinoma of the endometrium. Cancer 63: 2224–2228
20. Genest P, Drouin P, Erig L et al (1987) Prognostic factors in early carcinoma of the endometrium. Am J Clin Oncol 10: 71–77
21. Greven KM, Lanciano RM, Corn B et al (1993) Pathologic stage III endometrial carcinoma. Prognostic factors and patterns of recurrence. Cancer 71: 3697–3702
22. Hendrickson M, Ross J, Eifel P et al (1982) Uterine papillary serious carcinoma: a highly malignant form of endometrial adenocarcinoma. Am J Surg Pathol 6: 93–108
23. Hetzel DJ, Wilson TO, Keeney GL et al (1992) HER-2/neu expression: a major prognostic factor in endometrial cancer. Gynecol Oncol 47: 179–185
24. Iversen OE, Utaaker E, Skaarland E (1988) DNA ploidy and steroid receptors as predictors of disease course in patients with endometrial carcinoma. Acta Obstet Gynecol Scand 67: 531–537
25. Kadar N, Homesley HD, Malfetano JH (1992) Positive peritoneal cytology is an adverse factor in endometrial carcinoma only if there is other evidence of extrauterine disease. Gynecol Oncol 46: 145–149
26. Kadar N, Malfetano JH, Homesley HD (1992) Determinants of survival of surgically staged patients with endometrial carcinoma histologically confined to the uterus: implications for therapy. Obstet Gynecol 80: 655–659
27. Kadar N, Malfetano JH, Homesley HD (1993) Steroid receptor concentrations in endometrial carcinoma: effect on survival in surgically staged patients. Gynecol Oncol 50: 281–286

28. Kleine W, Maier T, Geyer H et al (1990) Estrogen and progesterone receptors in endometrial cancer and their prognostic value. Gynecol Oncol 38: 59–65
29. Lewis BV, Stallworthy JA, Cowdell R (1970) Adenocarcinoma of the body of the uterus. J Obstet Gynaecol Br Commonw 77: 343–348
30. Lurain JR, Rice BL, Rademaker AW (1991) Prognostic factors associated with recurrence in clinical stage I adenocarcinoma of the endometrium. Obstet Gynecol 78: 63–69
31. Lutz MH, Underwood PB, Kreutner A et al (1978) Endometrial carcinoma: a new method of classification of therapeutic and prognostic significance. Gynecol Oncol 6: 83–94
32. Morrow CP, Bundy BN, Kurman RJ et al (1991) Relationship between surgical-pathological risk factors and outcome in clinical stage I and II carcinoma of the endometrium: a Gynecologic Oncology Group study. Gynecol Oncol 40: 55–65
33. Rutledge F (1974) The role of radical hysterectomy in adenocarcinoma of the endometrium. Gynecol Oncol 2: 331–347
34. Sherman ME, Bitterman P, Rosenshein NB et al (1992) Uterine serous carcinoma: a morphologically diverse neoplasm with unifying clinicopathologic features. Am J Surg Pathol 16: 600–610
35. Symonds DA (1990) Prognostic value of pathologic features and DNA analysis in endometrial carcinoma. Gynecol Oncol 39: 272–276
36. Turner DA, Gershenson DM, Atkinson N et al (1989) The prognostic significance of peritoneal cytology for stage I endometrial cancer. Obstet Gynecol 74: 775–780
37. UICC International Union Against Cancer (1992) TNM classification of malignant tumours, 4th edn, 2nd rev. Springer, Berlin Heidelberg New York
38. Wilson TO, Podratz KC, Gaffey TA et al (1990) Evaluation of unfavorable histologic subtypes in endometrial adenocarcinoma. Am J Obstet Gynecol 162: 418–426

22 Fallopian Tube Carcinoma

A.C. Rosen and M.J. Klein

Introduction

Primary carcinoma of the fallopian tube is a very rare tumour. Worldwide, little more than 1500 cases have been published [8]. Fallopian tube carcinoma (FTC) is highly aggressive and has a poor prognosis. In the last few decades efforts were made to evaluate prognostic factors in clinical and pathological fields as well as the impact of therapy on survival. However, up to now, no multivariate analysis has been published.

Anatomic Extent of Disease

Anatomic extent of the disease at the time of diagnosis is the most powerful prognostic factor. The lack of generally approved staging criteria resulted in various and poorly comparable staging systems. Thus, Schiller and Silverberg followed the Dukes classification and showed it was of good prognostic value [11]. Erez, however, stated that tumour penetration through the serosa is significant in the early stage of the disease [2].

The FIGO (International Federation of Gynaecology and Obstetrics) TNM Classification for ovarian cancer was not found useful for FTC. Therefore, in 1991 a specific FTC FIGO classification was developed, taking anatomical as well as prognostic particularities into account [3] (Table 1). This classification was accepted as provisional by the UICC in 1993 and recommended for further testing before general acceptance [4].

In stage IA a 5-year survival rate of 56% was found. In the higher stages the 5-year survival rate declines from 27% (stage II) to 14% (stage III) and is statistically 0% in stage IV [5, 6, 9, 10]. Figure 1 shows a good correlation between these stage groupings and prognosis.

The prognostic importance of lymphatic spread is not clear. Some authors report early lymphatic dissemination which could precede abdominal spread and would be responsible for a high rate of recurrence and distant metastasis [13]. Other studies report lymph node spread to have only little prognostic value and no significant influence on overall survival as long as the intra-abdominal extent remains the same [5, 6].

Table 1. Summary of TNM classification and FIGO staging of fallopian tube carcinoma [4]

TNM	Fallopian tube	FIGO
T1	Limited to tube(s)	I
T1a	One tube, serosa intact	IA
T1b	Both tubes, serosa intact	IB
T1c	Serosa penetrated, malignant cells in ascites or peritoneal washings	IC
T2	Pelvic extension	II
T2a	Uterus, ovaries	IIA
T2b	Other pelvic structures	IIB
T2c	Malignant cells in ascites or peritoneal washings	IIC
T3 and/or N1	Peritoneal metastasis outside pelvis and/or regional lymph node metastasis	III
T3a	Microscopic peritoneal metastasis	IIIA
T3b	Macroscopic peritoneal metastasis ≤ 2 cm	IIIB
T3c and/or N1	Peritoneal metastasis > 2 cm and/or regional lymph node metastasis	IIIC
M1	Distant metastasis (excludes peritoneal metastasis)	IV

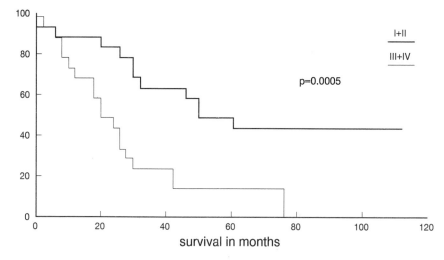

Fig. 1. Survival curves for 115 patients with carcinoma of the fallopian tube observed in Austria during the period 1980–1990. FIGO TNM stage I and II ($n = 67$) versus III and IV ($n = 48$) [9]

Ascites – a strong prognosticator in ovarian cancer – was found in only 22% of the women with stage III and IV disease and did not show any negative influence on survival in patients with cancer of the fallopian tube [9].

Histological Type and Grade

Carcinomas of the fallopian tube are adenocarcinomas. Pathological subclasses such as serous, papillary, mucinous, tubular or solid can be distinguished but have no impact on prognosis [9]. In contrast to this, histological grading distinguishing between G1 (well differentiated), G2 (moderately differentiated) and G3 (poorly differentiated) tumours seems to have some prognostic influence. On the whole, better differentiated tumours showed a trend to a more favourable outcome than G3 tumours. The median survival for patients with G1 tumours is about 45 months, whereas G2 and G3 tumours showed a poorer prognosis with a patient survival rate of only 29 months [7, 9].

Other Histological Factors

Lymphocytic infiltration of the tumour seems to be of prognostic influence in early stages of the disease. This was seen in approximately 70% of all tumours in stage I and II disease. Patients with this reaction showed a statistically significantly better outcome than patients without this feature (survival at the 75th quantile, 49.3 versus 19.4 months) [10].

Biological Factors

Oestrogen and progesterone receptors were recently demonstrated by immunohistology (26% ER positive, 42% PgR positive), but have failed to show any prognostic impact [10].

FTC shows a much higher rate of aneuploidy (>80%) compared to ovarian cancer [1, 11]. The only available data dealing with ploidy status of FTC show an equal distribution of diploid and aneuploid tumours among all FIGO stages and a better outcome of the diploid cases [11].

Conclusion

Primary carcinoma of the fallopian tube is so rare that data from single institutions cannot lead to any substantial conclusions regarding prognosis or therapy. The low number of cases, non-standardized staging systems and a variety of methods of treatment, particularly as far as postoperative therapy is concerned, make it difficult to compare results of different authors. Although tumour ploidy shows some prognostic value, at present, only anatomic extent and lymphocytic infiltration can be considered reliable prognostic factors.

References

1. Berchuk A, Boente MP, Kerns BJ, Kinney RB, Soper JT, Clarke-Pearson DL, Bast RC, Bacus SS (1992) Ploidy analysis of epithelial ovarian cancers using image cytometry. Gynecol Oncol 44: 61–65
2. Erez S, Kaplan AL, Wall JA (1967) Clinical staging of carcinoma of the uterine tube. Obstet Gynecol 30: 547–550
3. Creasman WT (1992) Revision in classification by the International Federation of Gynecology and Obstetrics. Am J Obstet Gynecol 167: 857–858
4. Hermanek P, Henson DE, Hutter RVP, Sobin LH (eds) (1993) TNM Supplement 1993. A commentary on uniform use. Springer, Berlin Heidelberg New York
5. Klein M, Rosen A, Lahousen M, Graf AH, Vavra N, Beck A (1993) Radical lymphadenectomy in the primary carcinoma of the Fallopian tube. Arch Gynecol Obstet 253: 21–25
6. Klein M, Rosen AC, Lahousen M, Graf AH, Vavra N, Beck A (1994) Lymphogenous metastases in the primary carcinoma of the fallopian tube and its impact on prognosis. Gynecol Oncol 55: 336–338
7. McMurray EH, Jacobs AJ, Perez CA, Camel HM, Kao MS, Galakatos A (1986) Carcinoma of the fallopian tube. Cancer 58: 2070–2075
8. Pfleiderer A (1989) Malignom der Tube. In: Wulf K, Schmidt-Matthiesen S (eds) Klinik der Frauenheilkunde und Geburtshilfe, vol XII. Urban and Schwarzenberg, Munich, pp 38–44
9. Rosen AC, Klein M, Lahousen M, Graf AH, Reiner A, Vavra N (1993) Primary fallopian tube carcinoma in Austria – retrospective multicenter study. Br J Cancer 68: 605–609
10. Rosen AC, Reiner A, Klein M, Lahousen M, Graf AH, Vavra N, Rosen HR (1994) Prognostic factors in primary fallopian tube carcinomas. Gynecol Oncol 53: 307–313
11. Rosen AC, Graf AH, Klein M, Lahousen M, Vaora N, Reiner A, Hacker GW (1994) DNA ploidy in primary fallopian tube carcinomas using cytometry. Int J Cancer 59: 1–4
12. Schiller HM, Silverberg SG (1971) Staging and prognosis in primary carcinoma of the fallopian tube. Cancer 28: 389–395
13. Tamimi HK, Figge DC (1981) Adenocarcinoma of the uterine tube: potential for lymph node metastases. Am J Obstet Gynecol 141: 132–137

23 Ovarian Cancer

A. Pfleiderer

The ovary is the site of a wide variety of tumours. Ovarian cancer is a term covering not one but many diseases with a range of biological manifestations. The number of prognostic factors for malignant germ cell and sex-cord stromal tumours is too small and their heterogeneity too great for multivariate analysis. Therefore, this chapter refers only to prognostic factors in epithelial ovarian carcinoma. The following will be discussed: (a) epithelial tumours of borderline malignancy (carcinomas of low malignant potential), (b) invasive stage I and II ovarian carcinomas and (c) invasive stage III and IV ovarian carcinomas.

Prognostic Factors in Borderline Epithelial Tumours of the Ovary

It is important to analyse patients with epithelial tumours of borderline malignancy separately, as these tumours have a different natural history to invasive carcinomas.

Histological Type

Serous and mucinous neoplasms are the two most frequent types of ovarian borderline carcinomas [12, 40]. Most serous borderline tumours show a remarkably constant and homogenous pattern throughout the neoplasm. The frequency of bilaterality is high, ranging from 26% to 50%. About 35% are associated with apparent extra-ovarian spread at the time of initial diagnosis as tumour implants on the pelvic peritoneum and infracolic omentum. It is unknown whether these peritoneal and omental lesions are true implantation metastases or autochthonous lesions arising in situ. Some of these secondary lesions will progress, albeit usually in an indolent fashion, recur after a long interval or even behave as a clearly malignant adenocarcinoma, but a considerable proportion will either remain stationary or regress after removal of the dominant ovarian neoplasm. Mucinous tumours of borderline malignancy, on the other hand, show a variety of patterns. Bilaterality of mucinous borderline tumours is much lower, averaging about 5%. A total of 10%–15% of these tumours show apparent extra-ovarian spread, nearly always taking the form of pseudomyxoma peritonei. Pseudomyxoma peritonei occurs almost invariably in association with the enteric type of ovarian borderline mucinous tumour [12]. Endometrioid, Brenner and clear cell tumours of borderline malignancy are very rare and data on prognostic factors are not available.

Anatomic Extent Expressed by TNM FIGO Stage Grouping (UICC 1992) [19]

Borderline ovarian tumours are associated with an excellent overall survival, yet a small fraction of patients die of the disease [26]. The 5-year survival rate for women with serous tumours of borderline malignancy is between 90% and 97%, and the 10-year survival rate between 75% and 90%. The 5- and 10-year survival rates of patients with stage I disease exceed 95%. Survival rates for patients with bilateral tumours (IB) and stage IIA are as good as for stage IA, whilst the 5-year survival rates for stages IIB or III have been reported to be between 65% and 87% [40]. A more effective staging technique, however, reveals far more peritoneal implants today [24, 26]. This suggests firstly that the prognosis for stage IIB, IIC and III borderline serous tumours may be rather better (Pettersson [35]: IIB and IIC, 93.5%; III, 90.3%) than that reported in older studies and secondly that stage, though of some clinical value, is of much less prognostic significance than is the case with invasive serous neoplasms. The overall 5- and 10-year survival rates for women with borderline mucinous tumours are 87% and 85%; for stage I 98% and 96%. The outlook for patients with pseudomyxoma peritonei is much more gloomy and probably no higher than 20%. The problem of formulating an individual prognosis, especially for the minority of patients who will succumb to their disease, is principally a matter for the pathologist, since clinical stage is of much lesser predictive value than is the case for invasive malignant tumours [12].

Ploidy

During the last two decades several studies have shown nuclear DNA content to be of prognostic value [13]. It has been demonstrated that the frequency of diploid tumours measured by flow cytophotometry is much higher in borderline tumours than in invasive cancer. In a retrospective study of 370 patients [21], prognostic significance of DNA ploidy in relation to clinical and histopathological factors was evaluated: 91% of the tumours were diploid and 9% aneuploid. Aneuploidy was associated with older age, more advanced disease and non-serous histological types. By multivariate analysis the only parameters with prognostic significance for death from disease were ploidy, stage, histological type and age. Patients with aneuploid tumours, regardless of histology and stage, had a 19-fold increased risk of dying of disease compared to patients with diploid tumours. However, Harlow et al. [16], in a population-based analysis of 61 cases, could not confirm these findings.

Age

Age was of prognostic value only concerning long-time survival [21]. In another study, 31.8% of the patients suffering from borderline tumours were younger than 40 years compared to 8.7% of the invasive cases [35].

Prognostic Factors in Invasive Carcinoma Stage I and II

Prognostic factors in localised invasive ovarian cancer are different from those of higher stage tumours.

Anatomic Extent Expressed by TNM FIGO Stage Grouping

The 5-year survival of patients with epithelial ovarian cancer is correlated with tumour stage. The 5-year survival rate for patients with stage I tumours is 80%–95% depending on tumour grade. The 5-year survival rate for stages II and IIIA is about 55% compared to only 35% for stage IIIB [35]. Current studies using comprehensive staging laparotomy [33] demonstrate a 90% 5-year survival rate of patients with stage I and 80% of the small group of patients with stage II [50]. Numerous multivariate analyses show the importance of stage for survival of patients suffering from invasive ovarian cancer [5, 8, 14, 25, 43, 44, 46].

Histological Grade

In stage I (and II), the second most important independent prognostic factor is tumour grade. Stage I patients with well- or moderately differentiated tumours have a greater than 90% 5-year survival rate if treated with surgery alone. Patients with stage I disease with poorly differentiated tumours have a significantly lower survival rate, and postoperative therapy is indicated [50]. In advanced-stage patients, however, most studies have failed to demonstrate a significant correlation between histological grade and survival [33]. Testing the validity of a prognostic classification in 1698 postoperative patients at the Princess Margaret Hospital [7] and in 410 patients with stage I and II disease by a Danish multicenter study group [4], prognostic factors of significance were found to be grade and stage. The prognostic value of histological grading of malignant epithelial neoplasms has been widely accepted, but is highly subjective and is, in practice, difficult to apply in any consistent manner [11]. It is often the case that the more advanced the stage of the neoplasm, the more likely it is to be less differentiated.

Histological Type

Among the invasive epithelial ovarian carcinomas, endometrioid carcinomas had the best prognosis as long as there were no signs of spread, followed by the mucinous, serous and undifferentiated tumours in that order [25]. Clear cell ovarian carcinoma was not worse than the other types, but patients with stage I disease did significantly worse at 5 and 10 years [31]. Dembo et al. [8] pointed out the importance of histological type in relation to grading: low risk, all grade I serous and clear cell tumours; intermediate risk, all mucinous and endometrioid tumours; high risk, grade 2 and 3 serous and clear cell tumours and all unclassified or undifferentiated tumours. A multivariate analysis including patients treated from 1979 to 1985, however, indicates that histological type has less importance [7].

Ploidy and DNA Index

Several flow cytometric studies have shown that advanced-stage tumours have a higher frequency of aneuploidy [13, 23, 36] and have confirmed the prognostic significance of tumour ploidy [17]. As far as serous ovarian cancer is concerned, the DNA index was a more important prognostic factor in a multivariate analysis than stage, grade or ploidy [23]. DNA histogram and histological type as well as FIGO stage in that order proved to be the most discriminating parameters for the prediction of clinical outcome in stage I ovarian cancer. However, even when combined with conventional clinicopathological factors, they failed to give the correct prognostic assessment in about 20% of patients [41].

Other Prognostic Factors

The analysis of prognostic factors concerning relapse risk in stage I ovarian cancer of 519 patients treated in Oslo and Toronto revealed that grade of differentiation was the most powerful factor, but dense adhesions and large-volume ascites were also important. Bilaterality (IB), cyst rupture (IC), capsular penetration (IC), tumour size, histological type, patient age and postoperative therapy were not of prognostic significance [9]. The results of this study contradict earlier studies showing that the prognosis for patients with stage IB and IC (rupture) of poorly differentiated lesions [49] is worse than that of stage IA. The serum CA 125 levels had no independent prognostic significance [27].

Combined Prognostic Groups

The following combinations should be considered as stage-independent prognostic factors: grade of tumour and performance status within stage I; the presence of residual disease and grade within stage II; and the presence of residual disease within stage III [45]. Using these factors as many as six prognostic groups could be developed within a given stage. Survival rates varied from 46% to 91% in patients within different risk groups in stage I and from 9% to 84% in stage II.

Prognostic Factors in Invasive Carcinoma Stage III and IV

Most analyses concerning prognostic factors deal with ovarian carcinoma stage III. Survival is affected by anatomic extent, bulk and growth rate of residual tumour, patient age and various histological and biological features.

Anatomic Extent Expressed by TNM FIGO Stage Grouping

Patients with stage III disease have a 5-year survival rate of 22.7% and those with stage IV, 8% [35]. There are significant differences in the 5-year survival rates of patients with stage IIIA (>58%), IIIB (>38%) and IIIC (>22%) [35]. Partridge et al. [34] and Tropé (1993, personal communication) confirmed these data. In addition, analysis of the Oslo cases revealed that cases of stage IIIC (without remaining residual tumour after surgery, i.e. R0) were significantly worse than R0 cases of stage IIIB and IIIA. This confirms the more prominent role of preoperative tumour load as a prognostic factor.

Residual Disease

The volume of residual disease after cytoreductive surgery is well known as the strongest prognostic factor in extended ovarian carcinoma [6-8, 10, 14, 15, 35, 36, 38, 39, 43, 45, 46]. Patients with optimal cytoreduction of disease have a 22-month improvement in the median survival time compared with patients not undergoing optimal resection [33]. Not only the size of residual tumour but also the number of sites of residual tumour is an important prognostic factor [18]. It has not yet been established, however, whether the poor prognosis associated with bulky disease is due to the presence of an increased tumour burden (in which case cytoreductive surgery would be of potential benefit) or whether bulky disease is associated with differences in tumour biology [32]. Meerpohl et al. [30] analysed 245 cases in a multicentre study with respect to tumour reduction. Multivariate analysis detected extension to the upper abdomen as the most relevant factor against success. An important prognostic factor therefore is the preoperative tumour burden [18].

Age

Analysis of six major randomised trials carried out by GOG (Gynecologic Oncology Group) including 2123 patients [47] and of 342 patients collected in studies by SWOG (Southwest Oncology Group) [1] revealed age as an important prognostic factor. Both trials found age, volume of residual disease and performance status as the three major prognostic factors: patients older than 69 and 65 years of age, respectively, exhibited poorer survival, but there was no evidence that older patients tolerated intensive schedules worse than younger patients. Age was the most significant variable related to survival in stages III and IV and could not be accounted for by differences in adequacy of surgery [28] or dose intensity of chemotherapy [28, 47].

Histological Type, Grade, Tumour Ploidy and Morphometry

The histological type has less prognostic significance than the other clinical factors such as stage, volume of disease and histological grade [33]. A univariate analysis of stage III and IV cases ($n = 181$) demonstrated a prognostic effect of histological grade, age, residual tumour, stage and ploidy; a multivariate analysis, however, revealed the size of the residual tumour after debulking and the age of the patient to be the only factors independently associated with survival; ploidy in stages III and IV is not an independent prognostic factor [37]. In an analysis of 73 cases, Baak et al. [2] showed that the statistically most significant prognostic combination consisted of mean nuclear area, presence or absence of bulky disease and FIGO stage (in order of decreasing importance). Högberg et al. [20] confirmed nuclear morphometry as a quantitative method to give objective and valuable prognostic information. By multivariate analysis, however, the age of the patient and the size of the residual tumour were shown to be the only independent prognostic factors. None of the morphological variables proved to be significant.

Growth Factors and Oncogene Amplification

Studies of the genes (proto-oncogenes, tumour suppressors, growth factors) involved in the development and progression of ovarian carcinomas suggest that activation of dominant oncogenes and the inactivation of tumour suppressors are the ultimate cause for the uncontrolled cell proliferation and other characteristics of ovarian carcinomas. For ovarian cancer the following seem to be relevant: transforming growth factor (TGF) alpha, epidermal growth factor (EGF), the cytokines colony-stimulating factor (CSF)-1, interleukin (IL)-6, tumour necrosis factor (TNF), the receptors for EGF, erbB-2, fms and IL-6, the nuclear transcript factors JUN, FOS and MYC and the suppressor genes P53, RB-1 and TGF beta. However, data are not yet reliable enough for prognosis [3, 22]. Slamon et al. [42]

reported the significance of amplification and overexpression of the Her-2/neu proto-oncogene in patients with ovarian cancer. Gene amplification was highly associated with survival. Analysing 38 cases of ovarian cancer, Marth et al. [29] could not confirm Her 2/neu amplification as prognostically relevant.

References

1. Alberts DS, Dahlberg S, Green SJ, Garcia D, Hannigan EV, O'Toole R, Stock-Novack D, Surwit EA, Malviya VK, Jolles CJ (1993) Analysis of patient age as an independent prognostic factor for survival in a phase III study of cisplatin-cyclophosphamide versus carboplatin-cyclophamide in stages III (suboptimal) and IV ovarian cancer. A Southwest Oncology Group study. Cancer 71[2 Suppl]: 618–627
2. Baak JP, Schipper NW, Wisse-Brekelmans EC, Ceelen T, Bosman FT, van Geuns H, Wils J (1988) The prognostic value of morphometrical features and cellular DNA content in cisplatin treated late ovarian cancer patients. Br J Cancer 57: 503–508
3. Bauknecht T (1993) Die Biologie maligner Ovarialtumoren: Fortschritte und Probleme. In: Meerpohl HG, Pfleiderer A, Profous CZ (eds) Das Ovarialkarzinom 1. Springer, Berlin Heidelberg New York, pp 3–6
4. Bertelsen K, Holund B, Andersen JE, Nielsen K, Stroyer I, Ladehoff P (1993) Prognostic factors and adjuvant treatment in early epithelial ovarian cancer. Int J Gynecol Cancer 3: 211–218
5. Breitenecker G, Bartl W, Schreiber V (1982) Die Bedeutung verschiedener morphologischer Parameter für die Prognose des Ovarialkarzinoms. In: Dallenbach-Hellweg G (ed) Ovarialtumoren. Springer, Berlin Heidelberg New York
6. Burghardt E, Lahousen M, Stetter H (1989) The significance of pelvic and para-aortic lymphadenectomy in the operative treatment of ovarian cancer. Baillieres Clin Obstet Gynaecol 3: 157–165
7. Carey MS, Dembo AJ, Simm JE, Fyles AW, Treger T, Bush RS (1993) Testing the validity of a prognostic classification in patients with surgically optimal ovarian carcinoma: a 15 year review. Int J Gynecol Cancer 3:24–35
8. Dembo AJ, Bush RS, Brown TC (1982) Clinico-pathological correlates in ovarian cancer. Bull Cancer (Paris) 69: 292–297
9. Dembo AJ, Davy M, Stenwig AE, Berle EJ, Bush RS, Kjorstad K (1990) Prognostic factors in patients with stage I epithelial ovarian cancer. Obstet Gynecol 75: 263–273
10. Di Re F, Fontanelli R, Raspagliesi F, Di Re E (1989) Pelvic and paraaortic lymphadenectomy in cancer of the ovary. Baillieres Clin Obstet Gynecol 3: 131–142
11. Fox H (1985) Pathology of surface epithelial tumours. In: Hudson CN (ed) Ovarian cancer. Oxford Medical, Oxford, pp 72–93
12. Fox H (1989) The concept of borderline malignancy in ovarian tumours: a reappraisal. Curr Top Pathol 78: 111–134
13. Friedlander ML, Taylor IW, Russell P, Musgrove EA, Hedley DH, Tattersall MH (1983) Ploidy as a prognostic factor in ovarian cancer. Int J Gynecol Pathol 2: 55–63
14. Gall S, Bundy B, Beechum J, Whitney C, Homesley H, Lifshitz S, Adcock LL (1986) Therapy of stage III (optimal) epithelial carcinoma of the ovary, with melphalan or melphalan plus corynebactericum parvum. A GOG study. Gynecol Oncol 25: 26–36
15. Griffiths CT (1986) Surgery at the time of diagnosis in ovarian cancer. In: Blackledge G, Chan KK (eds) Management of ovarian cancer. Butterworths, London, pp 60–75
16. Harlow BL, Fuhr JE, McDonald TW, Schwartz SM, Beuerlein FJ, Weiss NS (1993) Flow cytometry as a prognostic indicator in women with borderline epithelial ovarian tumours. Gynecol Oncol 50: 305–309
17. Hedley DW, Friedlander ML, Taylor IN (1985) Application of DNA flow cytometry to paraffin-embedded archival material for the study of aneuploidy and its clinical significance. Cytometry 6: 327–333
18. Heintz AP, Van Oosterom AT, Trimbos JB, Schabereg A, Van der Velde EA, Nooy M (1988) The treatment of advanced ovarian carcinoma (I): clinical variables associated with prognosis. Gynecol Oncol 30: 347–358

19. Hermanek P, Sobin LH (eds) (1992) UICC TNM classification of malignant tumours, 4th edn, 2nd rev. Springer, Berlin Heidelberg New York
20. Högberg T, Wang G, Risber B, Guerrieri C, Hittson J, Boeryd B, Kagedal B, Simonsen E (1992) Nuclear morphometry: a strong prognostic factor for survival after secondary surgery in advanced ovarian cancer. Int J Gynecol Cancer 2: 198–206
21. Kaern J, Tropé CG, Kristensen GB, Abeler VM, Pettersen EO (1993) DNA ploidy; the most important prognostic factor in patients with borderline tumours of the ovary. Int J Gynecol Cancer 3: 349–358
22. Kacinski B (1993) Ovarian carcinoma: tumour and molecular biology. In: Meerpohl HG, Pfleiderer A, Profous CZ (eds) Das Ovarialkarzinom 1. Springer, Berlin Heidelberg New York, pp 7–19
23. Klemi PJ, Joensuu H, Maenpaa J, Kiilholma P (1989) Influence of cellular DNA content on survival in ovarian carcinoma. Obstet Gynecol 74: 200–204
24. Kliman L, Rome RM, Fortune DW (1986) Low malignant potential tumours of the ovary: a study of 76 cases. Obstet Gynecol 68: 338–344
25. Kolstad P (1986) Clinical gynecologic oncology. Norwegian University Press, Oslo
26. Leake JF, Currie JL, Rosenshein NB, Woodruff JD (1992) Long-term follow-up of serous ovarian tumours of low malignant potential. Gynecol Oncol 47: 150–8
27. Makar AP, Kristensen GB, Kaern J, Bormer OP, Abeler VM, Tropé CG (1992) Prognostic value of pre- and postoperative serum Ca 125 levels in ovarian cancer: new aspects and multivariate analysis. Obstetr Gynecol 79: 1002–1010
28. Marchetti DL, Lele SB, Priore RL, McPhee ME, Hreshchyshyn MM (1993) Treatment of advanced ovarian carcinoma in the elderly. Gynecol Oncol 49: 86–91
29. Marth CH, Zeimet AG, Müller-Holzner E, Schatzer J, Cronauer MV, Ullrich A, Daxenbichler E (1993) Die Bedeutung des Onkogens HER 2 beim Ovarialkarzinom. In: Meerpohl HG, Pfleiderer A, Profous CZ (eds) Das Ovarialkarzinom 1. Springer, Berlin Heidelberg New York, pp 28–36
30. Meerpohl HG, Sauerbrei W, Schumacher M, Pfleiderer A (1990) Welche Parameter beeinflussen die Größe des postoperativen Tumorrestes beim Ovarialkarzinom? Gynaekol Geburtsh 127: 11–12
31. O'Brien MER, Schofield JB, Tan S, Fryatt I, Fisher C, Wiltshaw E (1993) Clear cell epithelial ovarian cancer (mesonephroid): bad prognosis only in early stages. Gynecol Oncol 49: 250–254
32. Ozols RF, Young RC (1987) Ovarian cancer. Curr Probl Cancer 11: 57–122
33. Ozols RF, Rubin SC, Dembo AJ, Robboy S (1992) Epithelial ovarian cancer. In: Hoskins WJ, Perez CA, Young RC (eds) Gynecologic oncology. Lippincott, Philadelphia, pp 731–781
34. Partridge EE, Gunter BC, Gelder MS, Alvarez RD, Soong S-J, Austin JM, Kilgore LC (1993) The validity and significance of substages of advanced ovarian cancer. Gynecol Oncol 48: 236–241
35. Pettersson F (ed) (1991) Annual report on the results of treatment in gynecological cancer, vol XXI. Int J Gynecol Obstetr 36 [Suppl]: 1–315
36. Pfisterer J, Kommoss F, Renz H, Sauerbrei W, Meerpohl HG, Teufel G, Pfleiderer A (1993) Die flowzytometrische Bestimmung des nuklearen DNA-Gehaltes bei malignen epithelialen Tumoren der Ovarien. In: Meerpohl HG, Pfleiderer A, Profous CZ (eds) Das Ovarialkarzinom 1. Springer, Berlin Heidelberg New York Tokyo, pp 111–118
37. Pfisterer J, Kommoss F, Sauerbrei W, Renz H, du Bois A, Pfleiderer A. (1994) Cellular DNA content and survival in advanced ovarian carcinoma. Cancer 74: 2509–2515
38. Pfleiderer A (1989) Tumour reduction and chemotherapy in ovarian cancer. Baillieres Clin Obstet Gynaecol 3: 119–128
39. Pfleiderer A (1989) Malignome des Ovars. In: Wulf KH, Schmidt-Matthiesen H (eds) Klinik der Frauenheilkunde und Geburtshilfe, vol 12: Spezielle gynäkologische Onkologie II. Urban and Schwarzenberg, Munich, pp 45–129
40. Piver MS (1987) Progress and treatment of borderline ovarian tumours. In: Piver MS (ed) Ovarian malignancies. Churchill Livingstone, Edinburgh, pp 203–214
41. Punnonen R, Kallioniemi OP, Mattila J, Koivula T (1989) Prognostic assessment in stage I ovarian cancer using a discriminant analysis with clinicopathological and DNA flow cytometric data. Gynecol Obstet Invest 27: 213–216
42. Slamon DJ, Godolphin W, Jones LA, Holt JA, Wong SG, Keith DE, Levin WJ, Stuart SG, Udove J, Ullrich A et al (1989) Studies of the HER-2/NEU protooncogene in human breast and ovarian cancer. Science 244: 707–712

43. Smith JP, Day TG Jr (1979) Review of ovarian cancer at the University of Texas systems cancer center, MD Anderson hospital and tumor institute. Am J Obstet Gynecol 135: 984–993
44. Swenerton KD (1992) Prognostic indices in ovarian cancer. Acta Obstet Gynecol Scand 71 [Suppl 155]: 67–74
45. Swenerton KD, Hislop TE, Spinell J, Le Riche JC, Yang N, Boyes DA (1985) Ovarian carcinoma: a multivariate analysis of prognostic factors. Obstet Gynecol 65: 264–269
46. Terashima Y, Ochiai K, Sasaki H, Yakushiji M, Hirabayashi K (1989) Individualisation of surgical treatment for ovarian cancer. Baillieres Clin Obstet Gynaecol 3: 73–82
47. Thipgen T, Brady MF, Omura GA, Creasman WT, McGuire WP, Hoskins WJ, Williams S (1993) Age as a prognostic factor in ovarian carcinoma. The Gynecologic Oncology Group experience. Cancer 71 [Suppl]: 606–614
48. Tropé C (1993) Cellular DNA content as a new prognostic tool in patients with borderline tumors of the ovary. A second look. In: Meerpohl HG, Pfleiderer A, Profous CZ (eds) Das Ovarialkarzinom. 1.Tumorbiologie. Springer, Berlin Heidelberg New York, pp 90–100
49. Webb MJ, Decker DG, Mossey E, Williams TJ (1973) Factors influencing survival in stage I ovarian cancer. Am J Obstet Gynecol 116: 222–228
50. Young RC, Walton LA, Ellenberg SS, Homesley HD, Wilbanks GD, Decker DG, Miller A, Park R, Major F Jr (1990) Adjuvant therapy in stage I and stage II epithelial ovarian cancer. Results of two prospective randomized trials (see comments). N Engl J Med 322: 1021–1027

24 Prostate Carcinoma

L.J. Denis, P.A. Catton, M.K. Gospodarowicz,
G.P. Murphy, P.O. Hedlund, and F.K. Mostofi

Both incidental and clinical carcinoma of the prostate increase in incidence with age. The aging of the populations of the industrial nations is the major reason that adenocarcinoma of the prostate became the most common cancer in men. This cancer is usually multifocal in origin and presents in all stages of its natural and treated history as a heterogeneous disease with different biological potential.

Independent prognostic factors are sometimes far more important for a specific outcome of the disease than any treatment. It is important to recognise and identify these factors before and after completion of a trial in order to arrive at valid conclusions on the effectiveness of therapy. This can also serve as an indication for more or less aggressive treatment, depending on the prognostic index score [12].

In this review we only report on fixed pretreatment covariates, analysed by multivariate analysis.

Adenocarcinoma of the prostate in its natural course is a single biological process with a usually slow but constant growth. The most important aspect at the time of initial diagnosis is the distinction between localised disease, in which cure remains a possibility, and metastatic disease, in which all treatment is focused on disease control and palliation. It is evident that specific pathological features and biological or molecular expressions of tumour activity play a major role in the prognosis of localised disease in contrast to the prognosis of generalised disease.

Tumour-Related Factors

Anatomic Extent of Disease

The TNM classification [6, 28] is now universally accepted and widely utilised by the major urological organisations to categorise patients [44]. Anatomic extent of cancer as defined by TNM categories has been shown to be an independent factor for survival [13, 30, 31]. The relationship between stage and tumour grade has not been established, but appropriate use of carefully obtained stage and grade maximises the accuracy of any given prognosis [25].

In a landmark analysis of the prognostic factors for prostate cancer in the Veterans Administration Cooperative Urological Research Group studies, in which correct methodology was emphasised, it was shown that grade according to the Gleason sum and the presence or absence of metastasis were the most powerful prognostic factors in localised or advanced disease [8, 24]. Combined grading and staging seems to identify groups of patients in their proposed category score ranging from 3 to 15 (stage I, patterns 1–1, and stage 5, patterns 5–5), measured by follow-up mortality data in 1032 patients. There were no cancer deaths in the lowest prognostic categories, while 50% of patients with the highest category died of cancer. The grading, the size of the primary tumour and the average serum levels of acid phosphatase in patients with localised disease allow the formation of three risk groups that respectively show progression in 5 years in 6.9%, 9.1% and 31.2% of the cases. In patients with metastatic disease and Gleason sum above 8, the patients who did not die from cancer only amount to 35.8% of cases.

Tumour size in localised disease correlates with pathological disease extent. A tumour volume of 1.0 cm^3 has the probability of progression in capsular invasion of 0.210, in seminal vesical invasion of 0.042 and metastases of 0.032, while these figures in a tumour of 10 cm^3 are 0.746, 0.460 and 0.295, respectively [7]. However, in a multivariate analysis on progression of disease after radical prostatectomy in 185 patients, the histological grade was the best predictor of progression [17], while in a retrospective study on 1035 patients with T3 disease again tumour grade and increasing tumour volume correlated multivariately with cause-specific survival and progression with respective p values of 0.0021 and less than 0.0001 [9]. It is evident that tumour extent, even as capsular penetration, had a high risk of progression [16], while the adverse effect of locally advanced disease becomes even more distinct in node-positive disease. In a study on 475 patients treated with radiotherapy after pelvic lymphadenectomy, the patients with negative nodes had a median time to recurrence of 92 months versus 43 months for a single microscopic positive node, while cancer mortality with a mean follow-up of 67 months was 7% for patients with node-negative disease versus 30% for node-positive disease [23]. Involvement of the seminal vesicles is recognised as an adverse prognostic factor in progression or recurrence of disease treated by radical prostatectomy [3]. The direct consequence is that tumour size is predictive of local control in patients treated by radiotherapy or radical surgery [7, 40].

The independent prognostic value of both factors has been confirmed in the trials of the National Prostatic Cancer Project (NPCP) and the European Organisation for Research and Treatment of Cancer (EORTC) on patients with advanced disease [12, 13, 15]. Additional factors of importance included performance status, acid and alkaline phosphatase, associated chronic disease, haemoglobin, age and sometimes, but rarely, treatment.

Attempts to divide the patients in risk groups, usually three, resulted in median survival differences from 1 to more than 3 years. Total tumour burden as identified by the number of hot spots has been recognised as an independent prognostic factor in a number of studies [10, 12, 18, 29].

Histological Grade

The histological grade of the tumour correlates positively with progression and survival in all stages of the disease as repeatedly shown [12, 13, 15, 17, 33, 40].

Prognostic index scores designed to categorise patients in good and poor risk groups in order to adjust clinical management include at least grade as an independent factor [12, 13, 45, 46]. Tumour grading proved to be of independent significance to predict progression in the earliest T categories of prostate carcinoma [1, 2, 35].

Conventional grading considers glandular differentiation, the presence of mitosis and/or nuclear anaplasia. Separate evaluation of these factors [43] and use of a mitotic index [19] have been reported to separate the large group of G2 tumours into different prognostic subgroups. Neuroendocrine cell-negative tumours have a significantly better prognosis for survival than do positive tumours [14].

Ploidy

A correlation of the content of deoxyribonucleic acid (DNA) in the tumour cells has been suggested as a possible additional prognostic parameter to grade assessed by cytology or histology. Low-grade tumours are mostly diploid and high-grade tumours mostly aneuploid [1, 34]. Ploidy was shown to enhance the prognostic value of grade, especially in the moderately differentiated tumours [36, 37]. However, other studies failed to confirm these results [27, 32, 41].

Despite a large number of published reports, few are comparable due to lack of uniformity in methodology and categorisation of patients and the value of ploidy to predict prognosis in prostate carcinoma remains unclear.

The concept emerges that ploidy may be of value in patients with localised disease as compared to patients with distant metastases, in whom knowledge of the ploidy status will hardly influence management. Further clinical investigation is needed in this area to establish the independent correlation of DNA ploidy analysis with prognostic indicators proven to have an effect on treatment decisions.

Prostate-Specific Antigen

Prostate-specific antigen (PSA) has emerged as a potent and the most widely used marker of tumour activity. The prediction of pathological stage was enhanced by adding serum PSA to the Gleason score and clinical stage [39]. Undetectable levels of serum PSA are expected after a complete eradication of the carcinoma by radical prostatectomy, and PSA is an independent prognostic factor to measure response to radiotherapy and subsequent failure [42]. Also, a rapid and maximal decrease in serum PSA after hormonal treatment predicted a more favourable prognosis [4], while increasing serum PSA levels in patients in remission indicated the onset of clinical progression in the majority of the patients [12]. The fact that the absolute serum value correlates strongly with tumour burden is reflected in the outcome of a study on 161 patients in which an initial serum PSA level over 15 ng/ml was a powerful predictor of probable failure [47].

Alkaline Phosphatase

High levels of alkaline phosphatase (ALP) reflect an increased activity of bone and have been shown to be an independent prognostic factor in all randomised prospective trials on patients with metastatic cancer. The role of ALP in predicting survival was also shown in hormone-resistant disease [21].

Haemoglobin/Anemia

Low haemoglobin levels were found to be associated with poor survival in treated patients with metastatic disease [38].

Serum Testosterone

The pretreatment value of serum testosterone has been correlated with survival in patients with locally advanced and metastatic disease treated with hormones. Low pretreatment values predicted poor survival [18, 27, 29], but they may be related to the performance status of the patient.

Patient-Related Factors

Older age, not surprisingly, has been identified as a negative prognostic factor for survival of patients with advanced and metastatic disease treated with hormones in prospective studies [12, 13, 15]. The presence of concomitant disease has been identified as a negative factor in patients with metastatic disease [12, 13]. Low socio-economic status resulting in late stage and high grade at presentation may explain the poor survival of African-Americans with prostate carcinoma [5, 11]. Sedimentation rate was statistically significant in the analysis of a study on 150 patients with a p value of less than 0.0001 [30]. In 224 patients with hormone-resistant progression and a 1-year survival rate of only 24%, the independent prognostic factors were performance status, serum creatinine, ALP and duration of response to primary treatment [21].

   Performance status at presentation has been identified as a most important prognostic factor in a number of randomised studies in patients with advanced disease [12, 15]. Obstructive symptoms and pain have both been identified as adverse prognostic factors for survival, independent of performance status, hormonal treatment and serum ALP [10, 15].

Treatment-Related Factors

Transurethral resection of the prostate (TURP) has been reported to adversely influence progression and survival in patients treated with external beam radiation [20, 33], while conflicting reports failed to identify TURP as an adverse factor [3, 22].

The duration of response to primary hormonal treatment merely reflects the hormone-responsive status of the tumour at initiation of endocrine treatment resulting in increased progression-free survival and subsequent overall survival. However, all patients with hormone-resistant cancer in relapse, regardless of previous responses, show a poor prognosis [21].

Discussion

The treatment of prostate carcinoma in all stages of the disease is still controversial. All of the cited literature used multivariate analysis in which single covariates were shown to have an independent effect on end points and outcome of disease. These end points, especially to progression of disease, were not always clear. We also focused attention on the influence of initial prognostic factors known at diagnosis and before treatment or when a new treatment was started.

It is evident that the covariates for localised disease are markedly different from those for metastatic disease. A list of the most important prognostic factors in both phases of the disease is presented in Table 1. Stage and grade clearly dominate the assessment in patients with localised disease, while host-related factors will predict not only cause-specific but also overall survival in patients with metastatic disease. In addition, old age means that the patients are more likely to die from some cause other than cancer.

A number of prospective trials where the known prognostic factors could be balanced in the different treatment arms suggest the feasibility of risk group formation that separates patients as to outcome of disease and diminishes pure statistical chance by counting on a group of independent covariates.

Prognostic index scores in metastatic disease included the following: ALP, T classification and associated disease [13]; ALP, pain, haemoglobin and grade [12]; or performance status, ALP, creatinine and hormone response duration in hormone-refractory patients [21]. These index scores allow a separation of a cohort of trial patients into different subsets with a wide variation of outcome, even survival. These observations should guide us, lead to the establishment of more stringent entry criteria and convince the medical community to launch multicentre studies with larger accrual to allow statistical analysis in these subsets of patients.

Table 1. Significant prognostic factors by multivariate analysis on patients with localised or metastatic prostate carcinoma predicting outcome as progression and cause-specific survival

Localised carcinoma	Metastatic carcinoma
Tumour-related factors	
Extent of disease	
T and volume	T4
N positive	Extent of M1 disease
Other pathological factors	
Grade	Grade
Ploidy	
Biochemical factors	
PSA	PSA, ALP, Hb
Patient-related factors	
	Socio-economic status
	Age
	Performance status
	Pain
	Chronic disease
Treatment-related factors	
Previous TURP	Duration of primary response to hormones in progressive disease

PSA, prostate-specific antigen; ALP, alkaline phosphatase; Hb, haemoglobin; TURP, transurethral resection of the prostate.

Conclusions

The anatomic extent of disease as expressed by the TNM classification and the histological grade are still the most important prognostic factors in prostate carcinoma. A number of studies have shown that the prognostic factors for localised disease depend essentially on tumour-related factors, of which volume and still unknown biological factors play a major role. The impact of the total tumour mass and its effect on the patient demonstrate the importance of defining the independent factors and using this definition to stratify subsets of patients with identical prognosis. The important prognostic factors are easily identified in prostate carcinoma in routine practice, but further studies are recommended to reach a practical consensus on the clinical value of new prognostic factors, the technology and the therapeutic decisions arising from this information. Teamwork and quality control are essential for future studies.

References

1. Adolfsson J, Rönström L, Hedlund P et al (1990) The prognostic value of modal deoxyribonucleic acid in low grade, low stage untreated prostate cancer. J Urol 144: 1404–1406
2. Adolfsson J, Carstensen J (1991) Natural course of clinically localised prostate adenocarcinoma in men less than 70 years old. J Urol 146: 96–98

3. Anscher MS, Prosnitz LR (1991) Multivariate analysis of factors predicting local relapse after radical prostatectomy – possible indications for postoperative radiotherapy. Int J Radiat Oncol Biol Phys 21: 941–947
4. Arai Y, Yoshiki T, Yoshida O (1990) Prognostic significance of prostate specific antigen in endocrine treatment for prostatic cancer. J Urol 144: 1415–1419
5. Aziz H, Rotman M, Thelmo W et al (1988) Radiation-treated carcinoma of prostate. Comparison of survival of black and white patients by Gleason's grading system. Am J Clin Oncol 11: 166–171
6. Beahrs OH, Henson DE, Hutter RVP, Kennedy BJ (eds) (1992) American Joint Committee on Cancer (AJCC): Manual for staging of cancer, 4th edn. Philadelphia, Lippincott
7. Bostwick DG, Lee F, Graham SD et al (1993) Staging of early prostate cancer: a proposed tumour volume-based prognostic index. Urology 41: 403–411
8. Byar D, Corle D (1984) Analysis of prognostic factors for prostatic cancer in the VACURG studies. In: Denis L, Prout G, Schröder F (eds) Controlled clinical trials in urologic oncology. Raven, New York, pp 147–168
9. Cheng WS, Frydenberg M, Bergstralh EJ et al (1993) Radical prostatectomy for pathologic stage C prostate cancer: influence of pathologic variables and adjuvant treatment on disease outcome. Urology 42: 283–291
10. Chodak GW, Vogelzang NJ, Caplan RJ et al (1991) Independent prognostic factors in patients with metastatic (stage D2) prostate cancer. The Zoladex Study Group. J Am Med Assoc 265: 618–621
11. Dayal HH, Polissar L, Dahlberg S (1985) Race, socioeconomic status, and other prognostic factors for survival from prostate cancer. J Natl Cancer Inst 74: 1001–1006
12. Denis L (1993) Staging and prognosis in prostate cancer. Eur Urol 24: 13–19
13. De Voogt H, Suciu S, Sylvester R et al (1989) Multivariate analysis of prognostic factors in patients with advanced prostatic cancer. Results from two EORTC trials. J Urol 141: 883–888
14. Di Sant'Agnese PA, de Messy Jensen KL (1987) Neuroendocrine differentiation in prostatic carcinoma. Hum Pathol 18: 849–856
15. Emrich LJ, Priore RL, Murphy GP et al (1985) Prognostic factors in patients with advanced stage prostate cancer. Cancer Res 45: 5173–5179
16. Epstein JI, Carmichael MJ, Pizov G et al (1993) Influence of capsular penetration on progression following radical prostatectomy: a study of 196 cases with long-term followup. J Urol 150: 135–141
17. Epstein JI, Carmichael M, Partin AW et al (1993) Is tumor volume an independent predictor of progression following radical prostatectomy? A multivariate analysis of 185 clinical stage B adenocarcinomas of the prostate with 5 years of followup. J Urol 149: 1478–1481
18. Ernst DS, Hanson J, Venner PM (1991) Analysis of prognostic factors in men with metastatic prostate cancer. J Urol 146: 372–376
19. Eskelinen M, Lipponen P, Majapuro R et al (1991) Prognostic factors in prostatic adenocarcinoma assessed by means of quantitative histology. Eur Urol 19: 274–278
20. Forman JD, Order SE, Zinreich ES et al (1986) The correlation of pretreatment transurethral resection of prostatic cancer with tumor dissemination and disease-free survival. A univariate and multivariate analysis. Cancer 58: 1770–1778
21. Fossa SD, Dearnaley DP, Law M et al (1992) Prognostic factors in hormone-resistant progressing cancer of the prostate. Ann Oncol 3: 361–366
22. Fowler JJ, Fisher HA, Kaiser DL et al (1984) Relationship of pretreatment transurethral resection of the prostate to survival without distant metastases in patients treated with 125 I-implantation for localized prostatic cancer. Cancer 53: 1857–1863
23. Gervasi LA, Mata JA, Scardino JA et al (1989) Prognostic significance of lymph node metastases in prostatic cancer. J Urol 142: 332–336
24. Gleason DF, Mellinger GT, Veterans Administration Cooperative Urological Research Group (1974) Prediction of prognosis for prostatic adenocarcinoma by combined histological grading and clinical staging. J Urol 111: 58–64
25. Grayhack JT, Assimos DG (1983) Prognostic significance of tumour grade and stage in the patient with carcinoma of the prostate. Prostate 4: 13–31
26. Harper M, Pierrepoint C, Griffiths K (1984) Carcinoma of the prostate: relationship of pretreatment hormone levels to survival. Eur J Cancer Clin Oncol 20: 477–482
27. Haugen OA, Mjölneröd O (1990) DNA-ploidy as prognostic factor in prostatic carcinoma. Int J Cancer 45: 224–228

28. Hermanek P, Sobin LH (eds) (1992) UICC: TNM classification of malignant tumours, 4th edn, 2nd rev. Springer, Berlin Heidelberg New York
29. Ishikawa S, Soloway MS, van der Zwaag R et al (1989) Prognostic factors in survival free of progression after androgen deprivation therapy for treatment of prostate cancer. J Urol 141: 1139–1142
30. Johansson JE, Adami HO, Andersson SO et al (1989) Natural history of localised prostatic cancer. A population-based study in 223 untreated patients. Lancet 1: 799–803
31. Johansson J, Andersson S, Holmberg L et al (1991) Prognostic factors in progression-free survival and corrected survival in patients with advanced prostatic cancer: Results from a randomized study comprising 150 patients treated with orchiectomy or estrogens. J Urol 146: 1327–1333
32. Jones E, McNeal J, Bruchovsky N et al (1990) DNA content in prostatic adenocarcinoma: a flow cytometry study of the predictive value of aneuploidy for tumour volume, percentage Gleason grade 4 and 5, and lymph node metastases. Cancer 66: 752–757
33. Leibel S, Hanks G, Kramer S (1984) Patterns of care outcome studies: results of the national practice in adenocarcinoma of the prostate. Int J Rad Oncol Biol Phys 10: 401–409
34. Lieber M (1992) DNA content/ploidy as prognostic factors in prostate cancer. Prostate [Suppl] 4: 119–124
35. Lowe BA, Listrom MB (1988) Incidental carcinoma of the prostate: an analysis of the predictors of progression. J Urol 140: 1340–1344
36. Miller J, Horsfall D, Marshall V et al (1991) The prognostic value of deoxyribonucleic acid flow cytometric analysis in stage D2 prostatic carcinoma. J Urol 145: 1192–1196
37. Montgomery BT, Nativ O, Blute ML et al (1990) Stage B prostate adenocarcinoma. Flow cytometric nuclear DNA ploidy analysis. Arch Surg 125: 327–331
38. Mulders PF, Dijkman GA, Fernandez et al (1990) Analysis of prognostic factors in disseminated prostatic cancer. An update. Dutch Southeastern Urological Cooperative Group. Cancer 65: 2758–2761
39. Partin AW, Yoo J, Carter HB et al (1993) The use of prostate specific antigen, clinical stage and Gleason score to predict pathological stage in men with localized prostate cancer. J Urol 150: 110–114
40. Pilepich MV, Krall JM, Sause WT et al (1987) Prognostic factors in carcinoma of the prostate – analysis of RTOG study 75–06. Int J Radiat Oncol Biol Phys 13: 339–349
41. Ritchie AW, Dorey F, Layfield LJ et al (1988) Relationship of DNA content to conventional prognostic factors in clinically localised carcinoma of the prostate. Br J Urol 62: 245–260
42. Russell K, Dunatov C, Hafermann M et al (1991) Prostate specific antigen in the management of patients with localized adenocarcinoma of the prostate treated with primary radiation therapy. J Urol 146: 1046–1052
43. Schröder FH, Hop WCJ, Blom JHM et al (1985) Grading of prostatic cancer. III. Multivariate analysis of prognostic parameters. Prostate 7: 13–20
44. Schröder FH, Hermanek P, Denis L et al (1992) The TNM classification of prostate cancer. Prostate [Suppl] 4: 129–138
45. Wilson DW, Harper ME, Jensen HM et al (1985) A prognostic index for the clinical management of patients with advanced prostatic cancer: a British Prostate Study Group investigation. Prostate 7: 131–141
46. Zagars GK, von Eschenbach AC, Ayala AG (1993) Prognostic factors in prostate cancer. Analysis of 874 patients treated with radiation therapy. Cancer 72: 1709–1725
47. Zietman AL, Coen JJ, Shipley WU, Willett CG, Efird JT (1994) Radical radiation therapy in the management of prostatic adenocarcinoma: the initial prostate specific antigen value as a predictor of treatment outcome. J Urol 151: 640–645

25 Testicular Germ Cell Tumors

M.K. Gospodarowicz and J.F.G. Sturgeon

Germ cell tumors account for 95% of testicular tumors and are the commonest malignant tumors in young men. The pathology of germ cell testis tumors is complex and the two most widely used classifications are those of WHO, based on the original Dixon-Moore system, and Pugh, used mainly in the United Kingdom. The WHO classification [31] uses the following categories:

1. Tumors of one histologic type
   a) Seminoma
   b) Spermatocytic seminoma
   c) Embryonal carcinoma
   d) Yolk sac tumor
   e) Polyembryoma
   f) Choriocarinoma
   g) Teratomas
      – Mature
      – Immature
      – With malignant transformation
2. Tumors of more than one histologic type
   a) Embryonal carcinoma and teratoma
   b) Choriocarcinoma and any other type
   c) Other combinations

The British Testicular Tumor Panel [32] uses the following classification:

1. Seminoma
2. Teratoma
   a) Differentiated (TD)
   b) Malignant intermediate (MTI)
   c) Malignant trophoblastic (MTT)
   d) Malignant undifferentiated (MTU)
3. Combined tumors (seminoma and teratoma coexisting)

There are two main groups of tumors, pure seminomas and others, referred to as nonseminomatous germ cell tumors, including mixed tumors of nonseminomatous components and mixed seminoma and nonseminoma (NSGCTT). Patients with seminomas routinely present with stage I disease and are extremely radiosensitive. In contrast, patients with nonseminomas tend to present more often with stage II-III disease and are less sensitive to treatment with radiation (RT). In the past there were substantial differences in the management and the outcome of these two diseases. With the introduction of effective chemotherapy, the recent interest in surveillance for clinical stage I disease, and the recognition of the occurrence of subsequent nonseminoma in patients treated for pure seminoma, the differences in the approach to these diseases are becoming less pronounced. However, since the management of seminoma is still based mainly on RT and NSGCTT largely on chemotherapy, the patterns of failure and prognostic factors differ. For the purposes of this review the prognostic factors for seminoma and NSGCTT will be discussed separately (Tables 1, 2).

Seminoma

The main prognostic factors in seminoma are stage and bulk of disease [3, 37, 38]. Although many other factors have been examined, none has been consistently identified as being of independent prognostic value. The overall prognosis for patients with seminoma is excellent. This is largely due to the tendency for patients to present with localized disease that is curable with orchiectomy alone. Since patients with seminoma present most often with early-stage disease and

Table 1. Prognostic factors in seminoma

Factor	Unfavorable variant
Anatomic extent	Stages II and III
Retroperitoneal bulk	More than 5–10 cm or palpable mass
Site of metastasis	Lung, liver
Histologic type	Anaplastic
Tumor markers	β-HCG more than 1000 IU/l
Biochemical markers	LDH more than twice normal

β-HCG, beta human chorionic gonadotrophin; LDH, lactate dehydrogenase.

Table 2. Prognostic factors in nonseminomatous germ cell tumors

Factor	Unfavorable variant
Age	More than 30–35 years
Anatomic extent	Stage III
Volume of metastatic disease	Number and size
Site of metastasis	Liver, brain, neck lymph nodes
Number of metastases	Lung: more than 20
Histologic type	Pure choriocarcinoma
Blood vessel invasion	In stage I
β-HCG level	More than 1000–10 000 IU/l
Alpha-fetoprotein level	More than 500–1000 ng/ml

β-HCG, beta human chorionic gonadotrophin.

have an excellent prognosis, only very large series are able to identify those at risk of relapse or death from disease.

Tumor-Related Factors

Anatomic Extent of Disease

Approximately 80%–85% of patients with seminoma present with disease localized to the testis. The traditional treatment of stage I seminoma is radical orchiectomy and postoperative radiotherapy to the retroperitoneal lymph nodes, and 95%–99% of those treated in this manner are cured [22, 37, 38]. In stage I seminoma, the extent of local disease is of no prognostic value, because of the high success rate of standard therapy with orchiectomy and postoperative RT. Recent studies of postorchiectomy surveillance in stage I seminoma suggest that the size of primary tumor predicts for disease progression. In the Danish experience, the risk of progression was 36% for patients with primary tumors larger than 6 cm, 18% for those with 3- to 6-cm tumors, and 6% for those with tumors smaller than 3 cm [44]. The independent prognostic impact of primary tumor size has not been confirmed by other studies, although in the Toronto series 12% of patients with tumors smaller than 4 cm progressed, compared to 27% of those with tumors of 4 cm or more [9, 45]. Within stage II [17], bulk of retroperitoneal disease, originally expressed by the presence of a palpable abdominal mass and more recently by the transverse diameter of the retroperitoneal mass as seen radiographically, has been identified as the most important prognostic factor for relapse and survival. Patients with masses greater than 10 cm in diameter have a very high relapse rate (more than 40%–50%) when treated with RT alone. Patients with retroperitoneal lymph node masses 5–10 cm in diameter have a relapse rate of 10%–30% and those with smaller nodal masses have relapse rates of less than 20% [3, 22, 26, 38, 39]. To date, insufficient experience has been accumulated to assess the impact of large tumor bulk in patients with stage II disease treated with chemotherapy [13, 18, 40]. A multivariate analysis of a large international data set of patients with seminoma treated with cisplatin chemotherapy identified neck lymph node and liver metastases as independent adverse prognostic factors for survival in advanced disease [27].

Histologic Features

There is no consensus regarding the prognostic impact of the histologic type of seminoma. Anaplastic histology has been associated with more extensive disease and was found to be associated with a higher risk of relapse in patients with stage I disease treated with adjuvant radiotherapy [5, 14]. However, the exact reporting of anaplasia in seminoma has been inconsistent with some investigators following the WHO criteria of three mitotic figures per ten high power fields and others using five mitoses per ten high power fields. In the Danish surveillance experience with stage I seminoma, 16% of those with typical seminoma and 35% of those with anaplastic seminoma developed progression of disease [44]. Spermatocytic seminoma is uncommon, but it is associated with excellent survival and, in surveillance series, with a very low risk of relapse.

The presence of blood vessel and/or lymphatic invasion has been investigated as a possible prognostic factor in stage I seminoma treated with orchiectomy alone, but the data are insufficient to conclude whether it has an impact on outcome. The presence of syncytiotrophoblastic elements in seminoma is well recognized. There is no evidence that this impacts on the prognosis of patients with pure seminoma [37, 38, 44].

Carcinoma in situ has been identified in the contralateral testis of patients with testis tumors and in random biopsies of testis in patients undergoing orchidopexy. The factors predictive of carcinoma in situ and therefore the risk of future testis tumor include: presence of contralateral testis tumor; cryptorchidism, especially when associated with testicular atrophy; infertility associated with testicular tumor; and dysgenetic gonads [12, 16, 25, 43].

Tumor Markers and Biochemical Factors

High levels of the beta subunit of human chorionic gonadotrophin (β-HCG) were found to be an unfavorable factor in a multivariate analysis of patients with advanced seminoma treated with cisplatin-based chemotherapy [27]. An elevated lactic dehydrogenase (LDH) level was found to be an adverse factor for survival in a multivariate analysis of patients with advanced seminoma treated with chemotherapy [27]. There is little information regarding the prognostic value of LDH in patients treated with radiation therapy alone.

Patient-Related Factors

There is little data exploring the impact of age on outcome in seminoma. However, age over 50 years was found to be an adverse prognostic factor in a large study of seminomas treated with chemotherapy. The prognostic impact of age was, however, not significant in a multivariate analysis [27]. In a series of patients with stage I seminoma treated with orchiectomy alone, patients less than 34 years had a 30% actuarial 5-year risk of disease progression, while those over the 34 years had a 9% risk of progression [45]. This finding has not been observed in the other surveillance series [9, 44]. In the past decades, several reports in the literature have suggested that the delay from diagnosis to treatment is associated with more advanced presentations and a higher failure rate, but in the modern era of effective systemic treatment there is no evidence that the ultimate outcome is affected.

Treatment-Related Factors

Scrotal or inguinal surgery alters the lymphatic drainage of the testicle and it may be predictive of a higher risk of inguinal relapse. However, providing this is recognized and considered in treatment, there is no evidence that it is a significant risk factor for survival [38].

Summary – Seminoma

The survival of patients with seminoma is excellent. With such high cure rates, prognostic factors are not as important as in NSGCTT. However, many patients who currently receive postoperative RT may be cured with orchiectomy alone. It is possible that further studies of surveillance may identify prognostic factors for progression and permit selective recommendations for adjuvant therapy in stage I seminoma [18, 37, 40]. Presentation with advanced disease is uncommon in seminoma but, although the overall results of therapy are good, some patients still die of this disease. The recognition of prognostic factors would help to identify patients for whom current standard therapy is ineffective and who might benefit from experimental approaches.

Nonseminomatous Germ Cell Tumors of the Testis

The advent of cisplatin-based chemotherapy in 1970 drastically altered the prognosis of patients with NSGCTT. In contrast to the pre-cisplatin era when fewer than 10% of patients with disseminated disease had long-term survival, over 70% are now cured [4, 19, 30]. Comprehensive analyses of prognostic factors in testicular tumors have been reported by the MRC Testicular Cancer Group in the United Kingdom, Indiana University and the South Eastern Cancer Study Group (SECSG), Memorial Sloan-Kettering Cancer Center (MSKCC), EORTC Genitourinary Cancer Group, Gustave-Roussy Institut, Danish Testicular Cancer Group (DATECA), MD Anderson Hospital, and the Swedish Norwegian Testis Cancer (SWENOTECA) project [1, 2, 4, 7, 8, 24, 34, 35, 41, 42]. Although the methods of recording data, the statistical analyses and the end points vary, in most instances the factors identified in multivariate analysis are similar.

Tumor-Related Factors

Anatomic Extent of Disease

Anatomic extent of disease is an important prognostic factor for relapse after surgical treatment of NSGCTT. An increasing pT category has been correlated with the risk of metastases identified at retroperitoneal lymph node dissection and an increased risk of disease progression on surveillance in patients with clinical stage I disease [20, 21]. In SWENOTECA experience, patients with pT1 tumors had 10.3% risk of progression on surveillance as compared to a 26.2% progression rate in those with pT2–4 tumors [21]. However, for patients treated with chemotherapy, stage alone is not an important prognostic factor [29]. Tumor volume, tumor biochemical markers and sites of metastatic involvement predict outcome far better than the current staging system, which is focused on predicting the outcome in localized disease. Indiana University investigators and the SECSG identified volume of disease, as measured by the size of metastases, and the presence and size of large retroperitoneal masses as the most important prognostic factors [4]. Two studies showed that retroperitoneal masses greater than 5 cm and greater than 10 cm in diameter are associated with adverse prognosis [2, 29]. The SWENOTECA investigators also noted that lung metastases greater than 3 cm in diameter are associated with an adverse outcome. Indiana University investigators and the SECSG identified the number of lung metastases (>20) as an adverse prognostic factor [4]. The prognostic importance of the number of metastases in lung and elsewhere has also been documented by the EORTC, MSKCC, and the MRC UK investigators [7, 28, 33]. In the MRC UK experience, 88% of patients with one to three lung metastases survived 3 years, while of those with multiple lung metastases more than 2 cm in diameter only 56% survived 3 years [30]. The results of the International Study of prognostic factors in NSGCTT identified the number of sites of metastases (more than three sites) as an important factor in patients treated with chemotherapy [28].

The site of metastatic involvement is also of importance in predicting outcome. Liver and bone involvement have been identified as being associated with a less favorable prognosis than involvement of lung or nodal sites [4, 29, 41]. In the MRC UK study, the 3-year survival was 37% for patients with and 78% for those without liver and/or bone involvement. Brain metastases, although uncommon, are associated with poor survival [4, 29]. The EORTC data also suggested an inferior outcome for patients with supraclavicular nodal metastases [33].

Histologic Features

Histologic features in the primary tumor have been identified as important risk factors for progression in patients with stage I NSGCTT treated with orchiectomy alone. Several studies examined factors predictive for the presence of occult metastatic disease in stage I patients [10, 11, 20, 21, 36]. Independent prognostic factors identified in multivariate analyses include: the presence of lymphatic or venous invasion in the primary tumor, embryonal histology, and the absence of teratomatous or yolk sac elements in the tumor. Patients with any of the above factors have at least a 35%–50% chance of progression, while in the others the risk of progression is 20% or less. Presentations with pure choriocarcinoma have been identified as being associated with less favorable survival than those with other histologic types of NSGCTT [24, 34, 41]. Since such presentations are uncommon, not all investigators recognize choriocarcinoma as being unfavorable, unless accompanied by high β-HCG levels. The presence of chorionic elements in mixed germ cell tumor does not impact on outcome.

Tumor Markers

It has been recognized that approximately 75% of patients with stage I NSGCTT are cured with orchiectomy alone. The presence of elevated levels of alpha-fetoprotein (AFP) at diagnosis was found to confer a lower risk of progression after orchiectomy, likely because the marker allowed exclusion of patients with subclinical disease from surveillance protocols [21]. The independent prognostic factors in metastatic NSGCTT identified by several groups of investigators have included the serum marker levels of β-HCG and AFP [4, 6, 8, 28, 33, 41, 42]. A large international study of prognostic factors in NSGCTT identified the presence of more than 1000 ng AFP/ml or more than 5000 IU β-HCG/l as adverse prognostic factors for survival in patients treated with cisplatin-based chemotherapy [27]. The presence of elevated β-HCG levels has been identified as an unfavorable prognostic factor by all major investigators. The MRC Group, EORTC, Institute Gustave Roussy, and MSKCC reported that a β-HCG level above 6000–10000 IU/l was associated with poor prognosis [4, 6, 8, 24, 28, 33]. In the MRC UK series, patients with β-HCG levels greater than 10000 IU/l had 53% 3-year survival, while those with β-HCG levels of less than 1000 IU/l had a 85% 3-year survival rate [30]. In the Institut Gustave-Roussy experience, the 2-year survival for patients with β-HCG levels of more than 6000 IU/l, 10–6000 IU/l, and less than 10 IU/l were 36%, 64%, and 72%, respectively [8]. A lower level of β-HCG (> 1000 IU/l) was identified by the DATECA, SWENOTECA, and Australian investigators as an adverse prognostic factor [2, 23, 41]. The presence of elevated AFP (> 1000 ng/ml) does not have as strong an impact on outcome as the very high β-HCG levels, but it was observed as an independent prognostic factor in all the major studies of prognostic factors [4, 6, 8, 28, 33]. In the MRC experience, patients with AFP levels of more than 1000 ng/ml had a 3-year survival of 64% as compared to 80% 3-year survival for those with AFP levels of less than 100 ng/ml [30]. The SWENOTECA investigators observed lower levels of AFP (> 500 ng/ml) as predictive of adverse outcome [2]. LDH levels correlate with the presence of advanced disease. LDH was first identified as an important prognostic factor in NSGCTT by the Memorial Sloan Kettering (MSKCC) investigators [7]. Although not recognized as an important factor by all, in a large study of patients treated with chemotherapy, an elevated LDH level has been found to be an independent prognostic factor associated with a lower complete response rate, lower progression-free survival, and poorer overall survival [27].

Patient-Related Factors

Increasing age at diagnosis (> 30 years versus ≤ 30 years) was found to be an adverse feature in the univariate and multivariate analyses of the MRC [28, 29]. However, because of uncertainty about why age affects outcome, age was not taken into account in the prognostic groupings developed by the MRC investigators. Age over 35 years has also been identified as an unfavorable factor in the DATECA and SWENOTECA experience [1, 2, 41]. Duration of symptoms prior to treatment was identified as a prognostic factor on univariate analysis of the MRC experience [29]. It was strongly associated with volume of disease and marker level and therefore was not found to have independent prognostic value in multivariate analysis. Age was not found to affect the outcome in the EORTC experience [34].

Treatment-Related Factors

There is little information regarding the impact of treatment-related factors on outcome, but a recent study from the United Kingdom suggested an improved outcome for patients treated in units specializing in treatment of testis tumors [15].

Summary – Nonseminoma

Based on the identification of prognostic factors, several institutions have proposed various prognostic classifications. The need for international agreement in the recording and analysis of prognostic factors in NSGCTT has been recognized, but to date such agreement has not been reached [34]. Anatomic extent of disease and tumor burden are the most important prognostic factors in nonseminomatous testicular tumors. However, describing the stage of disease alone does not provide adequate prognostic classification. Other parameters have been found to exert significant influence on outcome in these patients. Although there is no complete agreement regarding the exact extent to which each factor or combination of factors affects outcome in an individual patient, most would agree that a knowledge of the prognostic factors discussed above is essential to optimal patient management. To date, only clinical prognostic factors have been identified. There is little information on the possible influence of proliferative activity or molecular or genetic markers in testis tumors.

Recently the International Germ Cell Cancer Collaborative Group (IGCCCG) has proposed a prognostic index for germ cell tumors [27]. The unfavorable group with expected survival of 50% includes patients with non-pulmonary visceral metastases and any of the following marker levels: β-HCG greater than 10 000 IU/l, AFP greater than 10 000 IU/l, or LDH greater than 10 times the normal level. The favorable group of patients with survival greater than 90% includes all patients without non-pulmonary visceral metastases and low tumor marker levels: β-HCG less than 1 000 IU/l, AFP less than 1 000 IU/l, and LDH less than 1.5 times the normal level [28].

References

1. Aass N, Fossa SD, Ous S et al (1990) Prognosis in patients with metastatic non-seminomatous testicular cancer. Radiother Oncol 17: 285–292
2. Aass N, Klepp O, Cavallin-Stahl E et al (1991) Prognostic factors in unselected patients with nonseminomatous metastatic testicular cancer: a multicenter experience. J Clin Oncol 9: 818–826
3. Ball D, Barrett A, Peckham MJ (1982) The management of metastatic seminoma testis. Cancer 50: 2289–2294
4. Birch R, Williams S, Cone A et al (1986) Prognostic factors for favorable outcome in disseminated germ cell tumors. J Clin Oncol 4: 400–407
5. Bobba VS, Mittal BB, Hoover SV et al (1988) Classical and anaplastic seminoma: difference in survival. Radiology 167: 849–852
6. Bosl GJ (1993) Prognostic factors for metastatic testicular germ cell tumours: the Memorial Sloan-Kettering Cancer model. Eur Urol 23: 182–187
7. Bosl GJ, Geller NL, Cirrincione C et al (1983) Multivariate analysis of prognostic variables in patients with metastatic testicular cancer. Cancer Research 43: 3403–3407
8. Droz JP, Kramar A, Ghosn M, Piot G, Rey A et al (1988) Prognostic factors in advanced nonseminomatous testicular cancer. A multivariate logistic regression analysis. Cancer 62: 564–568
9. Duchesne GM, Horwich A, Dearnaley DP et al (1990) Orchidectomy alone for stage I seminoma of the testis. Cancer 65: 1115–1118
10. Dunphy CH, Ayala AG, Swanson DA et al (1988) Clinical stage I nonseminomatous and mixed germ cell tumors of the testis. Cancer 62: 1202–1206
11. Fossa SD, Stenwig AE, Lien HH et al (1989) Non-seminomatous testicular cancer clinical stage I: prediction of outcome by histopathological parameters. A multivariate analysis. Oncology 46: 297–300
12. Giwercman A (1992) Carcinoma-in-situ of the testis: screening and management. Scand J Urol Nephrol Suppl 148: 1–47
13. Gospodarowicz MK, Thomas GT, Sturgeon JFG (1991) The optimal treatment of patients with stage II seminoma with moderate size retroperitoneal metastases (5—10 cm). Curr Opin Urol 1: 76–79
14. Gospodarowicz MK, Warde PR, Panzarella T, Catton CN, Sturgeon JFG, Moore M, Jewett MAS (1994) The Princess Margaret Hospital experience in the management of stage I & II seminoma – 1981 to 1991. In: Jones WG, Harnden P, Appleyard I (eds) Proceedings of the Third International Germ Cell Tumour Conference. Advances in Bioscience, vol 91. Elsevier, Oxford, pp 177–185
15. Harding MJ, Paul J, Gillis CR et al (1993) Management of malignant teratoma: does referral to a specialist unit matter? Lancet 341: 999–1002
16. Harland SJ, Cook PA, Fossa SD et al (1993) Risk factors for carcinoma in situ of the contralateral testis in patients with testicular cancer. An interim report. Eur Urol 23: 115–118
17. Hermanek P, Sobin LH (eds) (1992) UICC: TNM classification of malignant tumours, 4th edn, 2nd rev. Springer, Berlin Heidelberg New York
18. Horwich A (1990) Questions in the management of seminoma. Clin Oncol 2: 249–253
19. Horwich A (1991) Current controversies in the management of testicular cancer. Eur J Cancer 27: 326–330
20. Hoskin P, Dilly S, Eastors P et al (1986) Prognostic factors in stage I non-seminomatous germ cell testicular tumours managed by orchidectomy and surveillance: implications for adjuvant therapy. J Clin Oncol 4: 1031–1036
21. Klepp O, Olsson AM, Henrikson H et al (1990) Prognostic factors in clinical stage I nonseminomatous germ cell tumors of the testis: multivariate analysis of a prospective multicenter study. J Clin Oncol 8: 509–518

22. Lederman GS, Herman TS, Jochelson M et al (1989) Radiation therapy of seminoma: 17 year experience at the Joint Center for Radiation Therapy. Radiother Oncol 14: 203–208
23. Levi JA, Thomson D, Sandeman T et al (1988) A prospective study of cisplatin-based combination chemotherapy in advanced germ cell malignancy: role of maintenance and long-term follow-up. J Clin Oncol 6: 1154–1160
24. Logothetis CJ, Samuels ML, Selig DE et al (1986) Cyclic chemotherapy with cyclophosphamide, doxorubicin and cisplatin plus vinblastine and bleomycin in advanced germinal tumors. Am J Med 81: 219–228
25. Loy V, Dieckmann KP (1993) Prevalence of contralateral testicular intraepithelial neoplasia (carcinoma in situ) in patients with testicular germ cell tumour. Results of the German multicentre study. Eur Urol 23: 120–122
26. Mason BR, Kearsley JH (1988) Radiotherapy for stage 2 testicular seminoma: the prognostic influence of tumour bulk. J Clin Oncol 6: 1856–1862
27. Mead GM, on behalf of the IGCCCG (1995) International Consensus Prognostic Classification for metastatic germ cell tumors treated with platinum based chemotherapy; final report of the International Germ Cell Cancer Collaborative Group (IGCCCG). Proc Am Soc Clin Oncol (in press.)
28. Mead GM, Stenning SP (1993) Prognostic factors in metastatic non-seminomatous germ cell tumours: the Medical Research Council studies. Eur Urol 23: 196–200
29. Mead GM, Stenning SP, Parkinson MC et al (1992) The second Medical Research Council study of prognostic factors in nonseminomatous germ cell tumours. J Clin Oncol 10: 85–94
30. Medical Research Council (1985) Prognostic factors in advanced non-seminomatous germ-cell testicular tumours: results of a multicentre study. Lancet i: 8–12
31. Mostofi FK, Sobin LH (1977) Histological typing of testis tumors. International histological classification of tumours, no 16. WHO, Geneva
32. Pugh RCB (1976) Pathology of the testis. Blackwell, Oxford
33. Stoter G, Sleijfer D, Kaye SB et al (1993) Prognostic factors in metastatic non-seminomatous germ cell tumours: an interim analysis of the EORTC GU-Group experience. Eur Urol 23: 202–206
34. Stoter G, Sylvester R, Sleijfer DT et al (1988) A multivariate analysis of prognostic factors in disseminated non-seminomatous testicular cancer. Prog Clin Biol Res 269: 381–393
35. Stoter G, Sylvester R, Sleijfer DT et al (1987) Multivariate analysis of prognostic factors in patients with disseminated nonseminomtous testicular cancer: results from a European Organization for Research on Treatment of Cancer multi-institutional phase III study. Cancer Res 47: 2714–2718
36. Sturgeon JF, Jewett MA, Alison RE et al (1992) Surveillance after orchidectomy for patients with clinical stage I nonseminomatous testis tumors. J Clin Oncol 10: 564–568
37. Thomas G (1990) Progress and controversies in the management of seminoma. In: Newling DWW, Jones WG (eds) Prostate cancer and testicular cancer. Wiley-Liss, New York, pp 217–224 (EORTC genitourinary group monograph 7)
38. Thomas G, Jones W, VanOosterom A et al (1990) Consensus statement on the investigation and management of testicular seminoma 1989. Prog Clin Biol Res 357: 285–294
39. Thomas G, Rider WD, Dembo AJ et al (1982) Seminoma of the testis: results of treatment and patterns of failure after radiation therapy. Int J Radiat Oncol Biol Phys 8: 165–174
40. Thomas GM, Sturgeon JF, Alison R et al (1989) A study of post orchidectomy surveillance in stage I testicular seminoma. J Urol 142: 313–316
41. Veth M, Schultz HP, Von der Maase H et al (1984) Prognostic factors in testicular germ cell tumours experiences from 1–58 consecutive cases. Acta Radiol 23: 271–286
42. Vogelzang NJ (1987) Prognostic factors in metastatic testicular cancer. Int J Androl 10: 225–237
43. von der Maase H, Rorth M, Walbom-Jorgensen S et al (1986) Carcinoma in situ of contralateral testis in patients with testicular germ cell cancer: study of 27 cases in 500 patients. Br Med J 293: 1398–1401
44. von der Maase H, Specht L, Jacobson GK et al (1993) Surveillance following orchidectomy for stage I seminoma of the testis. Eur J Cancer 29A: 1931–1934
45. Warde P, Gospodarowicz M, Goodman P et al (1993) Results of a policy of surveillance in stage I testicular seminoma. Int J Radiat Oncol Biol Phys 27: 11–15

26 Renal Cell Carcinoma

M.K. Gospodarowicz and J.E. Montie

The clinical presentation of renal cell carcinoma is often diverse and outcome is notoriously difficult to predict. The only therapy for renal cell carcinoma with curative potential is radical surgery for patients presenting with locoregional disease. To date there is no evidence that treatment affects the outcome of patients with surgically unresectable or distant metastatic disease. Therefore stage, which reflects the anatomic extent of disease, is the most important factor predicting survival [3, 15, 31, 33, 36].

Although prognostic factors in renal cell carcinoma have been studied extensively, there are relatively few studies which include adequate patient numbers, consider all possible factors and utilise multivariate analysis. Because of that, factors which have been generally accepted to be of prognostic value in renal cell carcinoma and which are listed below have not all been proven to be of independent significance (Tables 1 and 2). Appropriate studies with properly conducted multivariate analysis have either not been reported or, when done, have not been comprehensive.

Prognostic factors in renal cell carcinoma have been studied most often in patients undergoing radical nephrectomy. The other, less often studied group, was that of patients with distant metastatic disease. Although fewer in number, these studies have been more comprehensive and more frequently involved multivariate analysis.

Tumour-Related Factors

Anatomic Extent of Disease

Anatomic extent of disease represented by stage of disease [16] is the single most important indicator of prognosis in renal cell carcinoma [2, 17, 31]. The 5-year survival rates are 70%–80% for those with stage I renal cell carcinoma, 50%–70% for stage II, 30%–50% for stage III, and 0%–10% for stage IV (predominantly metastatic disease). However, most authors acknowledge that the prognostic value of stage only reflects a better outcome for patients with disease limited to the kidney rather than those with metastatic disease, either nodal or distant [37, 39]. The next major discriminant is the presence of surgically unresectable tumour, the situation which is commonly associated with the presence of nodal involvement.

Table 1. Prognostic factors in renal cell carcinoma (locoregional disease)

Factor	Unfavourable variant
Anatomic extent	T3 (perinephric tissues/extrarenal vein involvement)
Histological type	Sarcomatoid pattern
Presentation	Symptoms
Histological grade	G3–4
Sedimentation rate	More than 30 mm/h

Table 2. Prognostic factors in renal cell carcinoma (distant metastases)

Factor	Unfavourable variant
Number of metastases	More than one
Site of metastases	Liver
Histological type	Sarcomatoid pattern
Histological grade	G3–4
Anaemia	Hb <10 g/dl (female)/<12 g/dl (male)
Sedimentation rate	More than 30 mm/h
Performance status	ECOG 2–3
Weight loss	Present

Hb, haemoglobin; ECOG, Eastern Cooperative Oncology Group.

Extension of the tumour into the perinephric fat has been found to be associated with a higher incidence of nodal involvement and thus to be associated with worse prognosis. It is unclear whether this is related to difficulty in achieving complete tumour resection either locally or due to coexistent nodal disease or to the higher risk of occult distant metastases in patients with perinephric fat involvement.

Subdividing tumours limited to the kidney according to size of the primary tumour is of less value and has been questioned by some. It has been found to reflect prognosis in patients with stage I disease, but the size of the primary tumour was not an independent prognostic factor when all stages of the disease were considered [33]. Stage I tumours less than 5 cm in diameter have been shown, in multivariate analysis, to have a better outcome than the larger primary tumours [11]. The influence of tumour size was more pronounced in patients with low-grade tumours rather than those with higher-grade tumours.

Involvement of the renal vein by primary tumour was recognised as an adverse prognostic factor as early as in 1943 [26]. More recent studies confirmed this established observation [15, 18, 30, 35, 39]. There is no evidence that involvement of intrarenal veins affects survival, while involvement of extrarenal portion of the renal vein has been found to do so. Takashi documented an 85% 5-year survival rate for patients with no venous involvement, 71% with tumour involving smaller veins, 26% renal vein, and 0% for tumours involving the inferior vena cava [39]. A less favourable outcome has been associated with higher levels of venous involvement, but the ability to achieve complete resection of the tumour has been found to be of more importance than the actual extent of disease. Importantly, the level of renal vein involvement has not been proven to be an independent prognostic factor for survival. However, although renal vein involvement has been generally accepted to be of prognostic importance, several studies have not confirmed its presence to be an independent prognostic factor [33, 36, 38].

In patients with distant metastatic disease, the number of metastatic sites, the presence of metastases in the liver or multiple lung metastases have been identified as independent prognostic factors for overall survival [6, 9, 32].

Histological Type and Grade

Histological cell type and growth pattern have been thought to have some prognostic value. The sarcomatoid histological type in particular has been found to be associated with poor survival [28, 37, 38].

Histological grade has been found to be an independent prognostic factor for survival in patients with localised and also in those with distant metastatic disease [13, 32, 33, 35]. The prognostic impact of tumour grade is most pronounced in stage I disease, with a 5-year survival rate of 90% for those with grade 2 versus 70% for those with grade 3 tumours [11]. However, a report which questioned the independent prognostic value of tumour grade has also been published [22].

Biological and Molecular Factors

The measurement of tumour ploidy has been reported to influence prognosis, although there are conflicting reports on its value as an independent prognostic factor. Although evidence has been presented for diploid or near-diploid tumours being associated with better survival, some studies have failed to confirm independent prognostic value of ploidy, because of its close correlation with tumour grade [4, 5, 7, 12, 23, 24]. Increased mitotic activity, which may reflect proliferative activity of the tumour better than tumour grade, predicted for poorer prognosis [12, 13].

Nuclear organiser regions (NORs) are intranuclear structures demonstrable by silver techniques. There is evidence that the number of intranuclear NORs is indicative of the proliferative activity of the tissue being examined. Delahunt et al. have found a mean number of NORs to be a predictor for survival in renal cell carcinoma, independent of stage [8]. The value of number of NORs as a prognostic factor independent of tumour grade has not been assessed.

It is known that abnormalities on the short arm (3p) of chromosome 3 are often found in clear cell renal carcinoma and alterations on chromosomes 7,17,16 and Y in papillary renal cell carcinoma [1, 21]. Although a large number of cytogenetic studies have been performed, the prognostic implications of such factors have rarely been addressed and, to date, there is no adequate evidence to warrant their use in clinical practice. Similarly, so far, only a small number of studies have addressed the prognostic implications of oncogene or suppressor gene expression and there is not enough data to suggest their usefulness in clinical practice [19, 40, 41].

Haematological and Biochemical Factors

The presence of anaemia has been shown to be an independent prognostic factor associated with poor survival in at least one study of patients with various stages of renal cell carcinoma [31]. Erythrocyte sedimentation rate (ESR) has been studied mostly in patients with distant metastatic disease and infrequently in patients with localised disease. However, an elevated ESR has been found to be associated with poorer survival both in patients with and without demonstrable distant metastases [3, 6, 14, 18, 31, 37].

To date there is no useful biochemical marker predictive for outcome in patients with renal cell carcinoma. Several substances have been studied, but none is currently in clinical use. Pseudouridine is a modified transfer RNA that is excreted in the urine upon degradation of RNA and may be elevated in some tumours. In a study by Rasmuson, urinary excretion of pseudouridine was the only biochemical marker analysed by multivariate analysis, and the elevated urinary excretion in patients with localised and metastatic renal cell carcinoma was shown to have independent prognostic significance for survival, while tumour size, grade and age were not [34].

Patient-Related Factors

There is very little evidence that age is of independent prognostic importance in renal cell carcinoma [25, 33]. However, at least one study reported age as an independent prognostic factor for observed survival in patients without distant metastatic disease [36]. There is no consensus regarding the influence of gender on survival in patients with renal cell carcinoma. Several studies have indicated an improved survival for women, although most of these studies did not use multi-variate analysis [18, 20, 27]. Others who have analysed gender as a possible prognostic variable have not been able to confirm this finding [22, 25, 33, 36]. Elson has identified performance status, measured according to the ECOG (Eastern Cooperative Oncology Groups) scale, as an independent prognostic factor in patients with recurrent or distant metastatic renal cell carcinoma who were entered on phase II ECOG chemotherapy trials. The median survival of patients with an ECOG performance status of 0–1 was 10.7–6.7 months, as compared to 3.3–2.0 months for those with an ECOG performance status of 2–3 [9]. Several other studies have also found a good performance status to be associated with improved survival [6, 9, 25]. Weight loss has been measured more frequently than performance status and has been identified as a valuable prognostic factor in those with locally recurrent or distant metastatic disease. Several studies have made this observation, and in some it was a significant factor in multivariate analysis [6, 9, 22, 32, 36]. In Elson's study of patients with distant metastatic disease on chemotherapy protocols, the median survival for patients with weight loss was 4.1 months and 7.3 months for those without weight loss. However, at least one conflicting report suggesting a lack of significance of weight loss has also been published [31].

Renal cell carcinoma has been recognised for its association with a wide variety of paraneoplastic syndromes. However, despite this association, the prognostic impact of paraneoplastic syndromes has not been studied adequately. Unexplained fever at diagnosis was found to be an independent prognostic factor, and the presence of hypercalcaemia in patients with distant metastatic disease has been found to indicate poor survival in univariate analysis [10, 22]. An increased rate of detection of asymptomatic renal cell carcinoma has been associated with the widespread use of abdominal ultrasound and computed tomography (CT). Presentation of renal cell carcinoma as an incidental finding has been found to be an independent prognostic factor associated with a better survival (73% at 5 years for incidental versus 32% for symptomatic carcinoma) [31].

Treatment-Related Factors

Radical nephrectomy is the traditional surgical procedure performed for renal cell carcinoma. There is increasing interest in the use of kidney-sparing surgery, i.e. partial nephrectomy for small lesions in the kidney, usually discovered as an incidental finding during abdominal or renal ultrasonography or an abdominal CT scan. To date, results suggest a comparable outcome for small lesions (pT1–pT2) treated by partial and total nephrectomy [17, 29]. The data as to the prognostic impact of kidney-sparing surgery are few. Prospective randomised studies are required to address this issue.

Summary

The anatomic extent of disease as reflected by stage, particularly the presence of regional lymph node or distant metastases, is the most important determinant of prognosis in patients with renal cell carcinoma. After stage, tumour grade is the second most important prognostic factor. DNA cytometry appears to be another factor, which may contribute to the prognostic assessment. Other prognostic factors such as histological type, anaemia, ESR and symptoms such as weight loss, are of lesser, but possibly important additional value. Patient-related factors such as age and gender have not been found to be of major importance, although performance status appears to be the most important factor in patients with distant metastatic disease. Unfortunately, although prognostic factors in renal cell carcinoma have been studied extensively, there are few comprehensive studies with multivariate statistical analysis. In the future, data on oncogenes and suppressor genes, which with the availability of newer molecular techniques have been studied with increasing frequency, may provide additional prognostic information for patients with renal cell carcinoma.

References

1. Anglard P, Tory K, Brauch H et al (1991) Molecular analysis of genetic changes in the origin and development of renal cell carcinoma. Cancer Res 51: 1071–1077
2. Bassil B, Dosoretz DE, Prout GRJ (1985) Validation of the tumor, nodes and metastasis classification of renal cell carcinoma. J Urol 134: 450–454
3. Bottinger LE (1970) Prognosis in renal cell carcinoma. Cancer 26: 780–787
4. Chin JL, Pontas JE, Frankfurt OS (1985) Flow cytometric deoxyribonucleic acid analysis of primary and metastatic human renal cell carcinoma. J Urol 133: 582–585
5. Currin SM, Lee SE, Walther PJ (1990) Flow cytometric assessment of deoxyribonucleic acid content in renal adenocarcinoma: does ploidy status enhance prognostic stratification over stage alone? J Urol 143: 458–463
6. de Forges A, Rey A, Klink M et al (1988) Prognostic factors of adult metastatic renal carcinoma: a multivariate analysis. Semin Surg Oncol 4: 149–154
7. DeKernion JB, Mukamel E, Ritchie AWS et al (1989) Prognostic significance of the DNA content of renal cell carcinoma. Cancer 64: 1669–1673
8. Delahunt B, Ribas JL, Nacey JN et al (1991) Nucleolar organizer regions and prognosis in renal cell carcinoma. J Pathol 163: 31–37
9. Elson PJ, Witte RS, Trump DL (1988) Prognostic factors for survival in patients with recurrent or metastatic renal cell carcinoma. Cancer Res 48: 7310–7313
10. Fahn HJ, Lee YH, Chen MT et al (1991) The incidence and prognostic significance of humoral hypercalcemia in renal cell carcinoma. J Urol 145: 248–250
11. Gelb AB, Shibuya RB, Weiss LM et al (1992) Stage I renal cell carcinoma. A clinicopathologic study of 82 cases. Am J Surg Pathol 17: 275–286
12. Grignon DJ, Ayala AG, El-Naggar A et al (1989) Renal cell carcinoma. A clinicopathologic and DNA flow cytometric analysis of 103 cases. Cancer 64: 2133–2140
13. Grignon DJ, El-Naggar A, Green LK et al (1989) DNA flow cytometry as a predictor of outcome of stage I renal cell carcinoma. Cancer 63: 1161–1165
14. Hannisdal E, Bostad L, Grottum KA et al (1989) Erythrocyte sedimentation rate as a prognostic factor in renal cell carcinoma. Eur J Surg Oncol 15: 333–336
15. Hermanek P, Schrott KM (1990) Evaluation of the new tumor, nodes and metastases classification of renal cell carcinoma. J Urol 144: 238–242
16. Hermanek P, Sobin LH (eds) (1992) UICC International Union Against Cancer: TNM Classification of malignant tumours, 4th edn, 2nd rev. Springer, Berlin Heidelberg New York
17. Herr HW (1994) Partial nephrectomy for renal cell carcinoma with a normal opposite kidney. Cancer 73: 160–162
18. Hop WCJ, van der Werf-Messing BHP (1980) Prognostic indexes for renal cell carcinoma. Eur J Cancer 16: 833–840
19. Kakehi Y, Yoshida O (1989) Restriction fragment length polymorphism of the L-myc gene and susceptibility to metastasis in renal cell carcinoma. Int J Cancer 43: 391–394
20. Kjaer M (1987) The treatment and prognosis of patients with renal adenocarcinoma with solitary metastasis. 10 year survival results. Int J Radiat Oncol Biol Phys 13: 619–621
21. Kovacs G, Fuzesi L, Emanuel A et al (1991) Cytogenetics of papillary renal cell tumors. Genes Chromosom Cancer 3: 249–255
22. Lieber MM, Tomera FM, Taylor WF et al (1981) Renal adenocarcinoma in young adults: survival and variables affecting prognosis. J Urol 125: 164–168
23. Ljungberg B, Larsson P, Stenling R et al (1991) Flow cytometric deoxyribonucleic acid analysis in stage I renal cell carcinoma. J Urol 146: 697–699
24. Ljungberg B, Roos G (1990) Value of DNA analysis for treatment of renal cell carcinoma. Eur Urol 2: 31–32

25. Maldazys JD, deKernion JB (1986) Prognostic factors in metastatic renal carcinoma. J Urol 136: 376–379
26. McDonald JR, Priestley JT (1943) Malignant tumors of the kidney. Surg Gynecol Obstet 77: 295–306
27. McNichols DW, Segura JW, DeWeerd JH (1981) Renal cell carcinoma: long-term survival and late recurrence. J Urol 126: 17–23
28. Medeiros LJ, Gelb AB, Weiss LM (1988) Renal cell carcinoma. Prognostic significance of morphologic parameters in 121 cases. Cancer 61: 1639–1651
29. Moll V, Becht E, Ziegler M (1993) Kidney preserving surgery in renal cell tumors: indications, techniques and results in 152 patients. J Urol 150: 319–323
30. Montie JE, El Ammar R, Pontes JE et al (1991) Renal cell carcinoma with inferior vena cava tumor thrombi. Surg Gynecol Obstet 173: 107–115
31. Nacey JN, Delahunt B (1986) Renal cell carcinoma. I. Clinical indicators of prognosis. N Z Med J 99: 531–533
32. Neves RJ, Zincke H, Taylor WF (1988) Metastatic renal cell cancer and radical nephrectomy: identification of prognostic factors and patient survival. J Urol 139: 1173–1176
33. Nurmi MJ (1984) Prognostic factors in renal carcinoma. An evaluation of operative findings. Br J Urol 56: 270–275
34. Rasmuson T, Bjork GR, Hietala SO et al (1991) Excretion of pseudouridine as an independent prognostic factor in renal cell carcinoma. Acta Oncol 30: 11–15
35. Sanchez de la Muela P, Zudaire JJ, Robles JE et al (1991) Renal cell carcinoma: vena cava invasion and prognostic factors. Eur Urol 19: 284–290
36. Selli C, Hinshaw WM, Woodard BH et al (1983) Stratification of risk factors in renal cell carcinoma. Cancer 52: 899–903
37. Sene AP, Hunt L, McMahon RFT et al (1992) Renal carcinoma in patients undergoing nephrectomy: analysis of survival and prognostic factors. Br J Urol 70: 125–134
38. Skinner DG, Colvin RB, Vermillion CD et al (1971) Diagnosis and management of renal cell carcinoma. Cancer 28: 1165–1177
39. Takashi M, Nakano Y, Sakata T et al (1993) Multivariate analysis of prognostic determinants for renal cell carcinoma. Urol Int 50: 6–12
40. Weaver D, Michalski K, Miles J (1988) Cytogenetic analysis in renal cell carcinoma: correlation with tumor aggressiveness. Cancer Res 48: 2887–2889
41. Weidner U, Peter S, Strohmeyer T et al (1990) Inverse relationship of epidermal growth factor receptor and HER2/neu gene expression in human renal cell carcinoma. Cancer Res 50: 4504–4509

27 Urinary Bladder Carcinoma

M.K. Gospodarowicz

Urinary bladder carcinoma is a heterogenous disease with considerable variation in its natural history. The 5-year survival rate varies from 90% for patients with superficial, well-differentiated tumors to 0%–10% for those with locally extensive tumor invading the pelvic side wall. Many clinical and pathologic factors including stage, grade, tumor size, multiplicity, tumor growth pattern, vascular invasion, positive urine cytology, or coexistent carcinoma in situ (Tis) have been described to affect the outcome. There is, however, a relative paucity of information regarding the more fundamental immunologic, biochemical, and molecular factors which may be of considerable prognostic importance. Prognostic factors may be related to the tumor itself, the patient, and the treatment delivered. This discussion will focus mainly on disease-related factors. Treatment-related factors, such as the method and quality of treatment, will not be discussed in detail, as there is a paucity of reliable comparative data as to the impact of therapy on outcome. Relatively few studies of prognostic factors in bladder carcinoma incorporate comprehensive multivariate analysis – thus the references quoted below also include studies which demonstrate compelling evidence for certain factors by univariate analysis only.

Tumor-Related Factors

Anatomic Extent of Disease

The single most important factor affecting outcome in bladder carcinoma, the depth of bladder wall invasion, is expressed by the TNM classification and stage grouping. Due to differences in the natural history, prognosis, and therapeutic approach, bladder tumors are generally discussed under two main headings: superficial disease, including Tis, Ta and T1 tumors, and muscle-invasive disease, including T categories T2–T4 (Tables 1 and 2). Stage has been found to affect prognosis in both of the above groups [2, 3, 5, 6, 9, 11–13, 15–18, 21, 26, 30, 31, 36, 39]. The 5-year survival rate for patients with superficial disease ranges from 90% to 95% for Ta (noninvasive papillary carcinoma) tumors to 60%–70% for T1 tumors managed with transurethral resection [21, 22]. In superficial bladder cancer, patients with Ta tumors have a significantly smaller risk of recurrence and progression than those with T1 tumors [29, 42]. In muscle-invasive disease,

Table 1. Unfavorable prognostic factors in superficial transitional bladder carcinoma

Factor	Survival	Local recurrence
Age	More than 65 years	–
Anatomic extent	T1	T1
Number of tumors	–	More than three
Size	–	More than 3 cm
Histologic grade	3–4	3–4
Growth pattern	Solid	Solid

Table 2. Unfavorable prognostic factors in muscle-invasive transitional bladder carcinoma

Factor	Survival	Local recurrence
Anatomic extent	T3, T4	T3, T4
Extravesical mass	T3b,T4b	T3b,T4b
Histologic grade	3–4	3–4
Growth pattern	Solid	Solid
Lymphatic/blood vessel invasion	Yes	–
Obstructive uropathy	Yes	Yes
Age	More than 65 years	–
Anemia	Hb less than 10 g/dl	–
ESR	More than 30 mm/h	–
Proliferation indices	High S-phase %	–
	High BUDR index	–

ESR, erythrocyte sedimentation rate; Hb, hemoglobin; BUDR, bromodeoxyuridine.

the 5-year survival rate ranges from 40% to 80% for T2 tumors, from 15% to 50% for T3 tumors, and from 0% to 10% for T4 tumors [11, 21, 36]. In muscle-invasive disease, an adverse outcome is related to the presence of extravesical tumor extension with a 5-year survival rate of 40%–50% in T3a tumors (deep muscle invasion) and 15%–30% for T3b lesions (extravesical extension) [11, 36].

Patients may present with carcinoma in situ alone or in association with either superficial or muscle-invasive tumors. It is usually a high-grade lesion. The presence of coexistent Tis does not affect the stage designation and therefore has not been extensively studied as a prognostic factor. However, there is evidence that the presence of coexistent Tis is associated with a higher local relapse rate in patients with muscle-invasive disease treated with radiation therapy and is also associated with a lower complete response rate in patients treated with systemic chemotherapy. Positive urine cytology, which is an adverse prognostic factor in patients with superficial disease, may well be an indicator of coexistent Tis [6, 11, 47, 48].

Multiple tumors are often seen in superficial disease and are unusual in patients presenting with muscle-invasive disease. The number of tumors at presentation has been found to affect the risk of local recurrence. In the EORTC (European Organisation for Research on Treatment of Cancer) series of superficial disease, the recurrence rate on follow-up cystoscopies was almost three times greater for patients with more than three tumors than for those with solitary tumors [2]. The risk of progression to a muscle-invasive tumor is also higher with multiple tumors. The importance of tumor multiplicity was independent of stage and grade [2, 17, 37]. There is no evidence, however, that the presence of multiple tumors impacts adversely on survival.

In patients with superficial bladder cancer, tumor size greater than 3–4 cm as measured at cystoscopy is an adverse factor for local recurrence and to a lesser extent for progression to muscle-invasive disease. Tumor size, whether intravesical or extravesical (as expressed by the presence of a palpable mass), has also been associated with a poorer outcome in muscle-invasive disease. A lower local control rate has been observed in patients with a palpable mass treated with radiation and also a higher rate of distant metastases and lower survival regardless of therapy [2, 3, 7, 11–13, 15, 17, 22, 37].

The presence of obstructive uropathy is closely related to the presence of muscle-invasive and extravesical disease and in some series has been identified as an independent prognostic factor associated with poor survival [31, 39].

Other Histologic Features

Transitional cell carcinoma comprises 85%–90% of all histologic types of bladder cancer. A substantial number of patients with transitional cell tumors have associated squamous or glandular metaplasia. Pure squamous cell carcinoma occurs less frequently and is associated with an adverse outcome [21]. Pure adenocarcinoma of the bladder is very rare and there is little information regarding the impact of this histologic type on outcome. Most studies of prognostic factors deal with transitional cell carcinoma and their results may not pertain to tumors of other histologic types [3, 40].

In superficial bladder cancer, histologic grade 3–4 is associated with an increased risk of local recurrence and progression to muscle-invasive disease [42]. Although tumor grade is closely correlated with stage, it is also an independent adverse factor for survival in patients with muscle-invasive disease [2, 3, 5, 11, 13, 16, 22, 26, 29, 30, 36, 39]. In a large Scandinavian study, the morphometric grade together with the pattern of tumor growth described below were each described as having independent prognostic value in predicting progression of noninvasive tumors [28].

The pattern of tumor growth, papillary or solid, is strongly associated with stage and grade. Frequently, overlap exists between papillary and solid tumors and in some patients growth pattern may be difficult to classify, but it is the pure solid growth pattern which is associated with adverse prognosis. Ta tumors and most T1 tumors are papillary unless associated with a high tumor grade. In superficial disease, tumor growth pattern has been found to predict for recurrence and invasion, but not survival. In muscle-invasive tumors treated with radiation, solid growth pattern was an independent prognostic factor for survival [11, 16, 43]. At least one other large series of patients with both superficial and muscle-invasive tumors documented the favorable impact of papillary growth pattern on survival [26].

The presence of lymphatic and blood vessel invasion is closely correlated with grade, but has been shown to independently predict a higher risk of relapse, mainly due to the development of distant metastases and poorer survival [43, 46].

Biologic and Molecular Factors

To date, information regarding the independent prognostic significance of biologic factors in bladder carcinoma is incomplete. There is an expectation that proliferative activity, as measured by Ki-67 antigen expression or flow cytometric measurement of S-phase fraction, should be of more value than the traditional clinical and pathologic prognostic factors. However, evidence to support this is presently limited, with data in support of this contention originating mainly from one center [8, 25, 27, 33]. Bromodeoxyuridine-labeled cell index status (> 10%) was found to be an additional prognostic factor to stage and grade in predicting survival in patients with bladder carcinoma [45]. There is no agreement as to the impact of ploidy on prognosis, with some studies suggesting an improved prognosis for diploid tumors and others finding that ploidy is correlated with tumor grade and has no independent prognostic significance [4, 30, 34]. Increased expression of epidermal growth factor receptor in superficial tumors has been identified as a predictor of progression to muscle-invasive bladder carcinoma [35]. Studies of bladder carcinoma-associated antigens suggest that expression of some antigens may be of prognostic value. Preliminary data on T-138 antigen expression has shown it to be a prognostic factor for survival in muscle-invasive bladder carcinoma [8]. Overexpression of p53 nuclear oncoprotein was found to correlate with high histologic grade, nonpapillary growth pattern, aneuploidy, and high S-phase fraction, but was not found to be an independent prognostic factor in multivariate analysis [24]. Similarly, the overexpression of c-erbB-2 oncoprotein was found to be associated with high tumor grade, aneuploidy, and high S-phase fraction. The immunohistochemic demonstration of c-erbB-2 oncoprotein overexpression had no additional prognostic value over already established predictors in transitional cell bladder carcinoma including the T category, papillary growth pattern, and S-phase fraction [23]. Abnormalities have been identified on chromosomes 1,5,7,9,11, and 17, but so far this information has not been shown to be clinically useful. Blood group isoantigen expression has been extensively investigated in an attempt to predict invasive potential of superficial disease, but to date has not been found useful as a clinical prognostic factor [30, 38]. The finding of squamous metaplasia and beta human chorionic gonadotrophin (β-HCG) staining in transitional cell carcinoma was found to be an adverse prognostic factor for response to radiotherapy [20, 32]. Another study has failed to confirm an influence of β-HCG expression by bladder carcinoma cells on response to radiation [19].

Table 3. Unfavorable prognostic factors in metastatic transitional bladder carcinoma (M1)

Factor	Unfavorable variant
Performance status	Karnofsky scale less than 60
Alkaline phosphatase	Elevated
Age	More than 65–70 years

Patient-Related Factors

Advanced age (> 65 or 70 years) is an adverse prognostic factor, the effect of which is usually attributed to a decreased ability of older patients to tolerate treatment, rather than to inherent differences in the nature of disease in the elderly [10, 30]. Patient age was found to be an independent prognostic factor in a large cohort of patients with both superficial and advanced disease managed in Finland [26]. Low Karnofsky performance status (< 60) has been identified as one of the most important adverse prognostic factors for survival in patients with metastatic carcinoma of the bladder treated with systemic chemotherapy (Table 3) [10]. The impact of performance status has not been investigated to the same extent in patients with disease confined to the bladder or bladder and perivesical tissues.

A low serum hemoglobin associated with locally advanced tumors may be an indicator of occult dissemination of disease. In multivariate analysis of patients with muscle-invasive disease treated with radiotherapy, anemia has been defined as an independent adverse prognostic factor for both local control and survival [5, 11, 13]. An elevated erythrocyte sedimentation rate (ESR) has been identified as an independent prognostic factor for overall survival in patients with muscle-invasive bladder carcinoma treated with radiotherapy [14, 44]. There is no information as to the prognostic impact of ESR in patients treated with cystectomy or in patients with metastatic disease. The extent of alkaline phosphatase elevation has been identified as an independent adverse prognostic factor in a multivariate analysis of patients with metastatic bladder carcinoma treated with chemotherapy [10].

Summary

Although the heterogeneity of carcinoma of the bladder is widely recognized, knowledge of independent prognostic factors is incomplete. A paucity of large studies with consistent recording and analysis of potential prognostic variables compromises our ability to objectively assess the impact of each factor on outcome. Further elucidation of both clinical and biologic factors is required before many of the above factors can be accepted as independent determinants of outcome in patients with carcinoma of the bladder. Efforts directed towards standardized approaches to clinical trials in carcinoma of the bladder have played an important role in emphasizing the need for international consensus regarding the definition and application of prognostic factors [1, 41].

References

1. Aso Y, Anderson L, Soloway M et al (1986) Prognostic factors in superficial bladder cancer. In: Denis L, Niijima T, Prout G Jr et al (eds) Developments in bladder cancer. Liss, New York, pp 257–267
2. Dalesio O, Schulman CC, Sylvester R et al (1983) Prognostic factors in superficial bladder tumours. A study of the European Organization for Research on Treatment of Cancer: Genitourinary Tract Cancer Cooperative Group. J Urol 129: 730–733
3. Davidson SE, Symonds RP, Snee MP et al (1990) Assessment of factors influencing the outcome of radiotherapy for bladder cancer. Br J Urol 66: 288–293
4. deVere WR, Deitch AD, West B et al (1988) The predictive value of flow cytometric information in the clinical management of stage 0 (Ta) bladder cancer. J Urol 139: 279–282
5. Duncan W, Quilty PM (1986) The results of a series of 963 patients with transitional cell carcinoma of the urinary bladder primarily treated by radical megavoltage x-ray therapy. Radiother Oncol 7: 299–310
6. Flamm J, Havelec L (1990) Factors affecting survival in primary superficial bladder cancer. Eur Urol 17: 113–118
7. Fossa SD, Ous S, Berner A (1991) Clinical significance of the "palpable mass" in patients with muscle-infiltrating bladder cancer undergoing cystectomy after pre-operative radiotherapy. Br J Urol 67: 54–60
8. Fradet Y (1990) Biological markers of prognosis in invasive bladder cancer. Semin Oncol 17: 533–543
9. Fung CY, Shipley WU, Young RH et al (1991) Prognostic factors in invasive bladder carcinoma in a prospective trial of preoperative adjuvant chemotherapy and radiotherapy (see comments). J Clin Oncol 9: 1533–1542
10. Geller NL, Sternberg CN, Penenberg D et al (1991) Prognostic factors for survival of patients with advanced urothelial tumours treated with methotrexate, vinblastine, doxorubicin, and cisplatin chemotherapy. Cancer 67: 1525–1531
11. Gospodarowicz MK, Hawkins NV, Rawlings GA et al (1989) Radical radiotherapy for muscle invasive transitional cell carcinoma of the bladder: failure analysis. J Urol 142: 1448–1453
12. Gospodarowicz MK, Rider WD, Keen CW et al (1991) Bladder cancer: long-term follow-up results of patients treated with radical radiation. Clin Oncol 3: 155–161
13. Greven KM, Solin LJ, Hanks GE (1990) Prognostic factors in patients with bladder carcinoma treated with definitive irradiation. Cancer 65: 908–912
14. Hannisdal E, Fossa S, Host H (1993) Blood tests and prognosis in bladder carcinomas treated with definitive radiotherapy. Radiother Oncol 27: 117–122
15. Hendry WF, Rawson NSB, Turney L et al (1990) Computerisation of urothelial carcinoma records: 16 years' experience with the TNM system. Br J Urol 65: 583–588
16. Heney NM, Broppe K, Prout GR et al (1983) Invasive bladder cancer: tumour configuration, lymphatic invasion and survival. J Urol 130: 895–897
17. Heney NM, Ahmed S, Flanagan MJ et al (1983) Superficial bladder cancer: progression and recurrence. J Urol 130: 1083–1086
18. Herr HW, Jakse G, Sheinfeld J (1990) The T1 bladder tumour. Semin Urol 8: 254–261
19. Jacobsen AB, Nesland JM, Fossa SD et al (1990) Human chorionic gonadotropin, neuron specific enolase and deoxyribonucleic acid flow cytometry in patients with high grade bladder carcinoma. J Urol 143: 706–709
20. Jenkins BJ, Martin JE, Baithun SI et al (1990) Prediction of response to radiotherapy in invasive bladder cancer. Br J Urol 65: 345–348
21. Kantoff PW (1990) Bladder cancer. Curr Probl Cancer 14: 235–291
22. Kaubisch S, Lum BL, Reese J et al (1991) Stage T1 bladder cancer: grade is the primary determinant for risk of muscle invasion. J Urol 146: 28–31

23. Lipponen P (1993) Expression of c-*erb*B-2 oncoprotein in transitional cell bladder cancer. Eur J Cancer 29A: 749–753
24. Lipponen PK (1993) Over-expression of p53 nuclear oncoprotein in transitional-cell bladder cancer and its prognostic value. Int J Cancer 53: 365–370
25. Lipponen PK (1993) Stereologically measured nuclear volume in comparison to two-dimensional nuclear morphometry, mitotic index and flow cytometry in predicting disease outcome in bladder cancer. Anticancer Res 13: 529–532
26. Lipponen PK, Eskelinen M, Jauhiainen K et al (1993) Clinical prognostic factors in transitional cell cancer of the bladder. Urol Int 50: 192–197
27. Lipponen PK, Eskelinen MJ, Kiviranta J et al (1991) Classic prognostic factors, flow cytometric data, nuclear morphometric variables and mitotic indexes as predictors in transitional cell bladder cancer. Anticancer Res 11: 911–916
28. Lipponen PK, Eskelinen MJ, Kiviranta J et al (1991) Prognosis of transitional cell bladder cancer: a multivariate prognostic score for improved prediction. J Urol 146: 1535–1540
29. Lutzeyer W, Rübben H, Dahm H (1982) Prognostic parameters in superficial bladder cancer: an analysis of 315 cases. J Urol 127: 250–252
30. Malmstrom PU, Norloen BJ, Andersson B et al (1989) Combination of blood group ABH antigen status and DNA ploidy as independent prognostic factor in transitional cell carcinoma of the urinary bladder. Br J Urol 64: 49–55
31. Mameghan H, Fisher R (1989) Invasive bladder cancer. Prognostic factors and results of radiotherapy with and without cystectomy. Br J Urol 63: 251–258
32. Martin JE, Jenkins BJ, Zuk RJ et al (1989) Human chorionic gonadotrophin expression and histological findings as predictors of response to radiotherapy in carcinoma of the bladder. Virchows Arch [A] 414: 273–277
33. Mellon K, Neal DE, Robinson MC et al (1990) Cell cycling in bladder carcinoma determined by monoclonal antibody Ki67. Br J Urol 66: 281–285
34. Murphy WM, Chandler RW, Trafford RM (1986) Flow cytometry of deparaffinized nuclei compared to histological grading for the pathological evaluation of transitional cell carcinomas. J Urol 135: 694–697
35. Neal DE, Sharples L, Smith K et al (1990) The epidermal growth factor receptor and the prognosis of bladder cancer. Cancer 65: 1619–1625
36. Pagano F, Bassi P, Galetti TP et al (1991) Results of contemporary radical cystectomy for invasive bladder cancer: a clinicopathological study with an emphasis on the inadequacy of the tumour, nodes and metastases classification. J Urol 145: 45–50
37. Parmar MK, Freedman LS, Hargreave TB et al (1989) Prognostic factors for recurrence and follow-up policies in the treatment of superficial bladder cancer: report from the British Medical Research Council Subgroup on superficial bladder cancer (Urological Cancer Working Party). J Urol 142: 284–288
38. Pauwels RP, Schapers RF, Smeets AW et al (1988) Blood group isoantigen deletion and chromosomal abnormalities in bladder cancer. J Urol 140: 959–963
39. Quilty PM, Kerr GR, Duncan W (1986) Prognostic indices for bladder cancer: an analysis of patients with transitional cell carcinoma of the bladder primarily treated by radical megavoltage x-ray therapy. Radiother Oncol 7: 311–321
40. Reuter VE (1990) Pathology of bladder cancer: assessment of prognostic variables and response to therapy. Semin Oncol 17: 524–532
41. Richards B, Aso Y, Bollack C et al (1986) Prognostic factors in infiltrating bladder cancer. In: Denis L, Niijima T, Prout G Jr et al (eds) Developments in bladder cancer. Liss, New York
42. Sanchez de la Muela P, Rosell D, Aguera L et al (1993) Multivariate analysis of progression in superficial bladder cancer. Br J Urol 71: 284–289
43. Slack NH, Prout GR (1980) The heterogeneity of invasive bladder carcinoma and different responses to treatment. J Urol 123: 644–652
44. Smaaland R, Akslen LA, Tonder B et al (1991) Radical radiation treatment of invasive and locally advanced bladder carcinoma in elderly patients. Br J Urol 67: 61–69
45. Tachibana M, Deguchi N, Baba S et al (1993) Prognostic significance of bromodeoxyuridine high labelled bladder cancer measured by flow cytometry: does flow cytometric determination predict the prognosis of patients with transitional cell carcinoma of the bladder? J Urol 149: 739–743
46. Van der Werf Messing BHP, van Putten WLJ (1989) Carcinoma of the urinary bladder category T2-3NXM0 treated by 40 Gy external radiation followed by cesium-137 implant at reduced dose (50%). Int J Radiat Oncol Biol Phys 16: 369–371

47. Wolf H, Kakizoe T, Smith PH et al (1986) Bladder tumours. Treated natural history. Prog Clin Biol Res 221: 223–255
48. Wolf H, Olsen PR, Hojgaard K (1985) Urothelial dysplasia concomitant with bladder tumours: a determinant for future new occurrences in patients treated by full-course radiotherapy. Lancet i: 1005–1008

28 Ophthalmic Tumours

G.K. Lang, C.W. Spraul, and G.O.H. Naumann

Tumours of the eye and its adnexa are a disparate group including carcinoma, melanoma, sarcoma and retinoblastoma in the following locations: eyelid, conjunctiva, uvea, retina, orbit and lacrimal gland.

Eyelid

In tumours of the eyelid, histological type is the most important prognostic factor.

Basal Cell Carcinoma

This tumour accounts for 85%–95% of all malignant epithelial tumours of the eyelid. It primarily involves the lower lid and inner canthus of fair-skinned adults. Prolonged exposure to sunlight seems to be an important predisposing factor. Several clinico-histological types have been described: nodulo-ulcerative, pigmented, morphea or sclerosing, superficial basal cell carcinoma, fibroepithelioma, the nevoid basal cell carcinoma syndrome and the linear basal cell nevus.

Basal cell carcinoma hardly ever leads to metastasis and has therefore by far the best prognosis of all eyelid carcinomas.

Basosquamous Cell Carcinoma (Metatypical Carcinoma)

This tumour differs histologically from squamous cell carcinoma and the typical basal cell carcinoma. The frequency of metastasis has been estimated to range here from 0.028% to 0.55% [8]. The mean survival time after metastasising was 1.6 years [9].

Squamous Cell Carcinoma

Less than 5% of epithelial neoplasms of the eyelid are squamous cell carcinomas. They carry an intermediate prognosis, sometimes leading to metastasis. If the tumour is in the upper lid the preauricular nodes are involved, whereas if the tumour is in the lower lid, spread is to the submandibulary nodes [31, 44]. Prognostic factors other than anatomic extent of disease expressed in TNM [5, 15] and histological differentiation have not been established very well for the eyelid, but have been established for the integument (see Chap.16 on "Skin Carcinoma").

Sebaceous Gland Carcinoma

Sebaceous gland carcinoma comprises 1%–3% of all malignant lid tumours [44]. It has a worse prognosis than the above-characterised more common types, as it leads to frequent and early metastasis [27, 31, 34]. In the series of 95 cases reported by Rao et al. [35] the recurrence rate was 33%. Metastases to periauricular or cervical lymph nodes or both occurred in 23% and 22 (23%) patients died as a result of the tumour.

The following prognostic factors other than anatomic extent of disease expressed in TNM [5, 15] have been identified by univariate analyses. A bad prognosis is indicated by location of the tumour in the upper lid, size of 10 mm or more in maximal diameter, duration of symptoms for more than 6 months, an infiltrative growth pattern [35], and moderate to poor sebaceous differentiation. Additional findings indicating a poor prognosis include multicentric origin [35], intraepithelial carcinomatous changes (pagetoid involvement or bowenoid changes) of the conjunctiva, cornea or epidermis of the eyelid [17, 35] and invasion [44] of lymphatic channels, vascular structures and the orbit. Inflammatory presentation of the tumour precludes early diagnosis and therefore also has a bad prognosis [6]. Wide excision with intraoperative frozen section control is better than simple excision with or without radiation [35].

Merkel Cell Carcinoma

Merkel cell carcinoma is a rare tumour, which is also characterised by poor prognosis [18]. One third recurred locally after excision, and lymph node metastases occurred in 53% [44]. A total of 40%–50% of the patients died as a result of the tumour. Because of the small numbers of cases with lid involvement and incomplete follow-up data, prognostic factors other than anatomic extent of disease expressed in TNM [5, 15] are not available.

Malignant Melanoma of the Eyelid

For prognostic evaluation see Chap. 17 on "Malignant Melanoma of Skin" and the recent review of literature by Tahery et al. [46].

Conjunctiva

Squamous Cell Carcinoma

Most squamous cell carcinomas arise in the interpalpebral area of the perilimbal conjunctiva and grow in an exophytic fashion. They tend to be only superficially invasive and to have a relatively benign clinical course [47]. In a series of 87 cases [47] only one patient died from metastases. In another series of 27 cases [44] there were three patients with deep corneal invasion and two with intraocular extension. Four of the patients showed orbital invasion, and two exhibited spread to regional lymph nodes. One patient died from metastatic tumour.

Mucoepidermoid Carcinoma

Mucoepidermoid carcinomas are uncommon tumours composed of varying proportions of mucus-secreting cells, squamous cells and intermediate cells. They appear to be more aggressive in their local behaviour than conventional squamous cell carcinoma and exhibit a tendency to intraocular and intraorbital invasion as well as early recurrence if incompletely excised. Because of the small numbers of cases involving the conjunctiva and incomplete follow-up data, prognostic factors other than anatomic extent of disease expressed in TNM [5, 15] are not yet available.

Malignant Melanoma

Malignant melanomas of the conjunctiva are rare tumours which arise from a nevus, an acquired melanosis or de novo. They usually occur in the bulbar conjunctiva or at the limbus, and only rarely in the caruncle or in the palpebral conjunctiva. In sharp contrast with uveal melanomas, which never metastasise to the regional lymph nodes, conjunctival melanomas share with cutaneous melanomas a definite tendency to invade the lymphatics and spread initially to the regional lymph nodes. The conjunctiva is richly supplied with lymphatic channels, some of which are situated very superficially. Thus even minimally invasive melanomas have the potential for reaching the lymphatic circulation. The natural behaviour of these melanomas is not predictable, but there is reason to believe they are considerably less malignant than similar melanomas of the eyelids and skin [31]. In a series of 131 cases of conjunctival melanoma, 26% of the patients died of metastatic melanoma [44]. There are some prognostic factors other than anatomic extent of disease expressed in TNM [5, 15] which have been identified by univariate analyses. Origin from acquired melanosis or de novo carries a worse prognosis with 40% mortality versus 20% mortality if the tumour arises from a pre-existing nevus. A bad prognosis is further indicated by tumour thickness of more than 1.5–2 mm [25, 43], age under 70 years [3] and invasive malignant melanoma in contrast to atypical melanocytic hyperplasia (in situ malignant melanoma) [43]. A bulbar location confers a low risk of metastatic disease. None of the cytological characteristics appear to influence prognosis. Most authorities agree that exenteration for tumours in the fornix does not improve the survival rate.

Malignant Melanoma of the Uvea

Malignant melanoma of the uvea is the most frequent primary malignant intraocular tumour in adults. The frequency increases from anterior to posterior – from the iris to the posterior choroid. Because metastasis to regional lymph nodes is virtually unknown and metastatic disease prior to treatment is infrequent, the TNM system is less applicable in this entity. Overall adjusted cumulative survival rates of patients with malignant melanoma of the choroid have not changed significantly over the past few decades [50] in spite of different treatment procedures. The 5-year mortality rate is between 23% and 28%, the 15-year mortality rate between 42% and 47%.

There have been a number of univariate analyses on prognostic factors, but there are still questions about the clinical significance of these factors and about the natural history of this tumour. A review of the literature shows the following important prognostic factors. The prognosis becomes worse from anterior to posterior location of the tumour; the iris shows a favourable prognosis with only 5% metastasing in 15 years [4, 13, 28, 31, 33, 37, 40, 42, 45]. Mortality increases with tumour size [44]; small tumours (< 11 mm) show a 10-year mortality rate of 19%, medium tumours (11–15 mm) a 10-year mortality rate of 40% and large tumours (> 15 mm) a 10-year mortality rate of 65%. The prognosis of the tumour also depends on the cell type [7, 16, 28, 30, 31, 40, 44, 48]. The best prognosis is with the spindle cell type (spindle A somewhat better than spindle B) with a 5-year mortality rate of 2%–8%. An intermediate prognosis is associated with the mixed cell type with a 5-year mortality rate of 42%. The epithelioid cell type shows the worst prognosis with a 5-year mortality rate of 55%. A bad prognosis is further indicated by high mitotic activity [24, 28, 37, 48], i.e. a fatal outcome in 39% of tumours with one mitotic figure per high power field (40x) versus a fatal outcome in 71% with ten mitotic figures per high power field (40x). Other unfavourable prognostic factors include scleral invasion [28, 40], vortex vein invasion [28], invasion of the optic nerve [2, 28, 41], perforation of Bruch's membrane [24, 40], high standard deviation of nuclear size [29, 30, 38], high pigmentation of the tumour [7, 24, 28, 37, 40], lower content of reticulin fibres [24], diffuse versus circumscribed growth [20, 28, 31] and lymphocytic invasion and/or necrosis in spindle B malignant melanoma [22]. The "no-touch" enucleation technique has a favourable effect on the prognosis [32, 39].

Other possible independent prognostic factors for which further investigation and confirmation are needed are:

Table 1. Prognosis of patients with retinoblastoma; dependence on pT classification (UICC 1987 [14, 15])

pT	Survival rates (%)	
	Five-year	24-year
pT2 (>25% to 50%)	100.0	100.0
pT3a (>50% and/or cells in vitreous)	96.6	96.6
pT3b (optic nerve up to lamina cribrosa)	91.3	91.3
pT3c (anterior chamber and /or uvea and/or intrascleral)	92.9	87.3
pT4a (beyond lamina cribrosa not at resection line)	76.9	60.3
pT4b (other extraocular and/or at resection line)	22.2	22.2

Data from [25].

– Gender [16, 28]
– Age [12, 16, 28, 40]
– Location of anterior tumour margin [44]
– Host's immunological defence mechanisms [44]

Retinoblastoma

Retinoblastoma is the most frequent intraocular tumour in infants ranging from 1 in 15 000 to 1 in 34 000 live births. The 5-year mortality rate in retinoblastoma is between 10% and 24% due to new treatment procedures [1, 26]. The following compilation of mortality rates depending on TNM is predominantly based on an overview of prognosis published in 1992 by Lommatzsch et al. shown in Table 1 [26].

The following prognostic factors other than anatomic extent of disease [5, 15] have been identified by univariate analyses (unless otherwise stated). A poor prognosis is indicated by a flat, diffusely infiltrating growth pattern ([21], multivariate analysis [31]), association of intracranial ectopic retinoblastoma ("trilateral retinoblastoma") ([21], multivariate analysis [31, 49]), bilaterality, which is associated with a high frequency of nonocular cancers ([21], multivariate analysis [1]), secondary glaucoma [31], multiplicity of tumour [31] and high mitotic activity [32]. Highly differentiated tumours exhibiting many well-formed Flexner-Wintersteiner rosettes in almost all viable areas, with or without fleurettes, carry a favourable prognosis [31].

Rhabdomyosarcoma of the Orbit

This is the most frequent malignant tumour of the orbit. The superior orbit is predominantly involved. The prognosis of orbital rhabdomyosarcoma is generally better than that of rhabdomyosarcoma located elsewhere in the head/neck region [19]. With the introduction of radiotherapy and chemotherapy, local cure has progressed to over 90% per cent of cases, and survival has improved to about 80% of patients [44].

Histological type is the only well-established prognostic factor other than anatomic extent of disease expressed in TNM [5, 15]. The "differentiated" type is associated with the best prognosis, the "alveolar" type with the worst [19].

Carcinoma of the Lacrimal Gland

Three epithelial malignancies predominate: adenoid cystic carcinoma (50%–60%), malignant mixed tumour (8%–48%) and adenocarcinoma (< 20%). The prognosis of lacrimal gland tumours in general is worse than that of the histologically similar salivary gland tumours [11]. The 5-year mortality rate for example for the adenoid cystic carcinoma is about 50% [44], the 10-year mortality rate about 80%.

The following prognostic factors other than anatomic extent of disease expressed in TNM [5, 15] have been identified by univariate analyses. Histological type is an important factor, adenoid cystic carcinoma having a "somewhat better" prognosis than adenocarcinoma [10]. Diagnostic biopsy prior to tumour excision has a "negative impact" on the prognosis [36]. The pre-existing lesion is also an important factor for the final outcome: presence of a component of benign pleomorphic adenoma results in a "considerably better" prognosis than of a de novo carcinoma [10]. Finally, the surgical approach is a prognostic factor: transtemporal approach causes a less favourable prognosis than lateral orbitotomy [36].

Summary

In recent years there has been an improvement in survival and in preservation of vision in the treatment of ophthalmic tumours. Good examples are the retinoblastoma and the rhabdomyosarcoma in terms of survival and preservation of vision and malignant melanoma of the choroid in terms of preservation of vision.

Ophthalmic tumours are composed of different entities with very different prognosis. The main prognostic factors are the anatomic extent of disease expressed in TNM [5, 15] and the histological type of the tumour.

References

1. Abramson DH, Eilsworth RM, Kitchin FD, Tung G (1984) Second monocular tumours in retinoblastoma survivors. Ophthalmology 91: 1351–1355
2. Albert D, Gaasterland D, Caldwell J, Howard R, Zimmerman LE (1972) Bilateral metastatic choroidal melanoma, nevi and cavernous degenerations. Involvement of the optic nervehead. Arch Ophthal 87: 39–47

3. Allen AC, Spitz S (1953) Malignant melanoma: a clinico-pathological analysis of the criteria for diagnosis and prognosis. Cancer 6: 1
4. Augsburger JJ, Gamel JW (1990) Clinical prognostic factors in patients with posterior uveal malignant melanoma. Cancer 66: 1596–1600
5. Beahrs OH, Henson DE, Hutter RVP, Kennedy BJ (eds) (1992) AJCC manual for staging cancer, 4th edn. Lippincott, Philadelphia
6. Boniuk M, Zimmerman LE (1968) Sebaceous carcinoma of the eyelid, eyebrow, caruncle and orbit. Trans Am Acad Ophthalmol Otolaryngol 72: 619–629
7. Coleman DJ, Silverman RH, Rondeau MJ, Lizzi FL, McLean IW, Jakobiec FA (1990) Correlation of acoustic tissue typing of malignant melanoma and histopathologic features as predictor of death. Am J Ophthalmol 110: 380–388
8. Doxanas MT, Green WR (1979) Adult lid lesions: basal cell carcinoma. Presented at the 38th meeting of the Wilmers Residents' Association, Baltimore
9. Farmer ER, Helwig EB (1980) Metastatic basal cell carcinoma: a clinicopathologic study of seventeen cases. Cancer 46: 748–57
10. Font RL, Gamel JW (1978) Epithelial tumours of the lacrimal gland: an analysis of 265 cases. In: Jakobiec FA (ed) Ocular and adnexal tumours. Aesculapius, Birmingham, Alabama, chapter 53
11. Forrest AW (1979) Lacrimal gland tumours. In: Jones IS, Jakobiec FA (eds) Diseases of the orbit. Harper and Row, Hagerstown
12. Gragoudas ES, Egan KM, Seddon JM, Glynn RJ, Walsh SM, Finn SM, Wunzenrider JE, Spar MD (1991) Survival of patients with metastases from uveal melanoma. Ophthalmology 98: 383–389
13. Green WR (1986) The uveal tract. In: Spencer WH (ed) Ophthalmic pathology. An atlas and textbook. Saunders, Philadelphia, pp 1352–2024
14. Hermanek P, Sobin LH (eds) (1987) UICC TNM classification of malignant tumours, 4th edn. Springer, Berlin Heidelberg New York
15. Hermanek P, Sobin LH (eds) (1992) UICC TNM classification of malignant tumours, 4th edn, 2nd rev. Springer, Berlin Heidelberg New York
16. Jensen OA (1982) Malignant melanoma of the human uvea. 25-year follow-up of cases in Denmark, 1943–1952. Acta Ophthalmol (Copenh) 60: 161–182
17. Khan JA, Doane JF, Grove AS Jr (1991) Sebaceous and meibomian carcinomas of the eyelid. Recognition, diagnosis and management. Ophthal Plast Reconstr Surg 7: 61–66
18. Kivela T, Tarkkanen A (1990) The Merkel cell and associated neoplasms in the eyelids and periocular region. Surv Ophthalmol 35: 171–187
19. Knowles M (1978) The diagnosis and treatment of rhabdomyosarcoma of the orbit. In: Jakobiec FA (ed) Ocular and adnexal tumours. Aesculapius, Birmingham, Alabama, chapter 49
20. Kolb H, Vollmar F (1974) Beitrag zum flaechenhaften malignen Melanom der Chorioidea. Graefes Arch Klin Ophthalmol 191: 45–52
21. Kopelman JE, McLean IW (1983) Multivariate analysis of clinical and histological risk factors for metastasis in retinoblastoma. Invest Ophthalmol Vis Sci 24 [Suppl]: 50
22. Kremer I, Gilad E, Kahan E, Derazne E, Bar-Ishak R (1991) Necrosis and lymphocytic infiltration in choroidal melanomas. Acta Ophthalmol (Copenh) 69: 347–351
23. Lommatzsch P, Dietrich B (1976) The effect of orbital irradiation on the survival rate of patients with choroidal melanoma. Ophthalmologica (Basel) 173: 49–52
24. Lommatzsch PK (1989) Intraoculare Tumoren. Enke, Stuttgart
25. Lommatzsch PK, Lommatzsch RE, Kirsch I, Fuhrmann P (1990) Therapeutic outcome of patients suffering from malignant melanomas of the conjunctiva. Br J Ophthalmol 74: 615–619
26. Lommatzsch PK, Morgenstern B (1992) Effect of histological criteria (pTNM classification, degree of differentiation) on mortality of patients with retinoblastoma. Klin Monatsbl Augenheilkd 200(4): 284–288
27. Margo CE, Lessner A, Stern GA (1992) Intraepithelial sebaceous carcinoma of the conjunctiva and skin of the eyelids. Ophthalmology 99(2): 227–231
28. McLean IW, Foster WD, Zimmerman LE (1977) Prognostic factors in small malignant melanomas of choroid and ciliary body. Arch Ophthal 95: 48–61
29. McLean IW, Zimmerman LE, Evans M (1978) Reappraisal of Callender's spindle A type of malignant melanoma of the choroid and ciliary body. Am J Ophthalmol 86: 557–564
30. McLean IW, Foster WD, Zimmerman LE (1983) Modifications of Callender's classification of uveal melanomas at the Armed Forces Institute of Pathology. Am J Ophthalmol 96: 502–509

31. Naumann GOH, Apple DJ (1986) Pathology of the eye. Springer, Berlin Heidelberg New York
32. Niederkorn JY (1984) Enucleation-incuced metastasis of intraocular melanomas in mice. Ophthalmology 91: 692–700
33. Nowakowski VA, Ivery G, Gastro JR, Char DH, Linstadt DE, Ahn D, Phillips TL, Quivey JM, Decker M, Petti PL (1991) Uveal melanoma: development of metastases after helium ion irradiation. Radiology 178: 277–280
34. Richard DL, Jokobiec FA, Small P (1989) Sebaceous carcinoma of the eyelids. Ophthalmology 96: 1021–1026
35. Rao NA, McLean IW, Zimmerman LE (1978) Sebaceous carcinoma of eyelids and caruncle: Correlation of clinicopathologic features with prognosis. In: Jakobiec FA (ed) Ocular and adnexal tumors. Aesculapius, Birmingham, Alabama, chapter 32
36. Riedel KG, Markl A, Hasenfratz G, Kampik A, Stefani FH, Lund OE (1990) Epithelial tumours of the lacrimal gland: clinico-pathologic correlation and management. Neurosurg Rev 13: 289–298
37. Seddon JM, Albert DM, Lavin PT, Robinson N (1983) A prognostic factor study of diseases free interval and survival following enucleation for uveal melanoma. Arch Ophthalmol 101: 1894–1899
38. Seddon JM, Polivogianis L, Hsieh C-C et al (1987) Death from uveal melanoma. Arch Ophthalmol 105: 801–806
39. Seddon JM, Gragoudas ES, Egan KM et al (1990) Relative survival rates after alternative therapies for uveal melanoma. Ophthalmology 97(6): 769–777
40. Shammas HF, Plodi FC (1977) Prognostic factors in choroidal and ciliary body melanomas. Arch Ophthal 95: 63–69
41. Shammas HF, Plodi FC (1978) Peripapillary choroidal melanomas. Extension along the optic nerve and its sheaths. Arch Ophthalmol 96: 440–445
42. Shields JA, Sanborn GE, Augsburger JJ (1983) The differential diagnosis of malignant melanoma of the iris. Ophthalmology 90: 716–720
43. Silvers DN, Jakobiec FA, Freeman TR, Lefkowitch JH, Elie RC (1978) Melanoma of the conjunctiva: a clinicopathologic study. In: Jakobiec FA (ed) Ocular and adnexal tumors. Aesculapius, Birmingham, Alabama, chapter 41
44. Spencer WH (1986) Ophthalmic pathology. Saunders, Philadelphia
45. Sunba MSN, Rahi AHS, Morgan G (1980) Tumor of the anterior uvea. Metastasizing malignant melanoma of the iris. Arch Ophthal 98: 82–85
46. Tahery DP, Goldberg R, Moy RL (1992) Malignant melanoma of the eyelid. A report of eight cases and a review of the literature. J Am Acad Dermatol 27: 17–21
47. Zimmerman LE (1969) The cancerous, precancerous and pseudocancerous lesions of the cornea and conjunctiva (The Pocklington Memorial Lecture). Proceedings of the 2nd international corneo-plastic conference, London 1967. Pergamon, Oxford, p 547
48. Zimmerman LE (1980) Melanocytic tumours of interest to the ophthalmologist. Ophthalmology 87: 497–502
49. Zimmerman LE, Burns RP, Wankum G (1982) Trilateral retinoblastoma: ectopic intracranial retinoblastoma associated with bilateral retinoblastoma. J Pediatr Ophthalmol 19: 320–325
50. Zimmerman LE, McLean IW (1984) Do growth and onset of symptoms of uveal melanomas indicate subclinical metastasis? Ophthalmology 91: 685–691

29 Neuroepithelial Tumours of Brain

K. Nomura and A.B.M.F. Karim

Introduction

The prognostic factors that have been shown to be statistically significant in the survival of patients with brain tumours are: tumour type, histological grade of the tumour, tumour location, patient's age at diagnosis and patient's performance status [2, 5 ,29, 34, 35]. Out of these factors, histological type and grade provide the most important prognostic factors for survival. The prognostic factors for patients with brain gliomas are discussed below.

Tumour-Related Factors

Tumour Type

Brain tumours of neuroepithelial type consist mostly of gliomas which can be categorised into two groups: astrocytic and non-astrocytic tumours. Astrocytic tumours consist of low-grade gliomas (LGG), e.g. pilocytic, fibrillary, protoplasmic, gemistocytic types, and high-grade gliomas (HGG), e.g. anaplastic astrocytomas and glioblastomas. Each of these tumour groups has independent prognostic influence on survival [31]. Pilocytic astrocytoma of the cerebellum is the only glioma that may be completely cured by operative treatment alone.

Non-astrocytic glial tumours comprise oligodendrogliomas, ependymomas, medulloblastomas and other rare types. A special subgroup called mixed oligo-astrocytoma is increasingly being reported in the literature. In the LGG subgroup covering astrocytic as well as oligodendrocytic tumours, the frequency of mixed tumours may be around 10% [16]. Each of these tumour subclassifications for astrocytic and non-astrocytic tumours shows different prognostic variables [2]. Therefore, their prognostic factors should be analysed separately.

Histological grade

Astrocytic tumours are usually subdivided by their degree of malignancy using Kernohan's four grades [17]. They are termed grade 1–2 for low grade and 3–4 for high grade tumours. There is concern over the validity of histological criteria for grading [6, 15, 35]. This lack of definite criteria has resulted in a lack of uniformity. The earlier World Health Organization Histological Classification had problems concerning grade (I-IV, not consistent with the Kernohan grades) [35, 39]. Daumas-Duport's recent proposal [6] attempts to improve consistency. The revised WHO classification [20, 21] attempts to bring the modified Kernohan scheme [6] and the former WHO grading system [39] into accord. The recent WHO grades might be added as (WHO) I–IV to the pertinent diagnoses in an optional way.

Tumour Size

It is difficult to measure tumour size and infiltration with precision. Nevertheless, tumour size detected by computerised tomography (CT) or magnetic resonance imaging (MRI) [3, 28] is considered to be an effective prognostic factor for the survival of patients with LGG. A total of 228 supratentorial astrocytic tumours from the Brain Tumour Registry of Japan were analysed with regards to the size of tumour before operation (5 cm or less, $n = 51$; more than 5 cm, $n = 177$). This parameter was found to be a significant variable for survival in supratentorial astrocytic tumours along with histological typing, but a weak prognostic factor for malignant astrocytomas. In the data from the Brain Tumour Registry of Japan (unpublished), there was no prognostic significance indicated for glioblastomas by regression tree analysis. Others report that the size of tumour, as indicated by CT prior to operation, is not significant in terms of the length of survival of patients with low-grade astrocytomas [25], malignant astrocytic tumours [30, 34, 37] or medulloblastomas in multivariate analysis [14]. Important unpublished data on prognostic influence of tumour size are emerging from the EORTC (European Organisation for Research on Treatment of Cancer) randomised trial 22844 on LGG; it appears from a multivariate analysis that the size of the tumour (≤ 3 cm, >3–5 cm, >5–10 cm and > 10 cm) is a strong predictor ($p = 0.0007$) for overall survival and more so ($p = 0.00001$) for disease-free survival of patients with LGG, namely astrocytoma, oligodendroglioma and mixed oligoastrocytoma of adults.

Location of Tumours

The extent of surgical excision of gliomas is often limited by the site and the extent of the lesion. Winger [36] reports that tumour location is a significant independent variable only in respect to its accessibility for excision. The location of the tumour in the basal ganglia, thalamus, hypothalamus or brain stem may indicate limitation of applicable surgical approaches. The tumour location shows no difference in survival among patients with frontal, parietal, temporal or occipital tumours. In another report [2] on patients with malignant (anaplastic) gliomas, these locations indicate, to some extent, a difference in survival by univariate analysis. Ependymomas show different prognosis for survival dependent on location in the brain, supratentorial or infratentorial: the former has a higher mortality than the latter [24].

In the UICC (International Union Against Cancer) /AJCC (American Joint Committee on Cancer) TNM classification [1, 10], tumours encroaching upon the ventricular system have a high classification (T3). However, this is not always correct for gliomas. Ventricles may be easily the site of tumour invasion in medulloblastomas, ependymomas or any other deep tumour. Choroid plexus papillomas originate in the ventricles.

Pontine gliomas occur more frequently in children than in adults and have the same problems for prognostic ratings by location. Nazar et al. [27] have shown that the pattern of growth and the location of the tumour in the brain stem determined the prognosis of young patients. This means that tumours in these special locations should be independently analysed for prognostic purposes.

DNA Ploidy

DNA aneuploidy by flow cytometric analysis has been reported to be significant in predicting favourable prognosis for patients with medulloblastoma [38], but remains controversial for astrocytic tumours [7, 32].

Bromodeoxyuridine (BUdR) and Ki-67 Labelling Index

The development of monoclonal antibodies to BUdR and Ki-67 allows measuring the percentage of BUdR- or Ki-67-labelled cells. The labelling index (LI) may permit a correlation between the proliferative potential of an individual tumour and the survival of the host. In patients with low-grade astrocytomas, survival has been shown to be a function of the BUdR LI alone [12]. The Ki-67 LI also indicates the tumour's proliferative potential [13]. These techniques indicate that proliferative potential may be an independent prognostic factor for survival of patients even in a multivariate analysis.

Patient-Related Factors

Age

It has been frequently reported [28, 34, 36] that younger patients live longer than elderly adults with gliomas. This association between age and survival is a significant variable both in uni- and mutivariate analysis. The most highly significant decade in such analyses is 40–50 years of age. In ependymoma, this is also a highly significant prognostic factor for survival. Children with ependymoma have worse prognoses than adults by univariate analysis [23, 27].

Gender

There is no agreement on the role of gender as a prognostic factor. In some papers, gender is not predictive of survival for patients with astrocytomas and glioblastomas [9, 25, 33, 36], medulloblastomas [14] and ependymomas [11]. Others report significant gender associations for survival in astrocytomas [5, 6], the prognosis being more favourable for women ($p < 0.001$) in multivariate analysis [29].

Performance Status

There are several reports on the relationship between preoperative performance status and survival [5, 8, 18, 23, 26, 34, 36] based on the Karnofsky performance scale [19].

Preoperative Mental and Neurological Function Status

The presence of preoperative altered mental status is shown to indicate poor prognosis. The presence of a focal neurogenic deficit with normal mental status may not be significant for prognosis [22, 29]. However, neurological (function) status could be an important prognostic factor ($p = 0.00001$) in LGG as seen in preliminary unpublished data from the EORTC (European Organisation for Research on Treatment of Cancer).

Duration of Symptoms

Duration of symptoms appears to be a significant independent variable for survival in supratentorial anaplastic gliomas [5, 9, 36], although there are some exceptions reported [23, 26]. Duration of symptoms was not found to be an independent variable for survival in low-grade gliomas [29].

Treatment-Related Factors

With regard to residual tumour after surgery, reports are available on the significance between the amount of tumour removed and patient survival [11, 36, 37]. Patients with gross total excision of supratentorial anaplastic gliomas live longer than those with partial excisions [14, 15, 37]; however, Coffey et al. report no such relationship [4].

Conclusion

A variety of prognostic factors for gliomas have been discussed. Several factors remain controversial. Applying parameters uniformly is a problem, especially in applying histological grading. Multivariate analyses of these prognostic factors suggests that histological grade and tumour type are the most important prognostic factors, followed by the patient's age. Age remains an important factor in overall survival. Mental change most likely is a predictive factor for poor survival. Tumour size and location are also predictive factors for survival, their contributions depending on the histological grade and type of gliomas. For patients with LGG, T classification (size among other parameters) indicating volume of the tumour may be another important prognostic factor for overall and disease-free survival. However, this classification may not be suitable in determining the prognosis of all tumours due to the association of deep-seated location or brain stem gliomas with poor prognosis.

References

1. Beahrs OH, Henson DE, Hutter RVP, Kennedy BJ (eds) (1992) American Joint Commission on Cancer (AJCC): Manual for staging of cancer, 4th edn. Lippincott, Philadelphia
2. Brain Tumour Registry of Japan (1992) Part III: Results of treatment. Neurol Med Chir (Tokyo) 32: 469–487 (special issue)
3. Burger PC, Heinz ER, Shibata T et al (1988) Topographic anatomy CT correlations in the untreated glioblastoma multiforme. J Neurosurg 68: 698–704
4. Coffey RJ, Lunsford LD, Taylor FH (1988) Survival after stereotactic biopsy of malignant gliomas. Neurosurgery 22: 465–473
5. Curran WJ, Scott CB, Horton J et al (1993) Recursive partitioning analysis of prognostic factors in three radiation therapy oncology group malignant glioma trials. J Natl Cancer Inst 85: 704–710
6. Daumas-Duport C, Scheithauer B, O'Fallon J et al (1988) Grading of astrocytomas, a simple and reproducible method. Cancer 62: 2152–2165
7. Gaetani P, Danova M, Butti G et al (1988) Cell kinetics aspects of human malignant neuroepithelial tumours: a follow up study. Tumori 74: 145–150
8. Green S, Byar DP, Walker MD et al (1983) Comparison of carmustine, procarbazine, and high dose methylpredonisolone as addition to surgery and radiotherapy for the treatment of malignant glioma. Cancer Treat Rep 7: 121–132
9. Grigsby PW, Garcia DM, Simpson JR et al (1989) Prognostic factors and results of therapy for adult thalamic and brain stem tumours. Cancer 63: 2124–2129
10. Hermanek P, Sobin LH (eds) (1992) TNM classification of malignant tumours, 4th edn, 2nd rev. Springer, Berlin Heidelberg New York
11. Hoaley EA, Barnes PD, Kupsky WJ et al (1991) The prognostic significance of postoperative residual tumour in ependymoma. Neurosurgery 28: 666–672
12. Hoshino T (1991) Proliferative potential of astrocytoma and glioblastomas. In: Paoletti P, Takakura K, Walker MD et al (eds) Neurooncology. Kluwer Academic, Dorderecht, pp 33–39
13. Jaros E, Perry RH, Adam L et al (1992) Prognostic implication of P59 protein, epidermal growth factor receptor, Ki-67 labelling in brain tumours. Br J Cancer 66: 373–385
14. Jenkin DJ, Goddard K, Armstrong D et al (1990) Posterior fossa medulloblastoma in childhood: treatment results and a proposal for a new staging system. Int J Radiat Oncol Biol Phys 19: 265–274
15. Karim ABMF, Kralendonk JH (1991) Pitfalls and controversies in the treatment of gliomas. In: Karim ABMF, Laws ER Jr (eds) Glioma, principles and practice in neurooncology. Springer, Berlin Heidelberg New York, pp 1–16

16. Karim ABMF (1991) Cure and quality of life after treatment for glioma. In: Karim ABMF, Laws ER Jr (eds) Glioma, principles and practice in neurooncology. Springer, Berlin Heidelberg New York, pp 271–282
17. Kernohan JW, Mabon RF, Svien HJ et al (1949) A simplified classification of gliomas. Proc Staff Meet Mayo Clin 24: 71–75
18. Kimsella TJ, Rowland CJ, Klecker R et al (1988) Pharmacology and phase I/II study of continuous intra-venous infusions in patients with glioblastoma multiforme. J Clin Oncol 6: 876–879
19. Karnofsky DA, Abelmann WH, Craver LS et al (1948) The use of the nitrogen mustards in the palliative treatment of carcinoma; with particular reference to bronchogenic carcinoma. Cancer 1: 634–656
20. Kleihues B, Burger PC, Scheithauer BW (1993) Histological typing of tumours of the central nervous system, 2nd edn. WHO international histological classification of tumours. Springer, Berlin Heidelberg New York
21. Kleihues B, Burger PC, Scheithauer BW (1993) The new WHO classification of brain tumours. Brain Pathol 3: 255–268
22. Laws ER, Taylor WF, Bergstrahl EJ (1986) Neurosurgical management of low-grade astrocytoma. Clin Neurosurg 33: 575–588
23. Lyons MK, Kelly PJ (1991) Posterior fossa ependymomas: report of 30 cases and review of literature. Neurosurgery 28: 659–665
24. Marks JE, Adler SJ (1982) A comparative study of ependymomas by site of origin. Int J Radiat Oncol Biol Phys 8: 37–43
25. Medbery CA, Straus KL, Steinberg SM et al (1988) Low grade astrocytomas: treatment results and prognostic variables. Int J Radiat Oncol Biol Phys 15: 837–847
26. Miller PJ, Hassanein RS, Giri PGS et al (1990) Univariate and multivariate statistical analysis of high-grade gliomas: the relationship of radiation dose and other prognostic factors. Int J Radiat Oncol Biol Phys 19: 275–280
27. Nazar CB, Hoffman HJ, Becker LE et al (1990) Infratentorial ependymomas in childhood: prognostic factors and treatment. J Neurosurg 72: 408–417
28. Nazzaro JM, Neuwelt EA (1990) The role of surgery in the management of supratentorial intermediate and high grade astrocytomas in adults. J Neurosurg 73: 331–344
29. North CA, North RB, Epstein JA et al (1990) Low-grade cerebral astrocytomas. Cancer 66: 6–14
30. Reeves GI, Marks JE (1979) Prognostic significance of lesion size for glioblastoma multiforme. Radiology 132: 469–471
31. Russel DS, Rubinstein LJ (1989) Tumours of central neuroepithelial origin. In: Russel DS, Rubinstein LJ (eds) Tumours of the central nervous system, 5th edn. Arnold, London, pp 83–350
32. Salmon I, Kiss R, Dewitte D et al (1992) Histologic grading and DNA ploidy in relation to survival among 206 adult astrocytic tumour patients. Cancer 70: 538–546
33. Sandberg-Wollheim M, Malmstrom P, Stromblad LG et al (1991) A randomised study of chemotherapy with procarbazine, vincristine, and lomustine with and without radiation therapy for astrocytoma grade 3 and/or 4. Cancer 68: 22–29
34. Simpson JR, Horton J, Scott C et al (1993) Influence of location and extent of surgical resection on survival of patients with glioblastoma multiforme: results of three consecutive radiation therapy oncology group (RTOG) clinical trials. Int J Radiat Oncol Biol Phys 26: 239–244
35. Stam FC (1991) The problems of pathological diagnosis. In: Karim ABMF, Laws ER Jr (eds) Glioma, principles and practice in neuro-oncology. Springer, Berlin Heidelberg New York, pp 17–36
36. Winger MJ, Macdonald DR, Cairncross JG (1989) Supratentorial anaplastic gliomas in adults. The prognostic importance of extent of resection and prior low-grade gliomas. J Neurosurg 71: 487–493
37. Wood JR, Green SB, Shapiro WR (1988) The prognostic importance of tumour size in malignant gliomas: a computed tomographic scan study by the brain tumour cooperative group. J Clin Oncol 6: 338–43
38. Yasue M, Tomita T, Engelhard H et al (1989) Prognostic importance of DNA ploidy in medulloblastoma of childhood. J Neurosurg 70: 385–391
39. Zülch KJ (1986) Brain tumors: their biology and pathology, 3rd edn. Springer, Berlin Heidelberg New York, pp 258–276

30 Hodgkin Disease

M.K. Gospodarowicz, L. Specht, and S.B. Sutcliffe

Improvements in patient assessment and treatment of Hodgkin disease allow us now to cure the majority of patients with this disease. These improved results have minimised the impact of prognostic factors and, currently, prognostic factors are employed more frequently to select therapy than to estimate survival. Over the last three decades, numerous factors have been shown to affect the prognosis of patients with Hodgkin disease. Most of these factors are highly interrelated. Consequently, multivariate analyses are needed to determine which factors are merely related to better known prognostic factors, but are without independent prognostic significance. A large number of multivariate studies of prognostic factors in Hodgkin disease have been published. The differing conclusions may be attributed to variation with regard to factors being examined, patient assessment and treatment, and the methods of analysis employed in individual studies. A comprehensive review of the literature on prognostic factors in Hodgkin disease emphasised both the wealth of data and differences in opinion due to the differences in recording and analysis of prognostic factors [35].

Ideally, to study prognostic factors, one should have uniform measurement and recording in a cohort of previously untreated patients managed according to well-defined treatment policies. Unfortunately, such data are not always available and if analysis is confined to data obtained in prospective trials, one may omit important prognostic factors observed in retrospective analyses. Nevertheless, it is possible to identify the principal factors influencing prognosis in Hodgkin disease (Tables 1 and 2).

Clinical Features

Systemic symptoms ("B" symptoms) have been known for many years to influence the prognosis of patients with Hodgkin disease and were included in the Ann Arbor staging classification as either category A (no systemic symptoms) or B (systemic symptoms present). At the Ann Arbor conference, unexplained fever (> 38.5°C), weight loss exceeding 10% of normal body weight during the last 6 months and night sweats were considered to be of prognostic significance. Recent re-evaluations of systemic symptoms indicate that severe pruritus, although rarely encountered, also confers a particularly adverse prognosis [6, 11]. The presence of systemic symptoms is correlated with the extent of disease [15, 20, 22,

Table 1. Prognostic factors in stage I and II Hodgkin disease

Factor	Variants
Anatomic extent	I vs. II Ann Arbor classification
Symptoms	Fever (>38.5 °C), weight loss (>10%), night sweats
Histological type	LP and NS vs. MC and LD
Number of sites involved	Three or less sites vs. more than three sites
Tumour burden	Bulk and number of sites
Large mediastinal mass	None or small vs. large mass
Age	Up to 50 years vs. over 50 years
Gender	Male vs. female
Sedimentation rate	Up to 50 vs. more than 50 mm/h

LP, lymphocyte predominant; NS, nodular sclerosis; MC, mixed cellularity; LD, lymphocyte depleted.

Table 2. Prognostic factors in stage III and IV Hodgkin disease

Factor	Variants
Anatomic extent	III vs. IV Ann Arbor classification
Symptoms	Fever (>38.5 °C), weight loss (>10%), night sweats
Extent of extranodal involvement	One vs. multiple extranodal sites
Tumour burden	Bulk and number of sites
Age	Up to 50 years vs. over 50 years
Gender	Male vs. female
Anaemia[a]	Hb less than 10 g/l
Lymphocytopenia[a]	Less than 500–1000 per ml

[a] In stage IV disease only.
Hb, haemoglobin.

28, 48]. However, in multivariate analysis of the International Database on Hodgkin Disease, systemic symptoms were an important prognostic factor for cause-specific survival rates [15]. In multivariate analyses in which the extent of disease was analysed in greater detail, the presence of systemic symptoms was correlated with total tumour burden and was not of independent significance [39–41]. B symptoms are not easily quantifiable and may be subjective as patients differ in their awareness of them. Still, B symptoms seem to be independently significant unless the total extent of disease is very accurately evaluated.

Older age (> 40 years or > 50 years) has been associated with poor survival. Whilst the impact of age on overall survival has been considered in many reports, the independent prognostic influence on cause-specific survival rates has now been confirmed in several multivariate analyses [14, 15, 22, 28, 40, 42, 43]. Disease-free survival is influenced adversely by age in some but not all studies, but it is generally agreed that survival after relapse is adversely affected by age [15, 23, 35, 40, 42–44, 46, 48, 49]. It is still not established whether Hodgkin disease is a biologically more aggressive disease in older patients or whether the poorer prognosis results from an inability to tolerate intensive therapy.

The curious fact that Hodgkin disease seems to have a slightly more benign course in women remains unexplained. The influence of gender independent of other prognostic factors is, however, virtually negligible in large cohorts of patients [11, 14, 15, 22, 28, 37, 38, 46, 48].

Anatomic Extent of Disease

The Ann Arbor staging classification adopted by the UICC (International Union Against Cancer) [16] in a slightly modified version for Hodgkin disease is largely based on the anatomic extent of disease. The experience derived from the International Database on Hodgkin Disease has defined the 10-year overall survival rate for patients with stage I and II Hodgkin disease treated in the 1970s to be 80%, with a 70%–75% relapse-free survival. In stage III and IV disease the 10-year overall survival was 40%–66% [15]. The prognostic significance of the Ann Arbor classification has been confirmed over the last two decades [5, 11, 15, 20, 30, 31, 43]. However, clinical experience has shown that subgroups of patients with widely differing prognoses exist within individual Ann Arbor stages.

The extent of disease may vary considerably in stages other than stage I, and it has been demonstrated that the anatomic extent of disease within each stage has prognostic significance. The number of involved nodal regions has been found to be a significant factor in multivariate analysis of patients with stage I and II Hodgkin disease treated with radiotherapy alone or chemotherapy combined with mantle irradiation [15, 22, 28, 46, 48, 49]. In the EORTC (European Organisation for Research on Treatment of Cancer) data, involvement of more than two nodal regions was found to be an independent prognostic factor for overall survival and disease-free survival in patients treated with radiotherapy alone and in patients treated with combined modality therapy. An adverse impact on survival and disease-free survival was also demonstrated for patients with stage I-IIIA disease with involvement of three or more nodal regions in the multivariate analysis of the International Database on Hodgkin Disease. In a multivariate analysis of advanced disease, involvement of three or more nodal sites was also an adverse factor for disease-free survival [34].

Several studies have suggested that patients with stage III disease limited to the upper abdomen have a better outcome than those with lower abdomen and pelvis involvement [12, 27]. This finding was not confirmed by other investigators and may not be of as much importance for patients treated with effective chemotherapy. For patients with stage IV disease, involvement of more than two extranodal sites has been shown to adversely affect complete response rate, disease-free survival and overall survival rates [19, 23, 32, 33].

The volume of disease in individual regions is not considered in the Ann Arbor classification. However, tumour burden in a single region has been established as prognostically significant. The significance of a large mediastinal mass has been investigated most extensively. The size of the mediastinal mass has been expressed as the maximal width of the mass (greater than 7 cm or 10 cm), the ratio of the maximum mass width to maximum chest diameter (greater than a third), with the thoracic diameter defined at T5-6 level, the T6-7 vertebral level, the thoracic diameter at carina or as the volume of mediastinal disease on thoracic computed tomography (CT) scan [35, 43]. The original and most frequently used definition of a large mediastinal mass is that proposed by Mauch et al. [27] – the width of the mediastinal mass being greater than one third of the widest thoracic diameter. The presence of a large mediastinal mass has been associated with a greater number of sites of initial involvement, systemic symptoms, stage II disease, E-lesions and hilar involvement. However, even when other factors are taken into account in the multivariate analysis, a large mediastinal mass remains an important adverse prognostic factor for disease-free survival for patients treated with radiation, combined modality therapy or chemotherapy alone [1, 17, 29, 49]. Because of the small number of deaths in stage I and II Hodgkin disease, few studies have shown the presence of a large mediastinal mass to be a significant independent factor for overall survival [2, 29]. A large mediastinal mass has also been shown to adversely affect disease-free and overall survival in stage III and IV disease [4, 42].

A large tumour mass in a single region appears to be of definite prognostic importance only when located in the mediastinum. The prognostic value of a large tumour at a peripheral site is not well documented in any stage of Hodgkin disease, principally because such presentations are extremely uncommon [2, 4, 21, 43, 49].

In stage III Hodgkin disease, the amount of tumour in the spleen, specifically more than four splenic tumour nodules, has been shown to adversely influence disease-free survival in patients treated with irradiation alone [18]. In most centres laparotomy is now only performed in a minority of patients, thus limiting the usefulness of the extent of splenic involvement as a prognostic factor.

Extent and volume of disease have thus been shown to be very important for prognosis in Hodgkin disease. A measure of the total tumour burden, combining the total extent and volume of tumour in the body, has been shown to be a highly significant independent prognostic factor in Hodgkin disease [35–41].

Site of Disease

In general, there is no definite evidence to indicate that a particular localisation of Hodgkin disease significantly affects prognosis. Specific exceptions include upper neck involvement and bone marrow involvement. Nodal disease limited to the upper neck is uncommon, but when present carries a very low risk of relapse (<10%) even when treated with involved field radiation therapy alone. Conversely, bone marrow involvement, which is also rare, was associated with a 20% 5-year survival rate in Danish experience [10, 20, 38, 42, 43, 48]. The above situations may, however, be prognostically relevant by virtue of the total tumour burden rather than the specification of site of disease.

Histological Type

The Rye classification divides patients with Hodgkin disease into four types: lymphocyte predominance, nodular sclerosis, mixed cellularity and lymphocyte depletion [24]. The prognostic importance of histopathological type has been demonstrated in many studies, although its relevance in an era of high cure rates with therapy is modest [7, 8, 11, 25, 43, 47]. The presence of mixed cellularity Hodgkin disease is associated with a significantly increased risk of death from disease (RR, 1.37) and the presence of lymphocyte-depleted Hodgkin disease is associated with even greater risk of death (RR, 2.19) [15]. Histological type is correlated with extent of disease, age and sex. In many series the nodular sclerosis type constitutes up to 75% of cases, therefore limiting the value of the Rye classification. So far, proposals for a subdivision of nodular sclerosis have not been found to be consistently useful [3, 9, 26, 35]. Currently, histological type cannot be uniformly regarded as a strong and independent prognostic factor in Hodgkin disease other than in clinical stage I and II patients treated with radiation therapy alone. In this situation, the risk of relapse for mixed cellularity and lymphocyte-depleted Hodgkin disease is 30%–40% compared with 15%–25% risk of relapse at 5 years for patients with lymphocyte predominance and nodular sclerosis Hodgkin disease [13, 43].

Haematologic and Biochemical Indicators

An elevated erythrocyte sedimentation rate (ESR) adversely affects the prognosis in Hodgkin disease. Although an elevated ESR correlates with other factors, such as systemic symptoms, histology and stage, a number of studies have shown it to be an independent prognostic factor. ESR greater than 40–60 mm/h confers a poorer outcome in clinical stage I and II patients treated with irradiation alone as well as in those treated with combined modality [13–15, 45, 46, 48]. Others have found an elevated ESR to be associated with a less favourable outcome in patients with stage III and IV [11]. However, other studies taking extent of disease into account have not found the ESR to be an independent prognostic factor [38–42, 49].

Lymphocytopenia is associated with a poorer outcome but is correlated with other factors and has no independent prognostic impact except in advanced disease [14, 38, 40, 50]. Severe anaemia is uncommon in Hodgkin disease other than in stage III and IV. Although it has been associated with a worse prognosis, independent significance has only been defined in stage IV disease [42].

Numerous biochemical indicators have been shown to correlate with Hodgkin disease. An elevation in serum copper level, serum ceruloplasmin, ferritin, haptoglobin, beta-2 microglobulin or a decreased serum albumin level have been shown to be relevant, but their independent prognostic significance, when other factors are taken into account, has not been established. Serum lactic dehydrogenase has not been extensively investigated, but was found to be an independent prognostic factor in at least one multivariate analysis of outcome in patients with stage III and IV and would appear to correlate with tumour mass and prognosis in Hodgkin disease as in other malignancies [15, 35, 42].

Immunological indicators have not yet been generally accepted as prognostic factors in patients with Hodgkin disease. A high level of CD30 antigen has been shown to be associated with advanced disease and requires further evaluation as a possible prognostic variable. Cytogenetic studies, flow cytometry and HLA typing do not provide uniformly useful prognostic information [35].

Summary

Although Ann Arbor stage is a very important prognostic factor in Hodgkin disease, other factors, expressing either burden of disease or its biological potential, have been shown to affect outcome. These factors need to be considered along with stage for the optimal management of patients with Hodgkin disease. The introduction of systemic chemotherapy into the management of stage I and II disease associated with adverse prognostic factors has altered the impact of these factors. With the introduction of high-dose chemotherapy with bone marrow support into the management of patients who do not respond to standard chemotherapy, prognostic factors predictive for the success of this new treatment approach are being investigated.

References

1. Anderson H, Deakin DP, Wagstaff J et al (1984) A randomised study of adjuvant chemotherapy after mantle radiotherapy in supradiaphragmatic Hodgkin's disease PS IA-III: a report from the Manchester Lymphoma Group. Br J Cancer 49: 695–702
2. Anderson H, Jenkins JPR, Brigg DJ et al (1985) The prognostic significance of mediastinal bulk in patients with stage IA-IVB Hodgkin's disease: a report from the Manchester Lymphoma Group. Clin Radiol 36: 449–454
3. Bennett KH, MacLennan KA, Easterling MJ et al (1985) The prognostic significance of cellular subtypes in nodular sclerosing Hodgkin's disease: an analysis of 271 non-laparotomised cases (BNLI report no 22). Clin Radiol 34: 497–501
4. Bonadonna G, Valagussa P, Santoro A (1985) Prognosis of bulky Hodgkin's disease treated with chemotherapy alone or combined with radiotherapy. Cancer Surv 4: 439–458
5. Carbone PP, Kaplan HS, Musshoff K et al (1971) Report of the committee on Hodgkin's disease staging classification. Cancer Res 31: 1860–1861
6. Crnkovich MJ, Leopold K, Hoppe RT (1987) Stage I to IIB Hodgkin's disease: the combined experience at Stanford University and the Joint Center for Radiation Therapy. J Clin Oncol 5: 1041–1049
7. Davis S, Dahlberg S, Myers MH et al (1987) Hodgkin's disease in the United States: a comparison of patient characteristics and survival in the Centralized Cancer Patient Data System and the Surveillance, Epidemiology and End Results Program. J Natl Cancer Inst 78: 471–478
8. De Vita VT, Simon RM, Hubbard SM et al (1980) Curability of advanced Hodgkin's disease with chemotherapy. Ann Intern Med 92: 587–594
9. Ferry JA, Linggood RM, Convery KM et al (1993) Hodgkin disease, nodular sclerosis type. Implications of histologic subclassification. Cancer 71: 457–463

10. Fuller LM, Gamble JF, Schullenberger CC et al (1971) Prognostic factors in localized Hodgkin's disease treated with regional radiation. Clinical presentation and specific histology. Radiology 98: 641–654

11. Gobbi PG, Cavalli C, Federico M et al (1988) Hodgkin's disease prognosis: a directly predictive equation. Lancet I: 675–679

12. Golomb HM, Sweet DL, Ultmann JE et al (1980) Importance of substaging of stage III Hodgkin's disease. Semin Oncol 7: 136–143

13. Gospodarowicz MK, Sutcliffe SB, Clark RM et al (1992) Analysis of supradiaphragmatic clinical stage I and II Hodgkin's disease treated with radiation alone. Int J Radiat Oncol Biol Phys 22: 859–865

14. Haybittle JL, Haygoe FGJ, Easterling MJ et al (1985) Review of British National Lymphoma Investigation studies of Hodgkin's disease and development of prognostic index. Lancet I: 967–972

15. Henry-Amar M, Aeppli DM, Anderson J et al (1990) Workshop statistical report. In: Somers R, Henry-Amar M, Meerwaldt JK et al (eds) Treatment strategy in Hodgkin's disease. INSERM/John Libbey Eurotext, London, pp 169–422

16. Hermanek P, Sobin LH (eds) (1992) UICC TNM classification of malignant tumours, 4th edn, 2nd rev. Springer, Berlin Heidelberg New York

17. Hoppe RT, Coleman CN, Cox RS et al (1982) The management of stage I-II Hodgkin's disease with irradiation alone or combined modality therapy: the Stanford experience. Blood 59: 455–465

18. Hoppe RT, Cox RS, Rosenberg SA et al (1982) Prognostic factors in pathologic stage III Hodgkin's disease. Cancer Treat Rep 66: 743–749

19. Jaffe HS, Cadman EC, Farber LR et al (1986) Pretreatment hematocrit as an independent prognostic variable in Hodgkin's disease. Blood 68: 562–564

20. Kaplan HS (1980) Hodgkin's disease, 2nd edn. Harvard University Press, Cambridge

21. Liew KH, Easton D, Horwich A et al (1984) Bulky mediastinal Hodgkin's disease management and prognosis. Hematol Oncol 2: 45–59

22. Loffler M, Dixon DO, Swindell R (1990) Prognostic factors of stage III and IV Hodgkin's disease. In: Somers R, Henry-Amar M, Meerwaldt JK et al (eds) Treatment strategy in Hodgkin's disease. John Libbey Eurotext, Paris, pp 90–103

23. Longo DL, Young RC, Wesley M (1986) Twenty years of MOPP therapy for Hodgkin's disease. J Clin Oncol 4: 1295–1306

24. Lukes RJ, Craver LF, Hall TC et al (1966) Report of the Nomenclature Committee. Cancer Res 26: 1311

25. MacLennan KA, Bennett MH, Bosq J et al (1990) The histology and immunohistology of Hodgkin's disease: its relationship to prognosis and clinical behaviour. In: Somers R, Henry-Amar M, Meerwaldt JK et al (eds) Treatment strategy in Hodgkin's disease. John Libbey Eurotext, pp 17–25

26. Masih AS, Weisenburger DD, Vose JM et al (1992) Histologic grade does not predict prognosis in optimally treated, advanced-stage nodular sclerosing Hodgkin's disease. Cancer 69: 228–232

27. Mauch P, Goffman T, Rosenthal DS et al (1985) Stage III Hodgkin's disease: improved survival with combined modality therapy as compared with radiation therapy alone. J Clin Oncol 3: 1166–1173

28. Meerwaldt JH, Van Glabbeke M, Vaughan Hudson B (1990) Prognostic factors for stage I and II Hodgkin's disease. In: Somers R, Henry-Amar M, Meerwaldt JK et al (eds) Treatment strategy in Hodgkin's disease. John Libbey Eurotext, Paris, pp 37–50

29. Pavlovsky S, Maschio M, Santarelli MT et al (1988) Randomized trial of chemotherapy versus chemotherapy plus radiotherapy for stage I-II Hodgkin's disease. J Natl Cancer Inst 80: 1466–1473

30. Peters MV (1950) A study of survivals in Hodgkin's disease treated radiologically. Am J Roentgenol 63: 299–311

31. Peters MV, Middlemiss KCH (1958) A study of Hodgkin's disease treated by irradiation. Am J Roentgenol 79: 114–121

32. Pillai AN, Hagemeister FB, Velasquez WS (1985) Prognostic factors for stage IV Hodgkin's disease treated with MOPP, with or without bleomycin. Cancer 55: 691–697

33. Prosnitz LR, Farber LR, Kapp DS et al (1982) Combined modality therapy for advanced Hodgkin's disease: long-term follow-up data. Cancer Treat Rep 66: 871–879

34. Selby P, Patel P, Milan S et al (1990) Ch1VPP combination chemotherapy for Hodgkin's disease: long term results. Br J Cancer 62: 279–285

35. Specht L (1991) Prognostic factors in Hodgkin's disease. Cancer Treat Rev 18: 21–53
36. Specht L (1992) Tumour burden as the main indicator of prognosis in Hodgkin's disease. Eur J Cancer 28A: 1982–1985
37. Specht L, Lauritzen AF, Nordentoft AM et al (1990) Tumour cell concentration and tumour burden in relation to histopathologic subtype and other prognostic factors in early stage Hodgkin's disease. Cancer 65: 2594–2601
38. Specht L, Nissen NI (1988) Prognostic factors in Hodgkin's disease stage IV. Eur J Hematol 41: 359–367
39. Specht L, Nissen NI (1988) Prognostic factors in Hodgkin's disease stage III with special reference to tumour burden. Eur J Hematol 41: 80–87
40. Specht L, Nissen NI (1989) Hodgkin's disease and age. Eur J Hematol 43: 127–135
41. Specht L, Nordentoft AM, Soren S et al (1988) Tumor burden as the most important prognostic factor in early stage Hodgkin's disease. Cancer 61: 1719–1727
42. Straus DJ, Gaynor JJ, Myers J et al (1990) Prognostic factors among 185 adults with newly diagnosed advanced Hodgkin's disease treated with alternating potentially noncross-resistant chemotherapy and intermediate-dose radiation therapy. J Clin Oncol 8: 1173–1186
43. Sutcliffe SB, Gospodarowicz MK, Bergsagel DE et al (1985) Prognostic groups for management for localized Hodgkin's disease. J Clin Oncol 3: 393–401
44. Sutcliffe SB, Wrigley PFM, Peto J et al (1978) MVPP chemotherapy regimen for advanced Hodgkin's disease. Br Med J 1: 679–683
45. Tubiana M, Henry-Amar M, Burgers MV et al (1984) Prognostic significance of erythrocyte sedimentation rate in clinical stages I-II of Hodgkin's disease. J Clin Oncol 2: 194–200
46. Tubiana M, Henry-Amar M, Carde P et al (1989) Toward comprehensive management tailored to prognostic factors of patients with clinical stages I and II in Hodgkin's disease. The EORTC Lymphoma Group controlled clinical trials: 1964–1987. Blood 73: 47–56
47. Tubiana M, Henry-Amar M, Hayat M et al (1984) Prognostic significance of the number of involved areas in the early stages of Hodgkin's disease. Cancer 54: 885–894
48. Tubiana M, Henry-Amar M, Van der Werf-Messing B et al (1985) A multivariate analysis of prognostic factors in early stage Hodgkin's disease. Int J Radiat Oncol Biol Phys 11: 23–30
49. Verger E, Easton D, Brada M et al (1988) Radiotherapy results in laparotomy staged Hodgkin's disease. Clin Oncol 39: 428–431.
50. Wagstaff J, Gregory WM, Swindell R et al (1988) Prognostic factors for survival in stage IIIB and IV Hodgkin's disease: a multivariate analysis comparing two specialist treatment centres. Br J Cancer 58: 487–492

31 Non-Hodgkin Lymphomas

M.K. Gospodarowicz and M. Hayat

A diverse group of diseases is encompassed by the label "non-Hodgkin lymphomas". This diversity bedevils any attempt to put the assessment of prognostic factors on a rational basis. Nevertheless, some broad conclusions can be drawn. The Ann Arbor staging classification, developed for Hodgkin disease, is the accepted staging classification for non-Hodgkin lymphomas [3, 21]. Although the Ann Arbor classification has been shown to provide important prognostic information, other factors have equivalent, if not greater, influence on outcome in patients with non-Hodgkin lymphomas. It is known that systemic symptoms that are included in the Ann Arbor staging classification, histology, age, extent of nodal involvement, tumour bulk, extranodal involvement, erythrocyte sedimentation rate (ESR), lactic dehydrogenase (LDH), phenotype and proliferation rates, are all independent predictors of outcome in malignant non-Hodgkin lymphomas. This review considers factors with independent prognostic value documented in multivariate analysis. These factors have been identified in studies of non-Hodgkin lymphomas in adults. The childhood non-Hodgkin lymphomas have a different clinical and histological spectrum of disease and are not considered in this review. A summary of prognostic factors in non-Hodgkin lymphomas is given in Table 1.

Histological Type and Grade

Currently, a number of different histological classifications for non-Hodgkin lymphomas are in use. The two most commonly used are the Kiel classification introduced by Lennert in 1978 and updated in 1992, which is used widely in Europe, and the Working Formulation, which has replaced the previously popular Rappaport classification in North America [33, 62]. The Working Formulation was introduced in an attempt to standardise the reporting of the pathology of malignant lymphomas. Although it has been found to reflect the prognosis, it has not been universally accepted and has already been modified [64]. However, other classifications can be translated into the Working Formulation. Despite the known difficulties in the reproducibility of histopathological classification, the distinction between low-, intermediate- and high-grade lymphoma in the Working Formulation accurately reflects not only survival but also to a certain extent the curability of the disease [15, 52, 53]. Similarly, in the Kiel classification,

Table 1. Prognostic factors in non-Hodgkin lymphomas

Factor	Unfavourable feature	Significance
Age (years)	> 55–65	All
	> 40	Low-grade lymphoma
Gender	Male	Low-grade lymphoma
Performance status	Karnofsky < 60	All
	ECOG < 2	Primary brain lymphoma
Symptoms	B symptoms	All, especially age > 70 years
Anatomic extent	Ann Arbor stage III and IV	All
Tumour bulk	> 5 cm	Stage I and II treated with RT
	> 10–15 cm	All
	Large mediastinal mass	Stage III and IV
Number of sites	More than two sites involved	All
Extranodal disease	Brain, liver, bone marrow	All
	Intestine	GI lymphoma
Histological type	Large cell, high grade	All
	Non-MALT histology	GI lymphoma
LDH	Elevated	All
Beta-2 microglobulin	Elevated	All
Serum calcium	Elevated	T cell lymphoma – Japan
S-phase fraction	Elevated	All – Kiel classification
Ki-67 nuclear antigen	Increased expression	All
Immunophenotype	T cell lymphoma	Japan
Homing receptor	CD44 expression	All

LDH, lactate dehydrogenase; ECOG, Eastern Cooperative Oncology Group; MALT, mucosa-associated lymphoid tissue; RT, radiation treatment; GI, gastrointestinal tract.

centrocytic lymphomas represented in low-grade disease have a better survival rate than centroblastic lymphomas in the high-grade category [13]. In the last decade, lymphomas originating from mucosa-associated lymphoid tissue, so called MALT lymphomas, have been identified as distinct from other non-Hodgkin lymphomas [23]. In a multivariate analysis of gastrointestinal lymphomas, origin from MALT has been shown to be an independent prognostic factor associated with favourable outcome [41].

Clinical Features

Advanced age is an adverse prognostic factor in non-Hodgkin lymphomas regardless of stage and treatment. Patients over the age of 60 tend to have worse prognosis, as measured by overall survival and cause-specific survival rates. The main effect of age may be a reflection of a decreased tolerance to treatment beyond the age of 60. However, despite equivalent therapy, an increased risk of relapse has been noted in older patients treated with radiation alone for stage I and II disease [17, 20, 28, 35, 44, 52, 55, 56, 59, 60, 65, 66]. In a series of patients with stage I and II intermediate-grade lymphoma treated with radiation alone, the 5-year survival and freedom from relapse rates were 97% and 58% for patients less than 60 years old and 51% and 27% for those over 60 years old [28]. In a series of patients with low-grade lymphoma, age greater than 40 was associated with a poorer survival [14].

Male gender has been found to correlate with other adverse prognostic factors such as histology, stage, symptoms and, because of this correlation, in many series it was not considered to have an independent prognostic impact. However, male gender has been demonstrated to be an independently adverse prognostic factor in several reports of patients with low-grade non-Hodgkin lymphoma [14, 57, 60].

Low Karnofsky performance status has been shown to be an independent factor for adverse prognosis in patients with stage III and IV non-Hodgkin lymphomas [20, 30, 51, 52, 57]. It is, however, usually associated with other adverse factors such as advanced age and the extent of disease. Performance status was one of the main prognostic factors in patients with primary lymphomas of the brain [4].

Systemic symptoms including fever, night sweats and weight loss (B symptoms) are usually associated with stage III and IV disease, but their presence still has an independent prognostic effect after correction for Ann Arbor stage [17, 20, 22, 43, 59]. A large study of elderly patients with non-Hodgkin lymphomas identified B symptoms as one of the most important prognostic factors [13]. In this study patients with B symptoms had a 2.2 times higher risk of dying than those without B symptoms. The presence of B symptoms is generally correlated with stage III and IV disease, high tumour bulk and elevated LDH levels, all surrogates for high tumour burden.

In recent years there has been a constant rise in the incidence of human immunodeficiency virus (HIV)-related non-Hodgkin lymphomas [9, 29]. Also with the increase in kidney and heart transplantation, the number of immunosuppression-related non-Hodgkin lymphomas has also increased. These lymphomas usually present with a high or intermediate histological grade [9, 29]. Extranodal presentations are very frequent, especially primary central nervous system (CNS) and gastrointestinal (GI) lymphomas [6, 16, 25, 29]. The HIV-related lymphomas have a higher proliferation rate than their usual counterparts [39]. The prognosis of patients with HIV- or immunosuppression-related non-Hodgkin lymphomas relates more to the degree of immune defect than to stage and other prognostic factors identified for non-HIV- and non-immunosuppression-related lymphomas. In HIV-related lymphomas, the prognosis has been related mostly to the CD4 count, performance status and prior diagnosis of acquired immunodeficiency syndrome (AIDS) [16, 29]. The median survival of patients with HIV-related lymphomas associated with AIDS is less than 6 months [16, 29, 49]. The results of treatment and prognostic factors should be reported separately for HIV- and immunosuppression-related non-Hodgkin lymphomas.

Anatomic Extent of Disease

The Ann Arbor staging classification, developed for Hodgkin disease, is the accepted staging classification for non-Hodgkin lymphomas and is included in the AJCC (American Joint Committee on Cancer) and the UICC (International Union Against Cancer) manuals in a slightly modified version [3, 21]. Ann Arbor stage has been shown to be an independent prognostic factor in numerous studies of non-Hodgkin lymphomas [12, 20, 35, 57, 59]. In the Toronto experience with follicular lymphomas, the 10-year cause-specific survival rates for patients with stages I, II, III and IV were 68%, 56%, 42% and 18%, respectively [17]. However, although stage is an important factor, considerable variation of outcome exists within each stage. Therefore, further specification of tumour extent such as tumour bulk, number of involved sites and extranodal involvement are indispensable for predicting outcome in patients with non-Hodgkin lymphomas.

Tumour bulk or burden has been found to be one of the most important prognostic factors in non-Hodgkin lymphomas, whether localised (stage I and II) or advanced (stage III and IV) [17, 28, 38, 59, 65]. Tumour bulk predicts for relapse and survival in patients with localised disease treated with radiation alone and with combined chemotherapy and radiation. In patients treated with radiation therapy alone, tumour bulk greater than 5 cm or greater than 10 cm has been associated with a lower local control rate, higher risk of distant relapse and lower survival, independent of other prognostic factors. In patients with stage IA and IIA intermediate- and high-grade non-Hodgkin lymphomas treated with radiation alone, 39% of those with tumour bulk of less than 5 cm relapsed, while 62% of those with tumour bulk greater than 5 cm relapsed [59]. The impact of tumour bulk is greater in patients with intermediate- and high-grade histology than in those with low-grade non-Hodgkin lymphomas. Bulk greater than 10 cm is one of the most important factors in patients with stage III and IV disease treated with chemotherapy. Other definitions of high tumour burden, which have been associated with poor outcome, include the presence of a large mediastinal mass (more than one third of chest diameter), the presence of a palpable abdominal mass and a combination of para-aortic and pelvic node involvement in stage III and IV disease [17, 28, 38, 45, 47, 57, 59, 66, 67].

The number of sites of involvement, expressed either as the number of nodal regions involved in stage I and II disease or the number of nodal and extranodal sites involved in stage III and IV disease, has been found to be an independent prognostic factor for disease-free and overall survival in patients treated with chemotherapy alone or combined modality therapy [2, 28, 44, 47, 51, 66]. In a multivariate analysis of Vancouver patients with stage IIB-IV diffuse large cell lymphoma treated with chemotherapy, involvement of more than one extranodal site carried a relative risk of death of 3.3, and involvement of more than two nodal sites a relative risk of death of 3.7 [22].

Almost 50% of patients with stage I and II non-Hodgkin lymphomas present with disease in extranodal sites [5, 18, 28, 60]. Extranodal involvement is also very common in stage III and IV disease. There is confusion in the literature as to the precise definition of extranodal presentation versus extralymphatic disease as defined in the Ann Arbor classification. Some authors include lymphomas involving the Waldeyer ring as nodal, others as extranodal. The GI tract, in particular the stomach, is the commonest site of extranodal involvement. The intestine has been identified as an adverse site of extranodal presentation in multivariate analysis of early-stage patients due to the impact of locally advanced, bulky and unresectable disease not otherwise encountered in localised non-Hodgkin lymphomas [38]. Patients presenting with involvement of the Waldeyer ring and resectable GI lymphoma have been found in multivariate analysis to have better survival rates than those presenting in other extranodal sites [18, 52]. Other sites of extranodal involvement associated with poor outcome include liver, CNS and extensive bone marrow involvement [20, 47, 67]. Primary brain non-Hodgkin lymphomas are uncommon and are associated with a particularly poor outcome. The pattern of failure is mostly local and the main prognostic factors include degree of neurological impairment and performance status [25].

Haematologic and Biochemical Factors

Elevated serum LDH is one of the more important adverse prognostic factors in patients with non-Hodgkin lymphoma [61]. It is thought to reflect the tumour burden. While it correlates with stage and bulk, the serum LDH has been found to be one of the most important independent prognostic factors in both early and stage III and IV lymphomas [2, 12, 30, 35, 45, 56, 58, 66, 67]. Elevated serum calcium has been found to be an independent prognostic factor in patients with T cell lymphoma in Japan [51]. Other biochemical factors are important in special situations. For example, the level of the cerebrospinal fluid protein is an independent prognostic factor in patients with primary brain lymphomas [4].

A high beta-2 microglobulin level was found to be an independent prognostic factor for complete response rate and time to treatment failure in all stages of patients with low-grade non-Hodgkin lymphomas (Working Formulation) [37]. In the analysis of the high-grade lymphomas (Kiel classification), the level of beta-2 microglobulin was one of the most important prognostic variables for the response, disease-free and overall survival rates [27]. In this study of patients with high-grade non-Hodgkin lymphomas treated with chemotherapy, the 6-year survival rate for patients with high beta-2 microglobulin levels was 35%, while it was 70% for those with normal levels [27, 34].

Biological and Molecular Factors

A high proliferative activity has been associated with an adverse prognosis in non-Hodgkin lymphomas. The methods of measurement have not been standardised and, in some cases, only diploid cell populations have been examined. Results have not been systematically adjusted for histology and other known prognostic variables. However, the prognostic impact demonstrated in multiple studies should not be ignored. Methods measuring proliferation activity include: 3H-thymidine labelling index, Ki-67 antigen positivity, mitotic index, DNA malignancy grade and S-phase fraction. Studies quoted below have attempted to correlate the proliferation activity with other known prognostic factors.

The percentage of cells in S-phase as determined by flow cytometry strongly correlates with histological type and grade. In the Swedish experience, low-grade non-Hodgkin lymphomas (Kiel classification) had a lower frequency of S-phase cells (median, 4.1%) than high-grade lymphomas (median, 11.8%) [46]. However, a high proportion of cells in S-phase was shown to be an adverse prognostic factor in several studies and was independent of histological type and other prognostic factors [8, 24, 26, 32, 35, 46]. In the multivariate analysis of 106 patients with stage I-IV non-Hodgkin lymphomas reported by Rehn, S-phase of 4.5% or more was an independent adverse prognostic factor for low-grade lymphomas (Kiel classification), while S-phase of 16% or more was an adverse factor for survival in high-grade lymphomas [34, 46]. Others have observed a close correlation between the proliferation index (PI), histological type and complete response rate, but were unable to demonstrate the impact of PI on relapse-free or overall survival [11]. High proliferation activity as determined by Ki-67 expression in more than 60% of malignant cells was found to be a predictor of poor survival independent of age, stage, B symptoms, bulk and LDH [19, 54].

In at least one study the presence of chromosomal abnormalities was an adverse prognostic factor independent of age, stage, symptoms and LDH level [48].

Cellular immunophenotype was found to be an independent prognostic factor in patients with non-Hodgkin lymphomas in Japan [50]. In an analysis of patients with large cell non-Hodgkin lymphomas treated at Stanford, no such difference was evident. Other investigators have observed conflicting results, suggesting differences in patient populations being examined [1, 10, 31, 36]. HLA-DR-negative immune phenotype may predict poor survival, although the numbers of patients available for analysis are rather small and results are conflicting [40, 42, 54].

The identification of a homing receptor predicting the risk of occult dissemination in clinically localised presentations may be an interesting prognostic factor, although, as yet, its significance has not been adequately investigated. In recent studies, the expression of the lymphocyte homing receptor (CD44) correlated with stage of disease and outcome. Non-Hodgkin lymphomas showing no or weak reaction for CD44 were more often localised (stage I) and, in multivariate analysis, CD44 expression was found to be an independent prognostic factor [24].

Summary

Information regarding prognostic factors in non-Hodgkin lymphomas is more extensive than presented here. Major difficulties with the identification of independent prognostic factors result from a lack of standardisation in the

Table 2. Prognostic index for aggressive non-Hodgkin lymphomas [61]

Risk factors	Unfavourable feature	Risk Group	Number of unfavourable factors	Five-year survival rate (%)
Age	> 60 years	Low	0 or 1	75
LDH	> 1x normal	Low-intermediate	2	51
Performance status	Nonambulatory, ECOG 2–4	High-intermediate	3	43
Stage	III or IV Ann Arbor	High	4 or 5	26
Extranodal involvement	More than one site			

LDH, lactate dehydrogenase; ECOG, Eastern Cooperative Oncology Group.

recording and analysis of factors other than stage and histological type and grade, the analysis of factors in subgroups of patients rather than in the overall population and the paucity of studies incorporating multivariate analysis. With the recent interest in multiple prognostic factors, a prognostic index for large cell non-Hodgkin lymphomas has been proposed [61] (Table 2). This index incorporates clinical features that reflect the growth and invasive potential of the tumour (stage, LDH level and number of extranodal sites) and the patient-related factors (age and performance status). However, it is important to remember that proposals such as the PI presented here are based only on the data recorded in large numbers of patients and not necessarily on the optimal information available in an individual case. For example, the prognostic value of beta-2 microglobulin, S-phase and other biological factors could not be evaluated in the International Project due to the missing data [61]. Other proposals for consensus in the recording and reporting of prognostic factors in non-Hodgkin lymphomas have recently been presented and further efforts to standardise data collection may facilitate further research in this field [7, 63].

References

1. Armitage JO, Vose JM, Linder J et al (1989) Clinical significance of immunophenotype in diffuse aggressive non-Hodgkin's lymphoma. J Clin Oncol 7: 1783–1790
2. Bastion Y, Berger F, Bryon PA et al (1991) Follicular lymphomas: assessment of prognostic factors in 127 patients followed for 10 years. Ann Oncol 2: 123–129
3. Beahrs OH, Henson DE, Hutter RV et al (eds) (1992) American Joint Committee on Cancer: manual for staging of cancer, 4th edn. Lippincott, Philadelphia
4. Blay JY, Lasset C, Carrie C et al (1993) Multivariate analysis of prognostic factors in patients with non HIV-related primary cerebral lymphoma. A proposal for a prognostic scoring. Br J Cancer 67: 1136–1141
5. Bush RS, Gospodarowicz MK (1982) The place of radiation therapy in the management of patients with localized non-Hodgkin's lymphoma. In: Rosenberg SA, Kaplan HS (eds) Malignant lymphomas: etiology, immunology, pathology, treatment. Bristol Myers Cancer Symposia. Academic, New York, pp 485–502
6. Carbone A, Tirelli U, Vaccher E et al (1991) A clinicopathologic study of lymphoid neoplasias associated with human immunodeficiency virus infection in Italy. Cancer 68: 842–852

7. Child JA (1991) Prognostic factors in the non-Hodgkin's lymphomas – a time for consensus? (Editorial). Br J Cancer 63: 837–840
8. Christensson B, Lindemalm C, Johansson B et al (1989) Flow cytometric DNA analysis: a prognostic tool in non-Hodgkin's lymphoma. Leuk Res 13: 307–314
9. Clark WC, Dohan FCJ, Moss T et al (1991) AIDS-associated non-Hodgkin lymphoma. Lancet 337: 805–809
10. Cossman J, Jaffe ES, Fisher RI (1984) Immunologic phenotypes of diffuse, aggressive, non-Hodgkin's lymphomas. Correlation with clinical features. Cancer 54: 1310–1317
11. Cowan RA, Harris M, Jones M et al (1989) DNA content in high and intermediate grade non-Hodgkin's lymphoma – prognostic significance and clinicopathological correlations. Br J Cancer 60: 904–910
12. Cowan RA, Jones M, Harris M et al (1989) Prognostic factors in high and intermediate grade non-Hodgkin's lymphoma. Br J Cancer 59: 276–282
13. d'Amore F, Brincker H, Christensen BE et al (1992) Non-Hodgkin's lymphoma in the elderly. A study of 602 patients aged 70 or older from a Danish population-based registry. The Danish LYEO-Study Group. Ann Oncol 3: 379–386
14. Dana BW, Dahlberg S, Nathwani BN et al (1993) Long-term follow-up of patients with low-grade malignant lymphomas treated with doxorubicin-based chemotherapy or chemoimmuno-therapy. J Clin Oncol 11: 644–651
15. Ersboll J, Schultz HB, Hougaard P et al (1985) Comparison of the working formulation of non-Hodgkin's lymphoma with the Rappaport, Kiel, and Lukes and Collins classifications. Translational value and prognostic significance based on review of 658 patients treated at a single institution. Cancer 55: 2442–2458
16. Freter CE (1990) Acquired immunodeficiency syndrome-associated lymphomas. Monogr Natl Cancer Inst 10: 45–54
17. Gospodarowicz MK, Bush RS, Brown TC et al (1984) Prognostic factors in nodular lymphomas: a multivariate analysis based on the Princess Margaret experience. Int J Radiat Oncol Biol Phys 10: 489–497
18. Gospodarowicz MK, Sutcliffe SB, Brown TC et al (1987) Patterns of disease in localized extranodal lymphomas. Clin Oncol 5: 875–880
19. Grogan TM, Lippman SM, Spier CM et al (1988) Independent prognostic significance of a nuclear proliferation antigen in diffuse large cell lymphomas as determined by the monoclonal antibody Ki-67. Blood 71: 1157–1160
20. Hayward RL, Leonard RC, Prescott RJ (1991) A critical analysis of prognostic factors for survival in intermediate and high grade non-Hodgkin's lymphoma. Scotland and Newcastle Lymphoma Group Therapy Working Party. Br J Cancer 63: 945–952
21. Hermanek P, Sobin L (eds) (1992) UICC TNM classification of malignant tumors, 4th edn, 2nd rev. Springer, Berlin Heidelberg New York
22. Hoskins PJ, Ng V, Spinelli JJ et al (1991) Prognostic variables in patients with diffuse large-cell lymphoma treated with MACOP-B. J Clin Oncol 9: 220–226
23. Isaacson P (1990) Lymphoma of mucosa-associated lymphoid tissue. Histopathology 16: 627–649
24. Jalkanen S, Joensuu H, Klemi P (1990) Prognostic value of lymphocyte homing receptor and S phase fraction in non-Hodgkin's lymphoma. Blood 75: 1549–1556
25. Jellinger KA, Paulus W (1992) Primary central nervous system lymphomas – an update (editorial; review). J Cancer Res Clin Oncol 119: 7–27
26. Joensuu H, Klemi PJ, Söderström KO et al (1991) Comparison of S-phase fraction, working formulation, and Kiel classification in non-Hodgkin's lymphoma. Cancer 68: 1564–1571
27. Johnson PW, Whelan J, Longhurst S et al (1993) Beta-2 microglobulin: a prognostic factor in diffuse aggressive non-Hodgkin's lymphomas. Br J Cancer 67: 792–797
28. Kaminski MS, Coleman CN, Colby TV et al (1986) Factors predicting survival in adults with stage I and II large-cell lymphoma treated with primary radiation therapy. Ann Intern Med 104: 747–756
29. Kaplan LD (1990) AIDS-associated lymphoma. Ballieres Clin Haematol 3: 139–151
30. Kwak LW, Halpern J, Olshen RA et al (1990) Prognostic significance of actual dose intensity in diffuse large-cell lymphoma: results of a tree-structured survival analysis. J Clin Oncol 8: 963–977
31. Kwak LW, Wilson M, Weiss LM et al (1991) Similar outcome of treatment of B-cell and T-cell diffuse large-cell lymphomas: the Stanford experience. J Clin Oncol 9: 1426–1431

32. Lenner P, Roos G, Johansson H et al (1987) Non-Hodgkin lymphoma. Multivariate analysis of prognostic factors including fraction of S-phase cells. Acta Oncol 26: 179–183
33. Lennert K, Feller A (1992) Histopathology of non-Hodgkin's lymphomas (based on the updated Kiel classification), 2nd edn. Springer, Berlin Heidelberg New York
34. Lennert K, in collaboration with Mohri N, Stein H, Kaiserling E, Müller–Hermelink HK (1978) Malignant lymphomas other than Hodgkin's disease. In: Uehlinger E (ed) Handbuch der speziellen pathologischen Anatomie und Histologie, Bd I/3B. Springer, Berlin Heidelberg New York
35. Lindh J, Lenner P, Osterman B et al (1993) Prognostic significance of serum lactic dehydrogenase levels and fraction of S-phase cells in non-Hodgkin lymphomas. Eur J Hematol 50: 258–263
36. Lippman SM, Miller TP, Spier CM et al (1988) The prognostic significance of the immunotype in diffuse large-cell lymphoma: a comparative study of the T-cell and B-cell phenotype. Blood 72: 436–441
37. Litam P, Swan F, Cabanillas F et al (1991) Prognostic value of serum beta-2 microglobulin in low-grade lymphoma. Ann Intern Med 114: 855–860
38. Mackintosh JF, Cowan RA, Jones M et al (1988) Prognostic factors in stage I and II high and intermediate grade non-Hodgkin's lymphoma. Eur J Cancer Clin Oncol 24: 1617–1622
39. McDunn SH, Winter JN, Variakojis D et al (1991) Human immunodeficiency virus-related lymphomas: a possible association between tumor proliferation, lack of ploidy anomalies, and immune deficiency. J Clin Oncol 9: 1334–1340
40. Miller TP, Lippman SM, Spier CM et al (1988) HLA-DR (Ia) immune phenotype predicts outcome for patients with diffuse large cell lymphoma. J Clin Invest 82: 370–372
41. Morton JE, Leyland MJ, Vaughan Hudson G et al (1993) Primary gastrointestinal non-Hodgkin's lymphoma: a review of 175 British National Lymphoma Investigation cases. Br J Cancer 67: 776–782
42. O'Keane JC, Mack C, Lynch E et al (1990) Prognostic correlation of HLA-DR expression in large cell lymphoma as determined by LN3 antibody staining. An Eastern Cooperative Oncology Group (ECOG) study. Cancer 66: 1147–1153
43. O'Reilly SE, Hoskins P, Klimo P et al (1991) Long-term follow-up of ProMACE-CytaBOM in non-Hodgkin's lymphomas. Ann Oncol 1: 33–35
44. O'Reilly SE, Hoskins P, Klimo P et al (1991) MACOP-B and VACOP-B in diffuse large cell lymphomas and MOPP/ABV in Hodgkin's disease. Ann Oncol 1: 17–23
45. Prestidge BR, Horning SJ, Hoppe RT (1988) Combined modality therapy for stage I-II large cell lymphoma. Int J Radiat Oncol Biol Phys 15: 633–639
46. Rehn S, Glimelius B, Strang P et al (1990) Prognostic significance of flow cytometry studies in B-cell non-Hodgkin lymphoma. Hematol Oncol 8: 1–12
47. Romaguera JE, McLaughlin P, North L et al (1991) Multivariate analysis of prognostic factors in stage IV follicular low-grade lymphoma: a risk model. J Clin Oncol 9: 762–769
48. Schouten HC, Sanger WG, Weisenburger DD et al (1990) Chromosomal abnormalities in untreated patients with non-Hodgkin's lymphoma: association with histology, clinical characteristics, and treatment outcome. Blood 6: 1841–1847
49. Sebag MD, Makepeace AR, Spittle MF et al (1989) Non-Hodgkin's lymphoma associated with the acquired immune deficiency syndrome: a report of five cases. Radiother Oncol 14: 297–302
50. Shimizu K, Hamajima N, Ohnishi K et al (1989) T-cell phenotype is associated with decreased survival in non-Hodgkin's lymphoma. Jpn J Cancer Res 80: 720–726
51. Shimoyama M (1991) Peripheral T-cell lymphoma in Japan: recent progress. Ann Oncol 2 [Suppl 2]: 157–162
52. Shimoyama M, Ota K, Kikutchi M et al (1988) Major prognostic factors of adult patients with advanced B-cell lymphoma treated with vincristine, cyclophosphamide, prednisone and doxorubicin (VEPA) or VEPA plus methotrexate (VEPA-M). Jpn J Clin Oncol 18: 113–124
53. Simon R, Durrleman S, Hoppe RT et al (1988) The Non-Hodgkin Lymphoma Pathologic Classification Project. Long-term follow-up of 1153 patients with non-Hodgkin lymphomas. Ann Intern Med 109: 939–945
54. Slymen DJ, Miller TP, Lippman SM et al (1990) Immunobiologic factors predictive of clinical outcome in diffuse large-cell lymphoma. J Clin Oncol 8: 986–993
55. Soubeyran P, Eghbali H, Bonichon F et al (1988) Localized follicular lymphomas: prognosis and survival of stages I and II in a retrospective series of 103 patients. Radiother Oncol 13: 91–98
56. Stein RS, Greer JP, Cousar JB et al (1989) Malignant lymphomas of follicular centre cell origin in man. VII. Prognostic features in small cleaved cell lymphoma. Hematol Oncol 7: 381–391

57. Steward WP, Crowther D, McWilliam LJ et al (1988) Maintenance chlorambucil after CVP in the management of advanced stage, low-grade histologic type non-Hodgkin's lymphoma. A randomized prospective study with an assessment of prognostic factors. Cancer 61: 441–447
58. Straus DJ, Wong G, Yahalom J et al (1991) Diffuse large cell lymphoma. Prognostic factors with treatment. Leukemia 1: 32–37
59. Sutcliffe SB, Gospodarowicz MK, Bush RS et al (1985) Role of radiation therapy in localized non-Hodgkin's lymphoma. Radiother Oncol 4: 211–223
60. Taylor RE, Allan SG, McIntyre MA et al (1988) Low grade stage I and II non-Hodgkin's lymphoma: results of treatment and relapse pattern following therapy. Clin Radiol 39: 287–290
61. The International Non-Hodgkin's Lymphoma Prognostic Factors Project (1993) A predictive model for aggressive non-Hodgkin's lymphoma. N Engl J Med 329: 987–994
62. The Non-Hodgkin's Lymphoma Pathologic Classification Project (1982) National Cancer Institute sponsored study of classifications of non-Hodgkin's lymphomas. Summary and description of a working formulation for clinical usage. Cancer 49: 2112–2135
63. Tirelli U, Zagonel V, Monfardini S (1991) Prognostic factors in the non-Hodgkin's lymphomas – a time for consensus? (Editorial) Br J Cancer 63: 837–840
64. Urba WJ, Duffey PL, Longo DL (1990) Treatment of patients with aggressive lymphomas: an overview. J Natl Cancer Inst 10: 29–37
65. Velasquez WS, Fuller LM, Jagannath S et al (1991) Stages I and II diffuse large cell lymphomas: prognostic factors and long-term results with CHOP-bleo and radiotherapy. Blood 77: 942–947
66. Velasquez WS, Jagannath S, Tucker SL et al (1989) Risk classification as the basis for clinical staging of diffuse large-cell lymphoma derived from 10-year survival data. Blood 74: 551–557
67. Vitolo U, Bertini M, Brusamolino E et al (1992) MACOP-B treatment in diffuse large cell lymphoma: identification of prognostic groups in an Italian multicenter study. J Clin Oncol 10: 219–227

Subject Index

Springer-Verlag
and the Environment

We at Springer-Verlag firmly believe that an international science publisher has a special obligation to the environment, and our corporate policies consistently reflect this conviction.

We also expect our business partners – paper mills, printers, packaging manufacturers, etc. – to commit themselves to using environmentally friendly materials and production processes.

The paper in this book is made from low- or no-chlorine pulp and is acid free, in conformance with international standards for paper permanency.

Printing: Saladruck, Berlin
Binding: Buchbinderei Lüderitz & Bauer, Berlin